Rapid Medicine

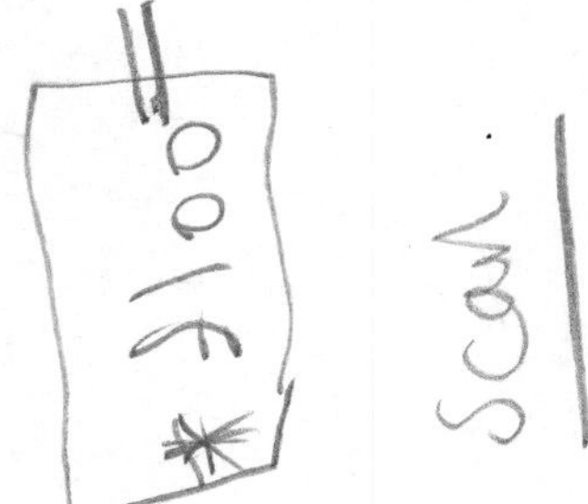

Rapid Medicine

Amir H. Sam
Cara R. Baker
James T.H. Teo
Saira Hameed
All of
Royal Free and University College Medical School,
University College London
London

EDITORIAL ADVISOR
Professor Roy Pounder
Professor of Medicine
Centre for Gastroenterology
The Royal Free Hospital
London

SERIES EDITOR
Amir H. Sam
Royal Free and University College Medical School,
University College London
London

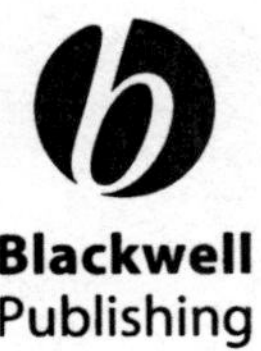

Blackwell
Publishing

Blackwell Publishing, Inc., 350 Main Street, Malden, Massachusetts 02148-5020, USA
Blackwell Publishing Ltd, 9600 Garsington Road, Oxford OX4 2DQ, UK
Blackwell Publishing Asia Pty Ltd, 550 Swanston Street, Carlton, Victoria 3053, Australia

First published 2003
6 2009

Library of Congress Cataloging-in-Publication Data
Rapid medicine/Amir H. Sam . . . [et al.].
p. ; cm.
ISBN 978-1-4051-0749-5
1. Internal medicine—Handbooks, manuals, etc.
[DNLM: 1. Clinical Medicine—Handbooks. WB 39 R218 2003] I Sam, Amir H.
RC55.R37 2003
616—dc21
2003002082

ISBN 978-1-4051-0749-5

A catalogue record for this title is available from the British Library

Set in 7.5pt/9.5pt Frutiger by Kolam Information Services Pvt. Ltd, India

Commissioning Editor: Vicki Noyes
Editorial Assistant: Nicola Ulyatt
Production Editor: Jonathan Rowley
Production Controller: Kate Charman

For further information on Blackwell Publishing, visit our website:
http://www.blackwellpublishing.com

Foreword

Rapid Medicine has been written by a group of enthusiastic and prize-winning clinical medical students at the Royal Free, some of whom are now working as house officers. They have identified the main conditions that encompass general medicine and its specialities, and they have then applied their 'system' to remember all the key features. This uniformity of approach not only means that they've forgotten nothing, but it should also help the reader to retain facts about each condition. Every topic has also been reviewed by a senior clinician; perhaps this could be considered a superior form of peer-review!

Students revising for MB BS and junior doctors preparing for MRCP will find *Rapid Medicine* an invaluable approach to learning and retention of medical knowledge. I can vouch that it certainly works for the authors, who stand-out as brilliant students and doctors! It should also help Registrars and Consultants, "I've just admitted a patient with . . ." might prompt a rapid and thorough revision of a topic using *Rapid Medicine*.

Roy Pounder MA MD DSc(Med) FRCP
January 2003

Preface

In the conception of this book, we envisioned a text presented in an easily accessible format on core conditions geared towards medical students. Students since time immemorial have been told to structure their knowledge. In this book, we have covered over 200 medical conditions using our own 'surgical sieve': Definition, Aetiology, Associations/Risk Factors, Epidemiology, History, Examination, Pathology/Pathophysiology, Investigations, Management, Complications and Prognosis. We hope that this will provide a useful pocketbook on the wards and in preparation for exams. We have included common conditions as well as rarities; thus, asthma sits alongside neurofibromatosis, but this is a reflection of our experience that unusual conditions may find their way into medical exams! We hope that you enjoy this book and use it to consolidate your ward-based learning. This is by no means a definitive textbook of medicine and we urge you to refer to more lengthy tomes to further explore topics that have caught your imagination.

This work would not have been possible without the invaluable enthusiasm and unwavering support of Professor Roy Pounder. We would also like to thank our teachers at the Royal Free Hospital particularly Professor Philip Hawkins, Dr Barbara Bannister, Dr Huw Beynon, Dr Pierre Bouloux, Dr Geraldine Brough, Dr Ian Cropley, Miss Claire Davey, Dr James Dooley, Dr Owen Epstein, Dr Lionel Ginsberg, Dr Mark Hamilton, Dr David Lipkin, Dr Marc Lipman, Dr Demitriou Mikhailidis, Dr Marsha Morgan, Dr Devi Nair, Dr David Patch, Dr Michael Potter, Dr Jonathan Robin, Dr Malcolm Rustin, Dr Frank Schafer and Dr Paul Sweny for their advice or help in reviewing our work.

Amir H. Sam
Cara R. Baker
James T.H. Teo
Saira Hameed
London, December 2002

ABG	Arterial blood gas
ABPA	Allergic bronchopulmonary aspergillosis
ACAG	Acute closed-angle glaucoma
ACE	Angiotensin-converting enzyme
ACh	Acetylecholine
ACTH	Adrenocorticotrophic hormone
ADH	Antidiuretic hormone
AF	Atrial fibrillation
AFP	Alpha feto-protein
AIDS	Acquired immune deficiency syndrome
AlkPhos	
ALA	δ-Aminolaevulinic acid
ALL	Acute lymphoblastic leukaemia
ALS	Amyotrophic lateral sclerosis
ALT	Alanine transaminase
AML	Acute myeloblastic leukaemia
ANA	Antinuclear antibody
ANCA	Anti-neutrophil cytoplasm antibody
APP	Amyloid precursor protein
APTT	Activated partial thromboplastin time
ARDS	Acute respiratory distress syndrome
ARF	Acute renal failure
5-ASA	5-Aminosalicyclic acid
ASD	Atrioseptal defect
ASM	Antismooth muscle antibody
AST	Aspartate aminotransferase
ATN	Acute tubular necrosis
AV	Atrioventricular
AXR	Abdominal X-ray
BCC	Basal cell carcinoma
BCG	Bacille Calmette–Guérin
BiPAP	Biphasic positive airway pressure
BMI	Body mass index
BP	Blood pressure
CABG	Coronary artery bypass graft
CAH	Congenital adrenal hyperplasia
c-ANCA	Cytoplasmic antineutrophil cytoplasmic antibodies
CAPD	Continuous ambulatory peritoneal dialysis
CEA	Carcinoembyonic antigen
CHD	Coronary heart disease
CK	Creatine kinase
CLL	Chronic lymphocytic leukaemia
CM	Cardiomyopathy
CML	Chronic myelocytic leukaemia
CMML	Chronic myelomonocytic leukaemia
CMV	Cytomegalovirus
CNS	Central nervous system
COAD	Chronic obstructive airway disease
COMT	Catechol-*O*-methyltransferase
COPD	Chronic obstructive pulmonary disease
CPAP	Continuous positive airway pressure
CPR	Cardiopulmonary resuscitation
CREST	Syndrome of calcinosis, Raynaud's, oesophageal dysmotility, sclerodactyly and telangiectasia
CRF	Corticotrophin-releasing factor/Chronic renal failure
CRH	Cortisol-releasing hormone
CRP	C-reactive protein
CSF	Cerebrospinal fluid
CSS	Churg–Strauss syndrome
CT	Computerized tomography
CTP	Carboxyterminal propeptide
CVA	Cerebrovascular accident
CVP	Central venous pressure
CVS	Chorionic villus sampling/Cardiovascular system
CXR	Chest X-ray

DCM	Dilated cardiomyopathy	**GBM**	Glomerular basement membrane
DDAVP	Desmopressin		
DHEA	Dehydroepiandrosterone	**GCA**	Giant cell arteritis
DHEAS	Dehydroepiandrosterone sulphate	**GCS**	Glasgow Coma Scale
		GFR	Glomerular filtration rate
DIC	Disseminated intravascular coagulation	**γ-GT**	γ-Glutamyl transferase
		GH	Growth hormone
DIDMOAD	Syndrome of diabetes insipidus, diabetes mellitus, optic atrophy and deafness	**GHRH**	Growth-hormone-releasing hormone
		GI	Gastrointestinal
		GnRH	Gonadotrophin-releasing hormone
DIP	Desquamative interstitial pneumonia/Distal interphalangeal	**G6PD**	Glucose-6-phosphate dehydrogenase
DKA	Diabetic ketoacidosis	**GTT**	Glucose tolerance test
DMD	Duchenne muscular dystrophy	**HAART**	Highly active antiretroviral treatment
DNA	Deoxyribonucleic acid	**HACEK**	Haemophilus, Actinobacillus, Cardiobacterium, Eikenella, Kingella
DOPA	Dihydroxyphenylalanine		
DPTA	Diethylenetriamine penta-acetate		
DVT	Deep vein thrombosis	**HAV**	Hepatitis A
EBV	Epstein–Barr virus	**Hb**	Haemoglobin
ECG	Electrocardiogram	**HBIG**	Hepatitis B immunoglobulin
EDTA	Ethylenediaminetetra-acetate	**HBV**	Hepatitis B virus
EEG	Electroencephalogram	**HCC**	Hepatocellular carcinoma
ELISA	Enzyme-linked immunoabsorbent assay	**hCG**	Human chorionic gonadotrophin
EMD	Electrical–mechanical dissociation	**HCM**	Hypertrophic cardiomyopathy
EMG	Electromyogram	**HCV**	Hepatitis C virus
ENT	Ear, nose and throat	**HDL**	High-density lipoprotein
ERCP	Endoscopic retrograde cholangio-pancreatography	**HDV**	Hepatitis D virus
		HEV	Hepatitis E
		5-HIAA	5-Hydroxyindole acetic acid
ESR	Erythrocyte sedimentation rate	**HIDA**	Hepatoiminodiacetic acid
ETT	Exercise tolerance test	**HIV**	Human immunodeficiency virus
FAB	French–American–British classification	**HLA**	Human leukocyte antigen
FBC	Full blood count		
***FEV*$_1$**	Forced expiratory volume in 1 s	**HNF**	Hepatocyte nuclear factor
		HONK	Hyperosmolar non-ketotic
FFP	Fresh frozen plasma		
FSH	Follicle-stimulating hormone	**HSP**	Henoch–Schönlein purpura
FVC	Forced vital capacity	**HSV**	Herpes simplex virus
GABA	Gamma-aminobutyric acid	**HTLV**	Human T-cell lymphoma virus
GAD	Glutamic acid decarboxylase	**HUS**	Haemolytic–uraemic syndrome

IBD Inflammatory bowel disease
IBS Irritable bowel syndrome
ICP Intracranial pressure
ICT Immunochromato-graphic test
IDDM Insulin-dependant diabetes mellitus
Ig Immunoglobulin
IGF Insulin-like growth factor
IHD Ischaemic heart disease
IL Interleukin
IM Intramuscular
INR International normalized ratio
IOP Intraocular pressure
IPPV Intermittent positive pressure ventilation
ITP Immune thrombocytopenic purpura
ITU Intensive therapy unit
IV Intravenous
IVIG Intravenous infusions of immunoglobulin
IVU Intravenous urogram
JVP Jugular venous pressure
KD Kawasaki's disease
KUB Abdominal radiograph of kidneys, ureter and bladder
LBBB Left bundle branch block
LDH Lactate dehydrogenase
LDL Low-density lipoprotein
LFT Liver function test
LH Luteinizing hormone/ Laparoscopic hysterectomy
LKM Liver/kidney microsomal (antibodies)
LMN Lower motor neurone
LMW Low molecular weight
MAO Monoamine oxidase
MCH Mean cell haemoglobin
MCP Metacarpal-phalangeal
MCV Mean cell volume
MEC Mixed essential cryoglobulinaemia
MEN Multiple endocrine neoplasia
MI Myocardial infarct
MIBG Meta-iodobenzyguanidine
MODS Multiple organ dysfunction syndrome
MODY Maturity-onset diabetes of the young
MP Microscopic polyangiitis
MPGN Membranoproliferative glomerulonephritis
MRCP Magnetic resonance cholangio-pancreography
MPTP 1-methyl-4-phenyl-1,2,3,6-tetrahydro-pyridine
MRI Magnetic resonance imaging
MS Multiple sclerosis
MSE Mental state examination
MSU Midstream urine
MTP Metatarsophalangeal
NAC *N*-acetylcysteine
NAPQI *N*-acetyl-*p*-benzoquinoneimine
NASH Non-alcoholic streatohepatitis
NIDDM Non-insulin-dependent diabetes mellitus
NK Natural killer
NSAIDs Non-steroidal anti-inflammatory drugs
NSIP Non-specific interstitial pneumonia
OGD Oesaphago-gastro-duodenoscopy
OTC Over-the-counter
PAF Platelet-activating factor
PAN Polyarteritis nodosa
pANCA Perinuclear antineutrophil cytoplasmic antibodies
PAS Periodic acid–Schiff
PBG Porphobilinogen
PCOS Polycystic ovarian syndrome
PCP *Pneumocystis carinii* pneumonia
PCR Polymerase chain reaction
PCS Primary sclerosing cholangitis
PCV Packed cell volume

List of Abbreviations continued

PCWP	Pulmonary capillary wedge pressure
PEEP	Positive end expiratory pressure
PEFR	Peak expiratory flow rate
PEG	Percutaneous endoscopic gastronomy
PET	Positron emission tomography
PIP	Peripheral-interphalangeal
PKD	Polycystic kidney disease
PKDL	Post kala azar dermal leishmaniasis
PMR	Polymyalgia rheumatica
POAG	Primary open-angle glaucoma
POEMS	Syndrome of polyneuropathy, endocrinopathy, monoclonal gammopathy and skin pigmentation
PPAR	Peroxisome proliferator-activated receptor
PPD	Purified protein derivative of tuberculin
PR	Per rectum
PSC	Primary sclerosing Cholangitis
PT	Prothrombin time
PTH	Parathyroid hormone
PUVA	Psoralen and ultraviolet A therapy
QBC	Quantitative buffy coat test
RA	Refractory anaemia
RAEB	Refractory anaemia with excess blasts
RAEB-t	RAEB in transformation
RAO	Retinal artery occlusion
RAPD	Relative afferent pupillary defect
RARS	Refractory anaemia with ring sideroblasts
RAST	Radio-allergosorbent test
RBBB	Right bundle branch block
RBC	Red blood cell
RCM	Restrictive cardiomyopathy
REAL	Revised American and European Lymphoma classification
RP	Relapsing polychondritis
RNA	Ribonucleic acid
RTA	Renal tubular acidosis
RUQ	Right upper quadrant
RVO	Retinal vein occlusion
SAA	Serum amyloid A
SAP	Serum amyloid P
SAPHO	Syndrome of synovitis, acne, palmoplantar pustulosis, hyperostosis, osteitis
SBP	Spontaneous bacterial peritonitis
SC	Subcutaneous
SCC	Squamous cell carcinoma
SHBG	Sex-hormone-binding globulin
SIADH	Syndrome of inappropriate ADH
SIRS	Systemic inflammatory response syndrome
SLE	Systemic lupus erythematosus
SMA	Smooth muscle antibody
SPECT	Single photon emission computerized tomography
SXR	Skull X-ray
$t_{1/2}$	Half-life
T_3	Tri-iodothyronine
T_4	Thyroxine
TA	Takayasu's disease
TB	Tuberculosis
t.d.s.	Three times per day
TEN	Toxic epidermal necrolysis
TFT	Thyroid function test
TIA	Transient ischaemic attack
TIBC	Total iron-binding capacity
TIPS	Transjugular intrahepatic portosystemic shunt
TLCO	Carbon monoxide transfer factor
TNF	Tumour necrosis factor
tPA	Tissue plasminogen activator
TPN	Total parenteral nutrition
TRAP	Tartrate-resistant acid phosphatase
TRH	Thyroid-releasing hormone
TSH	Thyroid-stimulating hormone

TTP Thrombotic thrombocytopenic purpura
UC Ulcerative colitis
U&E Urea and electrolytes
UIP Usual interstitial pneumonia
UMN Upper motor neurone
UTI Urinary tract infection
UV Ultraviolet
VCA Viral capsid antigen
VDRL Venereal disease research laboratory
VF Ventricular fibrillation
VLDL Very low-density lipoprotein
VQ Ventilation : perfusion ratio
VSD Ventriculoseptal defect
VT Ventricular tachycardia
vWF von Willebrand's factor
VZV Varicella zoster virus
VZIG Varicella zoster immunoglobulin
WCC White cell count
WG Wegener's granulomatosis
WHO World Health Organization

Symbols

$>$ Less than
$<$ Greater than
/ Or
↑ Increased
↓ Decreased
♀ Female
♂ Male

Rapid Series mnemonic

D:	Definition	*Doctors*
A:	Aetiology	*Are*
A/R:	Associations/Risk factors	*Always*
E:	Epidemiology	*Emphasizing*
H:	History	*History taking &*
E:	Examination	*Examining*
P:	Pathology/Pathogenesis	*Patients*
I:	Investigations	*In*
M:	Management	*Managing*
C:	Complications	*Clinical*
P:	Prognosis	*Problems*

Achalasia

D: A motor disorder of the oesophagus with aperistalsis and failure of lower oesophageal sphincter relaxation when swallowing.

A: Degeneration of ganglionic cells of myenteric plexus of the oesophagus disrupts the peristaltic coordination. Cause of the degeneration is unknown. Infection with *Trypanosoma cruzi* may produce a similar syndrome, but this is only common in South America (see Trypanosomiasis, American).

A/R: May rarely be associated with alacrimation and Addison's disease (triple A syndrome).

E: Annual UK incidence is 1 in 100 000. All age groups, but rare in childhood.

H: Intermittent dysphagia involving solids and liquids, food may be regurgitated (particularly at night), atypical/cramping retrosternal chest pain, weight loss.

E: Look for signs of complications.

P: **Micro:** Degeneration of intramural ganglionic cells of the oesophageal myenteric plexus. Degeneration of dorsal vagal nucleus in the brainstem medulla may also be seen.
Macro: Oesophagus can become severely dilated and elongated.

I: **CXR:** May show dilated oesophagus (double right heart border) and fluid level behind heart.
Barium swallow: Dilated body of oesophagus, which smoothly tapers down to the sphincter (beak-shaped), lack of peristalsis.
Oesophagoscopy: Excludes malignancy.
Manometry: Oesophageal and sphincter pressures. Abnormal sphincter resting pressure is > 30 mmHg.
Blood: Exclude Chagas' disease (serology for antibodies against *T. cruzi*), blood film might detect parasites.

M: **Medical:** Nifedipine or verapamil (calcium-channel antagonists) or isosorbide mononitrate as needed (for short-term relief). Endoscopic balloon dilation of lower oesophageal sphincter (80 % success rate, small risk of perforation). Endoscopic injection of botulinum toxin may be promising.
Surgery: Heller's cardiomyotomy of lower oesophageal sphincter via an abdominal or thoracic approach (can be complicated by reflux oesophagitis, so may be combined with a fundoplication procedure to prevent reflux).

C: If untreated, aspiration pneumonia, malnutrition and weight loss may result. 5 % risk of oesophageal malignancy regardless of treatment (on average $\sim$25 years after diagnosis).

P: Good if treated. If untreated, oesophageal dilation may worsen causing pressure on mediastinal structures.

Acne vulgaris

D: Inflammation of the pilosebaceous unit of the skin.

A: Increased production and impaired normal flow of sebum (caused by follicular hyperkeratinization and obstruction of the pilosebaceous duct) leading to inflammation and formation of closed or open comedones. The bacteria *Propionibacterium acnes*, *Staphylococcus epidermidis* and *Pityrosporum* yeast may be involved in pathogenesis.

A/R: Puberty or premenstrually, PCOS, cortisol excess (Cushing's syndrome), prolactinoma, late-onset adrenal hyperplasia, no dietary link proven.

E: Ubiquitous worldwide and across genders. Begins in puberty and tends to recede with age.

H: Usually self-diagnosed, acute onset, greasy skin, may be painful.

E: Open comedones (whiteheads: flesh-coloured papules), closed comedones (blackheads: the black colour is caused by oxidation of melanin pigment), papules, pustules, nodules, cysts and seborrhoea primarily affecting the face, neck, upper torso and back. Three grades: mild, moderate and severe.

P: Rarely biopsied.
Micro: Gross distension of the pilosebaceous follicle with neutrophil infiltration. Closed comedones may contain serous fluid. Severe acne can create fistulas between inflamed glands and cause scarring.

I: Normally none required, especially if experiencing puberty.
Blood: FSH, LH levels (to exclude PCOS), prolactin, sex-hormone-binding globulin, testosterone, 17-OH-progesterone (day 21 measurement).
Urine: 24-h urinary cortisol (if Cushing's syndrome suspected).
Imaging: Pelvic ultrasound (to exclude PCOS).

M: **Medical:** Start treatment early to prevent scarring.
For mild/moderate acne
- **OTC preparations:** containing benzoyl peroxide, azelaic acid.

For moderate/severe acne
- **Topical antibiotics** (clindamycin, erythromycin): consider if no response to other topical preparations (e.g. after 2 months). Side-effects: topical preparations may cause local irritation.
- **Topical vitamin A derivatives** (tretinoin): 3–4 months to work.
- **Combined topical:** benzamycin (benzoyl peroxide + erythromycin), or combined tretinoin and erythromycin.
- **Systemic antibiotics** (oxytetracycline, minocycline, erythromycin): for moderate/severe/inflammatory acne if topical treatment is not effective/tolerated or if there is a difficult site for topical application.

For severe acne
- **Oral vitamin A derivative** (isotretinoin): available only by specialist prescription. Side-effects: teratogenic, hyperlipidaemia.

Others: For females, oral contraceptive pill or cyproterone acetate reduce severity.
Advice: Counsel patients that an improvement may not be seen for at least a couple of months, use of non-greasy cosmetics, wash face daily.

C: Facial scarring (atrophic, 'ice pick', hypertrophic, keloidal), hyperpigmentation, secondary infection, psychological morbidity.

P: Generally improves spontaneously over months or years.

Acoustic neuroma

D: Benign schwannoma of the vestibular (VIII) nerve sheath.

A: The schwannoma expands from the internal acoustic meatus into the cerebellopontine angle, causing compression of structures (other cranial nerves and brainstem) in that region.

A/R: In type II neurofibromatosis (see Neurofibromatosis), bilateral acoustic neuromas are associated with meningiomas, gliomas, peripheral and spinal schwannomas. There have been reports of acoustic neuroma associated with acoustic trauma, e.g. chronic exposure to loud noise.

E: Incidence 1 in 100 000/year. Occurs at all ages, more common in 40–50 years (unilateral) or 20–30 years (bilateral). ♀ > ♂. Represents 8 % of all intracranial tumours in adults and 80–90 % of cerebellopontine angle tumours.

H: Unilateral hearing loss, vertigo.

E: Progressive unilateral sensorineural hearing loss. Nystagmus to the side opposite to tumour. Larger tumours compress: trigeminal (V) nerve (loss of corneal reflex, unilateral facial numbness); facial (VII) nerve (unilateral LMN facial palsy). Larger tumours can cause brainstem–cerebellar compression: bulbar cranial nerve palsies, reversal of the nystagmus, ipsilateral ataxia, obstruction at the level of the fourth ventricle: hydrocephalus, ↑ intracranial pressure, occipital headaches. Look for neurofibromas at other sites.

P: Arise from the Schwann cell perineural elements of the vestibular nerve and rarely the cochlear portion of the VIII nerve.
Micro: Zones of alternately dense and sparse cellularity ('Antoni A and B areas') are characteristic.

I: **Auditory evoked potentials:** This will show waveform delays, excluding lesions in the cochlea or the ear.
MRI: This will show the size and extent of the tumour. Gadolinium enhancement is particularly helpful to highlight the tumour clearly.

M: **Medical:** None.
Surgical: Suboccipital, translabyrinthine or middle fossa approach. Curative treatment; however, hearing is often permanently impaired. Morbidity depends on size of tumour. Radiosurgery may be considered for neuromas < 3 cm and in patients unfit for conventional surgery.
Advice: Patient may need to learn how to lip-read and use sign language, and should start practising before curative surgery is attempted.

C: Progressive compression of brainstem, pyramidal tracts and the fourth ventricle.

P: Hearing loss is often permanent. Treatment merely prevents further damage.

Acromegaly

D: Constellation of signs and symptoms caused by hypersecretion of GH in adults. (Excess GH before puberty results in gigantism.)

A: Most cases are a result of GH-secreting pituitary adenoma.
Rarely: Excess GHRH causing somatotroph hyperplasia from hypothalamic ganglioneuroma, bronchial carcinoid or pancreatic tumours.

A/R: MEN Type 1 seen in 6 % of patients.

E: *Rare*. Annual incidence: 5 in 1 000 000. Prevalence: 50 in 1 000 000. Age at diagnosis: 40–50 years.

H: Very gradual progression of symptoms over many years (often only detectable on serial photographs). May complain of rings and shoes becoming tight. ↑ Sweating, headache, carpal tunnel syndrome. Symptoms of hypopituitarism (hypogonadism, hypothyroidism, hypoadrenalism). Hyperprolactinaemia (irregular periods, ↓ libido, impotence). Visual disturbances (caused by optic chiasm compression).

E: **Hands:** Enlarged spade-like hands with thick greasy skin. Signs of carpal tunnel syndrome (see Carpal tunnel syndrome). Premature osteoarthritis (arthritis also affects other large joints, temporomandibular joint).
Face: Prominent eyebrow ridge (frontal bossing) and cheeks, broad nose bridge, prominent nasolabial folds, thick lips, ↑ gap between teeth, large tongue, prognathism, husky resonant voice (thickening vocal cords).
Visual field loss: Bitemporal superior quadrantanopia progressing to bitemporal hemianopia (caused by pituitary tumour compressing the optic chiasm).
Neck: Multinodular goitre.
Feet: Enlarged.

P: **Microscopy:** The most common cause is a pituitary adenoma consisting of acidophilic somatotrophs.

I: **Serum IGF-1:** Useful initial screening test as GH stimulates liver IGF-1 secretion (IGF-1 varies with age of patient and ↑ during pregnancy and puberty).
GTT: After 50–75 g oral glucose load, GH and glucose samples are taken every 30 min for 2 h. Serum GH levels are not suppressed in acromegaly (false-positive results are seen in anorexia nervosa, Wilson's disease, opiate addiction).
IV TRH, GnRH or dopamine agonists may produce 100–300 % rise in GH levels, but are not routinely performed.
Pituitary function tests (9 a.m. cortisol, LH and FSH): To test for hypopituitarism.
MRI of the brain: To image the pituitary tumour and effect on the optic chiasm.
Hand and feet X-ray (not commonly used): Tufting of terminal phalanges, osteophytes, ↑ joint space.
GHRH measurement: Detects GHRH-dependent acromegaly (rare).

M: **Surgical:** Hypophysectomy is the only curative treatment. Can be approached *trans*-sphenoidally (< 1 cm adenomas) or through a craniotomy (if inaccessible, *trans*-sphenoidally).
Radiotherapy: Adjunctive treatment to surgery.
Medical: Suitable for microadenomas that are not resectable, to improve symptoms.

SC somatostatin analogues (e.g. octreotide, lanreotide). Side-effects: abdominal pain, steatorrhoea glucose intolerance, gallstones, irritation at the injection site.
Oral dopamine agonists (e.g. bromocriptine, cabergoline). Side-effects: nausea, vomiting, constipation, postural hypotension (↑ dose gradually and take it during meals), Raynaud's phenomenon, psychosis (rare).
GH antagonist (e.g. pegvisomant): new therapy is promising.
Monitor: Pituitary function tests, echocardiography, regular colonoscopy and blood glucose.

C: **CVS:** Cardiomyopathy, hypertension.
Respiratory: Obstructive sleep apnoea.
GI: Colonic polyps.
Reproductive: Hyperprolactinaemia (30 %).
Metabolic: Hypercalcaemia, hyperphosphataemia, renal stones, diabetes mellitus, hypertriglyceridaemia.
Psychological: Depression, psychosis (resulting from dopamine agonist therapy).
Complications of surgery: Nasoseptal perforation, hypopituitarism, adenoma recurrence, CSF leak, infection (meninges, sphenoid sinus).

P: Good with early diagnosis and treatment, although physical changes are irreversible.

Acute respiratory distress syndrome (ARDS)

D: Characterized by acute respiratory failure, non-cardiogenic pulmonary oedema, reduced lung compliance and refractory hypoxaemia. Also known as acute lung injury.

A: Severe insult to the lungs or other organs (systemic illness) induces the release of neutrophil inflammatory mediators which increase capillary permeability and cause pulmonary oedema. Virtually any major insult can cause ARDS; common ones are:

1 sepsis;
2 pancreatitis;
3 pre-eclampsia;
4 hypovolaemic shock;
5 pneumonia;
6 tumour lysis syndrome;
7 severe burns;
8 major trauma;
9 DIC.

A/R: Often associated with multiorgan failure.

E: Annual UK incidence $\sim$1 in 6000.

H: Rapid deterioration of respiratory function; respiratory distress, cough; symptoms of aetiology.

E: Cyanosis, tachypnoea, tachycardia, widespread inspiratory crepitations. Hypoxia refractory to oxygen treatment. Signs are usually bilateral but may be asymmetrical in early stages.

P: **Macro:** Heavy, red and boggy lungs.
Micro: Diffuse alveolar and endothelial cell damage. Three phases:

1 Early exudative phase with inflammatory infiltrates, oedema in the interstitium and alveolar spaces.
2 Fibroproliferative phase as the alveolar exudates undergoes organization, with proliferation of type II pneumocytes and production of collagen by fibroblasts.
3 Final fibrotic phase emerges after 3–4 weeks, alveoli coalesce and adopt a 'honeycomb' appearance. Resolution of fibrosis is slow with gradual lung remodelling.

I: **CXR:** Bilateral alveolar and interstitial shadowing. Usually indistinguishable from pulmonary oedema.
Blood: FBC, U&E, LFT, ESR/CRP, amylase, clotting, ABG, blood culture, sputum culture.
Swan–Ganz catheterization: Monitoring of cardiac output and intracardiac pressures (particularly PCWP). If < 18 mmHg, ARDS is more likely than pulmonary oedema.
Mechanical ventilation: Lungs are less compliant, requiring high inflation pressures.

M: **Should be managed in ITU.**
Respiratory support: 40–60 % O_2 given with either:

1 CPAP to prevent alveolar collapse; or
2 mechanical ventilatory support, if patient is too weak to breathe for themselves.

If $PaO_2 < 8$ kPa despite O_2 or $PaCO_2 > 6$ kPa, intubate and give *IPPV* which delivers O_2 at a set tidal volume and rate. *PEEP* may be applied to prevent alveolar collapse. Newer techniques reduce peak airway pressure and complications of PEEP.

Inverse ratio ventilation: Inspiratory phase is longer than expiratory phase, so that the tidal volume is delivered over a longer period but at a lower pressure.

High-frequency jet ventilation: Delivers small volumes as a jet of gas at high frequencies.

Steroids: May be beneficial in the proliferative phase.

Cardiovascular support: Inotropes (e.g. dobutamine) to maintain cardiac output, blood transfusion for anaemia.

Treat the cause (e.g. antibiotics for sepsis, blood for shock).

Fluid balance: Treat pulmonary oedema (fluid restriction, diuretics to maintain urine output, inhaled nitric oxide acting as a pulmonary vasodilator), haemofiltration (also for renal failure).

Nutritional support: Enteral or parenteral while on the ventilator, stress ulcer protection.

C: Respiratory failure and death.

Complications of ventilation: secondary infections, upper airway trauma.

Complications of PEEP:

1 Lung overdistension can cause surgical emphysema from barotrauma.
2 High O_2 pressures and concentrations cause microvascular damage.
3 Pulmonary vessel compression, reduced venous return and cardiac output.

P: Highly variable depending on cause but generally poor. Mortality ~60 % (mostly from sepsis). A prolonged period of ventilation may be required with long convalescence.

Adrenal insufficiency

D: Deficiency of adrenal cortical hormones (e.g. mineralocorticoids, glucocorticoids and androgens).

A: **Primary:** (Addison's disease): Autoimmune (>70%).
Infections: Tuberculosis, meningococcal septicaemia (Waterhouse–Friderichsen syndrome), CMV (HIV patients), histoplasmosis.
Infiltration: Metastasis (e.g. lung, breast, melanoma), lymphomas, amyloidosis.
Infarction (thrombophilia, e.g. lupus anticoagulant syndrome).
Inherited: Adrenoleucodystrophy,* ACTH receptor mutation.
Surgical: After bilateral adrenalectomy.
Secondary: *Pituitary or hypothalamic* disease.
Iatrogenic: Sudden cessation of long-term steroid therapy which causes hypothalamic–pituitary–adrenal suppression.

A/R: Addison's disease is associated with pernicious anaemia, Hashimoto's thyroiditis, Graves' disease, HLA-DR3 and HLA-DR4. Addison's disease may be part of a syndrome (e.g. triple A syndrome of achalasia and alacrimation) or in polyglandular deficiencies.†

E: Most common cause is iatrogenic. Primary causes are rare (annual incidence of Addison's is 8 in 1 000 000).

H: **Chronic presentation:** Non-specific vague symptoms such as dizziness, anorexia, weight loss, diarrhoea, vomiting, abdominal pain, lethargy, weakness, depression.
Acute presentation of an Addisonian crisis: Acute adrenal insufficiency with major haemodynamic collapse often precipitated by stress (e.g. infection or surgery).

E: **Postural hypotension.**
Increased pigmentation: Generalized but more noticeable on buccal, scars, skin creases, nails, pressure points (resulting from melanocytes being stimulated by ↑ ACTH levels).
Loss of body hair in women (androgen deficiency).
Associated autoimmune conditions: e.g. vitiligo.
Addisonian crisis: Hypotensive shock, tachycardia, pale, cold, clammy, oliguria.

P: **Autoimmune:** Atrophic adrenal glands with lymphocytic infiltration. Adrenal medullas are spared.
Tuberculosis: Adrenal glands are enlarged with epithelioid granulomas and caseation. Later, they calcify.
Waterhouse–Friderichsen syndrome: Bilateral adrenal haemorrhage, beginning in the medulla.
Secondary: Adrenal cortical atrophy with sparing of the zona glomerulosa.

*Adrenoleucodystrophy is an X-linked inherited disease characterized by adrenal atrophy and demyelination.
†Polyglandular syndromes:
Type I (autosomal recessive): Addison's disease, chronic mucocutaneous candidiasis, hypoparathyroidism.
Type II (Schmidt's syndrome): Addison's disease, diabetes mellitus Type 1, hypothyroidism, hypogonadism.

I: **Blood:** *FBC* (neutrophilia), *U&E* (↑ urea, ↓ Na^+, ↑ K^+), *ESR or CRP* (↑ in acute infection), *Ca^{2+}* (may be ↑), *glucose* (↓), *blood cultures, serum cortisol* (may be ↓ but a Synacthen test is needed to make diagnosis), *ACTH* (↑ in primary disease and ↓ in secondary disease), *autoantibodies* (e.g. against 21-hydroxylase), *TFT*.

Urine: Urinalysis, culture and sensitivity (UTI may have triggered the crisis).

CXR: May identify cause (e.g. tuberculosis, carcinoma) or precipitant of crisis (e.g. infection).

Short Synacthen test: IM 250 μg tetracosactrin (synthetic ACTH) is given. Serum cortisol levels are measured at 0, 30 and 60 min. Serum cortisol < 550 nmol/L at 30 min indicates adrenal failure ('flat' short Synacthen test).

Long Synacthen test: 1 mg tetracosactrin is given and cortisol is measured at 0, 30, 60, 90 and 120 min then at 4, 6, 8, 12 and 24 h. In secondary adrenal failure, cortisol rises after ~24 h, but not in primary adrenal failure ('flat' response).

Abdominal ultrasound, CT or MRI: Visualizes structural lesions of the adrenal glands.

Adrenal biopsy: For microscopy, culture, PCR.

M: **Addisonian crisis:** Rapid IV fluid rehydration (0.9% saline, 1 L over 30–60 min, 2–4 L in 12–24 h). 50 mL of 50 % dextrose to correct hypoglycaemia. IV 200 mg hydrocortisone bolus followed by 100 mg 6 hourly (until BP is stable). Treat the precipitating cause (e.g. antibiotics for infection). Monitor temperature, pulse, respiratory rate, BP, sat O_2 and urine output.

Medical: *Hydrocortisone* (20 mg in morning, 10 mg in evening): dosage needs to be increased during acute illness or stress. IM hydrocortisone needed preoperatively. If associated with hypothyroidism, give hydrocortisone before thyroxine.

Fludrocortisone (synthetic mineralocorticoid).

Advice: Steroid warning card, Medicalert bracelet, emergency hydrocortisone ampoule, patient education.

C: Hyperkalaemia. Death during an Addisonian crisis.

P: Adrenal function rarely recovers, but normal life expectancy can be expected if treated.

Alcohol dependence

D: **Alcohol dependence** is characterized by three or more of:
- compulsion to drink;
- neglect of other interests;
- increased tolerance;
- difficulty controlling onset;
- difficulty controlling termination or the levels of alcohol use;
- physiological withdrawal state on cessation of alcohol or its use to avoid withdrawal symptoms; and
- persisting use despite awareness of the nature and extent of the harm that it is causing.

Problem drinker: An individual experiencing alcohol-related harm.

A: Alcohol is an amphiphilic molecule that non-competitively opens neuronal $GABA_A$ receptors to produce tolerance, dependence and addictive behaviour. Alcohol is a liver enzyme-inhibitor acutely, but chronic abuse induces liver enzymes.

A/R: Family history (~1 in 3 'alcoholics' have a parent with alcohol-related problems) and twin studies have shown that genetic factors have a role. Environmental factors include cultural, parental and peer group influences, availability of alcohol, occupation (e.g. ↑ risk in publicans, doctors, lawyers). Associated with depressive, anxiety states and antisocial personality disorder.

E: Common. According to the UK General Household Survey 1994:
13 % ♀ and 27 % ♂ drink more than recommended limits (14 and 21 units per week, respectively);
2 % ♀ and 6 % ♂ drink very high levels (>36 and >51 units per week, respectively).
(1 unit = 8 g alcohol: 1 glass wine or 1/2 pint of beer.)

H: **Acute intoxication:** Amnesia, ataxia, dysarthria, palpitations, flushing, disorientation and coma. Alcohol history and **CAGE** screening questions:
Cut-down: '... felt that you should cut-down on intake?
Annoyed: '... felt annoyed by criticism of your drinking?
Guilt: '... felt guilty about how much you drink?
Eye-opener: '... feel that you need a drink when you wake up?
A drinking diary is useful to record how much, what, when and with whom alcohol is taken.

Symptoms of withdrawal: Nausea, sweating and tremor, restlessness, agitation, visual hallucination, fever, tachycardia, confusion, seizures.

E: **Signs suggestive of chronic alcohol misuse:** Spider naevi, telangiectasia, facial mooning, Dupuytren's contracture, palmar erythema, bilateral parotid enlargement, gynaecomastia, bruising, smell of alcohol.
Signs of complications: (See Alcoholic hepatitis and Liver failure.)

P: There is a spectrum of alcohol-related liver injury from a fatty liver, enlarged with triglycerides deposited in hepatocytes, to alcoholic hepatitis and cirrhosis where the liver becomes shrunken with the architecture distorted by fibrous bands and nodule formation.

I: **Blood:** Commonly used markers are MCV (↑), γ-GT (↑), transaminases (↑). Other less specific markers include ↑ uric acid, ↑ triglycerides or markers of end organ damage (e.g. bilirubin, albumin, PT in liver).

Acute overdose: Blood alcohol, glucose, ABG (risk of ketoacidosis or lactic acidosis), U&E, toxic screen (e.g. barbiturates, paracetamol).
Liver biopsy: For assessment and staging of liver disease.

Ultrasound or CT imaging of liver.
Upper GI endoscopy: To look for oesphageal varices and treat them prophylactically.
Electroencephalogram: Not routine, but useful if uncertain if mental state is caused by encephalopathy.

M: **Acute intoxication:** Monitor and support of airway, breathing, circulation. Intubation and ventilation if severe respiratory depression, IV fluids and careful monitoring of urine output, blood glucose (as may ↓), U&E and blood gases.
Management of withdrawal: IV vitamin B complex (Pabrinex) and reducing doses of clomethiazole. Close attention to dehydration, electrolyte imbalances and infections. Nutritional support important as often malnourished. Lactulose and phosphate enemas may help any encephalopathy.
Advice and intervention: Using motivational interviewing techniques in those at risk of alcohol-related problems; counselling and community-based services, self-help groups (e.g. AA), alcohol treatment units for those with established problems, detoxification period is necessary for those physically dependent.
Medical: Acamprosate reduces craving. Disulfiram (an aldehyde dehydrogenase inhibitor) causes patient to develop vasomotor symptoms, nausea, abdominal pain when drinking alcohol.

C: **Withdrawal effects:** Fits, delirium tremens (48–72 h after cessation: coarse tremor, agitation, fever, tachycardia, confusion, delusions and hallucinations).
GI: Oesophagitis, Mallory–Weiss tears, varices, gastritis, peptic ulcers, acute or chronic pancreatitis.
Liver: Fatty change, alcoholic hepatitis, cirrhosis (see Alcoholic hepatitis and Liver failure).
Neurological: Acute intoxication. Chronic complications include cerebral atrophy and dementia, cerebellar degeneration, optic atrophy, peripheral neuropathy, myopathy. Indirect effects include hepatic encephalopathy, thiamine deficiency causing Wernicke's encephalopathy* or Korsakoff's psychosis.†
Drug interactions: e.g. oral contraceptive pill.
Teratogenicity: Fetal alcohol syndrome.
Haematological: Anaemia (vitamin B_{12} or folate deficiency, iron deficiency if caused by GI bleeding), thrombocytopenia (↓ maturation or ↑ destruction).
Respiratory: depression, inhalation of vomitus.
Cardiac: hypertension, cardiomyopathy, arrhythmias.
Psychosocial: depression, anxiety, deliberate self-harm. Domestic, employment and financial problems.

P: Alcoholic fatty liver is reversible on abstinence from alcohol. In general, 5-year survival rates in those with alcoholic cirrhosis who stop drinking are 59–75 %, but < 40 % in those who continue.

***Wernicke's encephalopathy** is nystagmus, ophthalmoplegia and ataxia, together with apathy, disorientation and disturbed memory. Treat urgently with thiamine or may progress to Korsakoff's psychosis.†
†**Korsakoff's psychosis** is characterized by profound impairment of retrograde and anterograde memory with confabulation, as a result of damage to the mammillary bodies and the hippocampus. Irreversible.

Alcoholic hepatitis

D: Inflammatory liver injury caused by chronic heavy intake of alcohol.

A: One of the three forms of liver disease caused by excessive intake of alcohol (see Alcohol dependence), a spectrum that ranges from alcoholic fatty liver (steatosis) to alcoholic hepatitis and chronic cirrhosis.

A/R: Females more susceptible than males. Binge drinking more likely to lead to hepatitis.

E: 10–35 % of heavy drinkers develop this form of liver disease.

H: May remain asymptomatic and undetected unless they present for other reasons.
May be **mild illness** with nausea, malaise, epigastric or right hypochondrial pain and a low-grade fever.
May be **more severe** with jaundice, abdominal discomfort or swelling, swollen ankles or GI bleeding. Women tend to present with more florid illness than men. There is a history of heavy alcohol intake (~ 15–20 years of excessive intake necessary for development of alcoholic hepatitis). There may be trigger events (e.g. aspiration pneumonia or injury).

E: **Signs of alcohol excess:** Malnourished, palmar erythema, Dupuytren's contracture, facial telangiectasia, parotid enlargement, spider naevi, gynaecomastia, testicular atrophy, hepatomegaly, easy bruising.
Signs of severe alcoholic hepatitis: Febrile (50 % of patients), tachycardia, jaundice (> 50 % of patients), bruising, encephalopathy (e.g. hepatic foetor, liver flap, drowsiness, unable to copy a five-pointed star, disoriented), ascites (30–60 % of patients), hepatomegaly (liver is usually mild–moderately enlarged and may be tender on palpation), splenomegaly.

P: Precise mechanism of ethanol-induced damage is unclear but appears to involve free radical and immunological damage. In alcoholic hepatitis, the liver histopathology shows centrilobular ballooning degeneration and necrosis of hepatocytes, steatosis, neutrophilic inflammation, cholestasis, Mallory hyaline inclusions (eosinophilic intracytoplasmic aggregates of cytokeratin intermediate filaments) and giant mitochondria.

I: **Blood:** *FBC:* ↓ Hb, ↑ MCV, ↑ WCC, ↓ platelets.
LFT: ↑ transminases but more marked with AST, ↑ bilirubin, ↓ albumin, ↑ AlkPhos, ↑ γ-GT.
U&E: Urea and K^+ levels tend to be low, unless significant renal impairment.
Clotting: Prolonged PT is a sensitive marker of significant liver damage.
Immunoglobulins: ↑ IgA and IgM.
Ultrasound scan: To exclude other causes of liver impairment (e.g. malignancies).
Upper GI endoscopy: To investigate for varices.
Liver biopsy: Percutaneous or transjugular, in the presence of coagulopathy.
Electroencephalogram: For encephalopathy.

M: **Acute:** Thiamine, folic acid and multivitamins. Monitor and correct K^+, Mg^{2+}, PO_4^- and glucose abnormalities. Ensure adequate urine output. Treat encephalopathy with oral lactulose and phosphate enemas. Ascites is managed by diuretics (spironolactone with or without frusemide (furosemide)) or therapeutic paracentesis. Nutrition: nasogastric feeding. Glypressin and *N*-acetylcysteine for hepatorenal syndrome.

Steroid therapy: If discriminant function >32 and no evidence of infection, and haemodynamically stable >48 h and no evidence of renal insufficiency:
Discriminant function $=$ (bilirubin/17) $+$ (prolongation of PT $\times$ 4.6).
Long-term: (See Alcohol dependence). Abstinence from alcohol is the key, with involvement of psychosocial support services. Naltrexone and acamprosate have been used to reduce craving. Negative reinforcement: disulfiram. Nutritional supplementation and vitamins (B group, thiamine, folic acid).

C: Acute liver decompensation, hepatorenal syndrome (renal failure secondary to advanced liver disease), cirrhosis (see Liver failure).

P: Mortality in first month is about 10 %, 40 % in first year. If alcohol intake continues, progression to cirrhosis within 1–3 years. If abstinent, it may slowly resolve.

α_1-Antitrypsin deficiency

D: Low levels or absence of α_1-antitrypsin that can lead to lung emphysema or liver cirrhosis.

A: α_1-Antitrypsin is a liver-derived protein which acts as an inhibitor of tissue proteases, in particular neutrophil elastase. The α_1-antitrypsin gene (*PiMM* is normal) is on chromosome 14. Numerous variant forms ranging from heterozygotes (*PiMZ* or *PiMNull*) to homozygotes; e.g.

- *PiZZ:* normally translated but peptide not properly folded in hepatocytes endoplasmic reticulum; and
- *PiNull-Null:* total absence of α_1-antitrypsin production.

A/R: Associated with bronchiectasis, panniculitis (adipose tissue inflammation).

E: Common. 1 in 2500 in northern Europe are homozygous for the *PiZZ* variant. Up to 1 in 10 carry a gene mutation but disease manifestations are very variable. Emphysema is the most common, but takes decades to become apparent. Liver disease may become evident in childhood, and is present in ~15 % by 50 years.

H: It is rare for both liver and lung disease to affect the same patient.
Lung: Breathlessness, wheeze, cough, sputum (75 % have respiratory symptoms, but < 1 % COPD is caused by α_1-antitrypsin deficiency).
Liver: Jaundice, confusion, ascites (distended abdomen), haematemesis.

E: **Signs of emphysema:** Barrel chest, intercostal recession, use of accessory muscles, ↓ expansion, hyper-resonant chest, ↓ dullness of heart and liver regions, wheeze, prolonged expiration phase.
Signs of cirrhosis: Shrunken liver, nodular liver edge, jaundice, ascites, altered mental state, bruising and clotting abnormalities.

P: Low levels of α_1-antitrypsin results in ↑ elastase activity. In the lung, there is ↑ breakdown of elastin and reduced mucociliary clearance leading to emphysema and chronic bronchitis. α_1-Antitrypsin accumulation in hepatocytes appears to be responsible for liver damage, but the mechanism is unclear. PAS staining and electron microscopy visualizes the protein as hepatocyte inclusions (in dilated rough endoplasmic reticulum).

I: **Blood:** LFTs (all enzymes may be ↑).
Plasma electrophoresis: α_1 Band is missing or lowered (< 2 g/L).
CXR: See COPD, bullae may predominate in the lower zones.
Pulmonary function tests: FEV_1 : FVC ratio (↓), PEFR (↓), gas transfer coefficient of CO (↓).
Liver biopsy: staining with PAS to detect α_1-antitrypsin accumulation and assess degree of liver damage.

M: **Advice:** Stop smoking and ↓ alcohol intake, genetic counselling.
Lung: Bronchodilators, if severe, assessment for long-term oxygen therapy or single lung transplantation. IV infusion of α_1-antitrypsin has not been assessed in clinical trials.
Liver: Liver transplantation for end-stage disease.
Panniculitis: Dapsone or IV α_1-antitrypsin replacement.

C: Emphysema, chronic bronchitis, pulmonary hypertension, cor pulmonale, recurrent pneumonias (*Strep. pneumoniae*, *H. influenzae*), secondary polycythaemia, liver cirrhosis and hepatocellular carcinoma.

P: Overall, lifespan is shortened by 10–15 years: 75 % have respiratory symptoms; 10–15 % develop cirrhosis by 50 years.

Alzheimer's disease

D: Primary chronic progressive neurodegenerative dementia* characterized histologically by β-amyloid plaques and neurofibrillary tangles.

A: APP (on chromosome 21) is secreted and cleaved by neuronal membrane secretases into β-amyloid peptide. The role of β-amyloid peptides in the plaques or that of intracellular neurofibrillary tangles is not clear.
Genetic factors: Risk of early onset include genes on chromosomes 1, 14, 19 and apoE4 lipoprotein allele.
Environmental factors: Previous head injury, role of aluminium exposure is controversial.

A/R: Younger age of onset (30s–40s) in Down's syndrome (↑ risk of amyloid synthesis from their extra copy of the *APP* gene on chromosome 21). Family history: 10–30 % chance of developing Alzheimer's disease amongst first-degree relatives of a patient.

E: Most common cause of dementia in all age groups. Affects 5 % of those >65 years. Accounts for 60–80 % of all dementias. ♂ = ♀.

H: History is usually obtained from relative. Gradual deterioration of cognitive functions: memory loss, difficulty in learning and retaining new information, change of personality, apathy, loss of concentration, disorientation. May be accompanied with extrapyramidal or psychiatric manifestations (hallucinations and delusions). Finally, amnesia, aphasia, apraxia, agnosia, behavioural disturbances, incontinence and loss of independence.

E: Mini-Mental State Exam will show global loss of cognitive abilities (orientation, memory, language).

P: **Micro:** Extracellular β-amyloid plaques, intracellular neurofibrillary tangles (composed of paired helical filaments), ↓ neurone count particularly in hippocampus, temporal neocortex and frontal lobe (nucleus basalis of Meynert), cholinergic neurones are particularly affected.
Macro: Cerebral atrophy particularly affecting the temporal lobe.

I: Exclude treatable causes of dementia.
Blood: FBC, U&E, LFT, ESR/CRP, TFT (exclude myxoedema), vitamin B12 deficiency, copper and caeruloplasmin (exclude Wilson's disease), syphilis and HIV serology.
***Dementia** is the significant impairment of memory and >1 other domain of cognition in a setting of clear consciousness (other domains are language, visuospatial skills, praxis, personality, social behaviour).
CT/MRI: Usually normal, assesses cerebral atrophy, exclude tumours, infarcts, subdural haematoma.
Psychometric testing: Global deficit rather than focal deficit.

M: **Conservative:** Medicalert bracelet, memory aids (diaries, labels).
Social: manage psychological impact of disease on carer and patient. Nursing and institutional care in the later stages or for respite.
Medical: Licensed medical therapies are only for mild to moderate disease and provide only temporary improvement, e.g. rivastigmine, donepezil, galantamine (acetylcholinesterase inhibitors). Treatment of systemic illness or infection that may exacerbate the disease, avoid sedative drugs, alcohol.

C: ↓ Quality of life, loss of independence, devastating effect on family.

P: Mean survival 7 years.

Amyloidosis

D: Heterogeneous group of diseases characterized by extracellular deposition of protein in a characteristic amyloid fibrillar conformation.

A: Classified according to fibril proteins. Can be systemic (generalized) or localized.

Type of amyloid	Fibril protein	Underlying disorders
AA	Serum amyloid A protein	Chronic inflammatory diseases (e.g. rheumatoid arthritis, seronegative arthritides, Crohn's disease, familial Mediterranean fever*), chronic infections (TB, bronchiectasis, osteomyelitis), malignancy (e.g. Hodgkin's disease, renal cancer)
AL	Monoclonal immunoglobulin light chains	Subtle monoclonal plasma cell dyscrasias usually, but sometimes multiple myeloma, Waldenström's macroglobulinaemia, B-cell lymphoma
ATTR (familial amyloid polyneuropathy)	Genetic-variant transthyretin	Autosomal dominantly transmitted mutations in the gene for transthyretin (*TTR*). Variable penetrance. Hereditary amyloidosis is also associated with other variant proteins

Localized amyloid: In pancreatic islets of Langerhans (see Diabetes mellitus Type II).
In brain and cerebral vessels (see Alzheimer's disease).
In bones and joints (in long-term dialysis caused by $A\beta_2M$ protein).

A/R: (see Aetiology). Individual susceptibility to developing amyloid varies substantially for largely unknown reasons.

E: **AA amyloidosis:** Lifetime incidence of 1–5 % among patients with chronic inflammatory diseases.
AL amyloidosis: Estimated annual incidence of about 3000 cases in the US and 300–600 cases in the UK.
Hereditary amyloidosis: Present in ≈5 % of patients with systemic amyloidosis; family history often absent.

H & E: **AA:** *Renal:* Proteinuria, nephrotic syndrome, renal failure. *Organomegaly:* Spleen, liver. *GI:* diarrhoea.
AL: *Renal:* (see AA amyloid). *GI:* Macroglossia, gut dysmotility, malabsorption, obstruction, perforation, weight loss, wasting. *Heart:* Restrictive cardiomyopathy, heart failure, arrhythmia. *Skin:* Purpura around eyes, plaques and nodules. *Neurological:* Autonomic, motor and sensory neuropathy, carpal tunnel syndrome. *Joints:* Painful asymmetrical large joints, 'shoulder pad' sign (bilateral swelling).
ATTR: Peripheral or autonomic neuropathy, frequent cardiac conduction problems, vitreous deposits. Wasting.

*Familial Mediterrenean fever is characterized by recurrent attacks of fever, serositis (peritonitis and pleurisy), caused by mutations in *MEFV* gene, which encodes pyrin, a protein involved in neutrophil regulation. Familial Mediterrenean fever is common in certain ethnic groups (Arabs, Ashkenazi Jews, Armenians and Turks).

Aβ_2M: Carpal tunnel syndrome, arthralgia, pathological fractures, bone cysts (see Renal failure, chronic).

P: **Micro:** Amorphous homogenous extracellular deposits which stain red with Congo red stain and give green birefringence under cross-polarized light.

Macro: Organs may be enlarged, firm and have a rubbery appearance.

Pathogenesis: Amyloid fibrils are formed when certain proteins present in excessive amounts or abnormal forms, misfold and assemble to a β-pleated sheet structure. They associate with glycosaminoglycans and SAP, and deposition progressively disrupts the structure and function of normal tissue.

I: **Tissue biopsy** (Congo red stain and immunohistochemistry): To diagnose amyloidosis and identify amyloid fibril protein. Reliable in AA, often poor for AL.

Urine: Proteinuria, free immunoglobulin light chains in AL.

Blood: CRP or ESR, rheumatoid factor, immunoglobulin levels and electrophoresis, LFT, U&E. SAA levels vital for monitoring treatment in AA.

^{123}I-SAP scan: Radiolabelled SAP localizes to the deposits enabling quantitative imaging of amyloidotic organs throughout the body.

Bone marrow, echocardiography and other investigations including DNA analysis for underlying disorders.

M: **Medical:** Reduction in the supply of the respective amyloid fibril precursor protein (e.g. chemotherapy for monoclonal hyperimmunoglobulinaemia, colchicine in familial Mediterranean fever, anti-inflammatory drugs in rheumatoid arthritis). Dialysis, management of hypertension, arrhythmias and symptomatic treatment.

Surgical: Organ transplantation in selected cases. Liver transplantation is effective in hereditary ATTR because this particular genetically variant precursor protein is produced in hepatocytes.

C: Failure of single or multiple organ systems, most commonly kidneys and heart (in AL type).

P: Without effective treatment: **AA:** 50 % die within 10 years of diagnosis; **AL:** 80 % die within 2 years. Survival can be prolonged substantially by treatment in at least 50 % of patients.

Anaemia, aplastic

D: Deficiency of all blood cell elements (pancytopenia) associated with bone marrow aplasia.

A: **Idiopathic** (> 40 %): May be mediated by T-cell immunological suppression of myeloid stem cells.
Acquired: Drugs (chloramphenicol, gold, alkylating agents, methotrexate), chemicals (DDT, benzene), radiation, viral infection (B19 parvovirus, CMV, HIV, measles), paroxysmal nocturnal haemoglobinuria.
Inherited: Fanconi's anaemia,* dyskeratosis congenita (rare sex-linked disorder with skin and nail atrophy).

A/R: Fanconi's anaemia.

E: Annual incidence: 2–5 in 1 000 000. Can occur at any age or either sex, slightly more common in males.

H: Slow (months) or rapid (days) onset.
Anaemia: Tiredness, lethargy and dyspnoea.
Thrombocytopenia: Easy bruising, bleeding gums, epistaxis.
Leukopenia: ↑ Frequency and severity of infections.

E: **Anaemia:** Pale.
Thrombocytopenia: Petechiae, bruises.
Leukopenia: Multiple bacterial or fungal infections. No hepatomegaly, splenomegaly or lymphadenopathy.

P: **Macro:** Pale or white bone marrow.
Micro: Hypocellular bone marrow composed of empty marrow spaces, fat cells, fibrous stroma and isolated foci of lymphocytes and plasma cells. Classic 'chicken wire' appearance.

I: **Blood:** FBC (↓ Hb, platelets, WCC, normal MCV, low or absent reticulocytes).
Blood film: To exclude leukaemia or myelomas.
Bone marrow trephine biopsy: For diagnosis and exclusion of other causes (bone marrow infiltration: lymphoma, leukaemia, malignancies, myeloma, myelofibrosis; see Pathology).
Chromosomal analysis: ↑ Random breaks in peripheral lymphocytes in Fanconi's anaemia.
Ham's test: For paroxysmal nocturnal haemoglobinuria, measures sensitivity of affected red blood cells to lysis by complement following activation in acidified serum.

M: **Treat the underlying cause:** e.g. review the causative drugs taken by patient.
Supportive: Blood and platelet transfusions, antibiotics for infections, consider antibiotic prophylaxis.
Immunosuppressive therapy: Steroids, ciclosporin A, antithymocyte globulin, androgens (oxymetholone) in patients > 45 years.
Bone marrow transplant (allogeneic): From HLA-matched sibling in patients < 20 years.
Patients between 20 and 45 may receive immunosuppressive therapy followed by bone marrow transplant.

*Farconi's anaemia: rare autosomal recessive genetic disorder caused by an error of DNA repair. Characterized by familial aplastic anaemia with bone abnormalities, microcephaly, hypogonadism, renal tract defects and brown pigmentation of skin.

C: Bleeding, infections. 10 % of those with Fanconi's anaemia may develop acute myeloid leukaemia. Complications of bone marrow transplantation (e.g. infection, graft-vs.-host disease).

P: Poor, although transplantation may be curative. Prognosis depends on the patient age and severity of the pancytopenia. Poor prognostic features include:

1 platelets $< 20 \times 10^9$/L;
2 neutrophils $< 0.5 \times 10^9$/L; or
3 reticulocytes $< 40 \times 10^9$/L.

Mortality of 50 % with these features lasting > 3 weeks.

Anaemia, haemolytic

D: Premature erythrocyte breakdown causing shortened erythrocyte life-span (< 120 days) and anaemia.

A: **Hereditary:**
Membrane defects: Hereditary spherocytosis,* elliptocytosis (elliptical erythrocytes).
Metabolic defects: G6PD deficiency.† Pyruvate kinase deficiencies (autosomal recessive).
Haemoglobinopathies: Sickle cell disease, thalassaemia (see Sickle cell anaemia and Thalassaemias).
Acquired:
Immune: *Autoimmune:* Warm or cold antibodies‡ attach to erythrocytes causing intravascular haemolysis and extravasular haemolysis in the spleen.
Isoimmune: Transfusion reaction, haemolytic disease of the newborn.
Drugs: Penicillin, quinine (through formation of drug–antibody–erythrocyte complex).
Non-immune: *Trauma:* Microangiopathic haemolytic anaemia caused by red cell fragmentation in abnormal microcirculation (e.g. haemolytic uraemic syndrome, DIC, malignant hypertension, pre-eclampsia), artificial heart valves.
Infection: Malaria, sepsis.
Paroxysmal nocturnal haemoglobinuria: ↑ Complement-mediated lysis caused by ↓ synthesis of protein cellular anchor of complement-degrading proteins.

A/R: (see Aetiology).

E: Common. Genetic causes are prevalent in African, Mediterranean, Middle Eastern populations. Hereditary spherocytosis is the most common inherited haemolytic anaemia in northern Europe.

H: Jaundice, haematuria, anaemia. Ask about systemic illness; family, drug and travel history.

E: Pallor (anaemia), jaundice, hepatosplenomegaly, features of the cause.

P: **Micro:** (see Investigations).

I: **Blood:** FBC (↓ Hb, ↑ reticulocytes, ↑ MCV, also ↑ unconjugated bilirubin, ↓ haptoglobin), U&E, folate.
Blood film: Leucoerythroblastic picture, macrocytosis, nucleated erythrocytes or reticulocytes, polychromasia. Identifies specific abnormal cells, such as spherocytes, elliptocytes, sickle cells, fragmented erythrocytes, malarial parasites, erythrocyte Heinz bodies (denatured Hb, stained with methyl violet seen in G6PD deficiency).

*Hereditary spherocytosis is an autosomal dominant condition where ↓ spectrin (a structural membrane protein) causes ↓ deformability of erythrocytes.
†G6PD deficiency (X-linked): G6PD is important in the hexose monophosphate shunt and maintains glutathione in reduced state. Deficiency results in susceptibility to oxidative stress (e.g. precipitated by sulphonamides, nitrofurantoin, dapsone, fava beans).
‡'Warm' antibodies (IgG) agglutinate erythrocytes at 37°C. Associated with SLE, lymphomas or methyldopa. 'Cold' antibodies (IgM) agglutinate erythrocytes in at room temperature or colder. Associated with infections (e.g. *Mycoplasma*, EBV) or lymphomas.

Urine: ↑ Urobilirubinogen. If intravascular haemolysis, there is haemoglobinuria and haemosiderinuria.

Direct Coombs' test: Identifies erythrocytes coated with antibodies (agglutinins) using antihuman globulin. Warm agglutinin and cold agglutinin.‡

Osmotic fragility test or Spectrin mutation analysis: To identify membrane abnormalities.

Ham's test: Lysis of erythrocytes in acidified serum in paraxosymal nocturnal haemoglobinuria.

Hb electrophoresis or enzyme assays: When other causes excluded.

Bone marrow biopsy (rarely required): Erythroid hyperplasia.

M: Treat underlying cause and avoid the contributing factor (e.g. cold exposure for cold agglutinins).

Spherocytosis: Folate supplement, splenectomy (postponed until >5 years old), lifetime penicillin, vaccination against encapsulated organisms (e.g. pneumococcus, *Haemophilus influenzae* and meningococcus).

Autoimmune (warm agglutinins): Prednisolone, splenectomy, azathioprine or cyclophosphamide.

Paroxysmal nocturnal haemoglobinuria: Blood transfusions (leucocyte-depleted). Anticoagulants (e.g. warfarin) for thrombotic episodes. Bone marrow transplantation has been successful in some patients.

C: Depends on cause. All can cause acute renal failure.

Spherocytosis: Gallstones. Aplastic, megaloblastic and haemolytic crises, leg ulcers.

Paroxysmal nocturnal haemoglobinuria: can transform to aplastic anaemia or leukaemia.

P: Mostly normal life expectancy, may be reduced in sickle cell anaemia, β-thalassaemia major and paroxysmal nocturnal haemoglobinuria.

Anaemia, macrocytic

D: Anaemia associated with a high MCV of erythrocytes (> 100 fl in adults). Subclassified into megaloblastic or non-megaloblastic.

A: **Megaloblastic:** Deficiency of B_{12} or folate required for DNA synthesis.
Vitamin B_{12}: ↓ *absorption:* Post-gastrectomy, pernicious anaemia*, terminal ileal resection or disease, coeliac disease, Crohn's disease, TB, tropical sprue, bacterial overgrowth, fish tapeworm.
↓*intake:* in vegans.
abnormal metabolism: Transcobalamin II deficiency (congenital), nitrous oxide (inactivates B_{12}).
Folate: ↓ *intake:* Alcoholics, elderly, anorexia.
↑ *demand:* Pregnancy, lactation, malignancy, chronic inflammation, chronic haemolytic anaemia, haemodialysis.
↓ *absorption:* Jejunal disease, e.g. coeliac disease, tropical sprue.
drugs: e.g. phenytoin, sulphasalazine, trimethoprim.
Non-megaloblastic: Pregnancy, alcohol excess, liver disease, myelodysplasia, hypothyroidism, haemolysis, drugs, e.g. hydroxyurea, azathioprine.

A/R: ↑ Incidence of pernicious anaemia with blood group A. Pernicious anaemia is associated with other autoimmune diseases (e.g. vitiligo and hypothyroidism).

E: Common finding on routine blood tests. More common in the elderly and females. Annual worldwide incidence of pernicious anaemia in over-40-year-olds is ~25 in 100 000. Most common cause of vitamin B_{12} deficiency in the West.

H: **Non-specific signs of anaemia:** Tiredness, lethargy, dyspnoea. Family history of autoimmune disease. Previous history of gastrointestinal surgery. Symptoms of the cause, e.g. weight loss, diarrhoea, steatorrhea in coeliac disease.

E: **Sign of anaemia** e.g. pallor, tachycardia, dyspnoea. There may be signs of the cause, e.g. malnutrition, jaundice, hypothyroid appearance.
Signs of pernicious anaemia: Lemon-tinted skin (mild jaundice), glossitis (red sore tongue), angular stomatitis (cheilitis), weight loss.
Signs of vitamin B_{12} deficiency: Symmetrical peripheral neuropathy, subacute combined degeneration of the spinal cord,† optic atrophy, dementia.

P: **Megaloblastic anaemia:** Nuclear maturation of developing erythrocytes lags behind cytoplasmic maturation, as a result of defective DNA synthesis. Leucocytes may also be affected causing low WCC and hypersegmented neutrophil nuclei (> 5 lobes).

I: **Blood:** FBC (by definition, ↓ Hb and ↑ MCV), LFT (↑ bilirubin as a result of ineffective erythropoiesis and ↑ Hb breakdown), ESR, TFT, serum vitamin B_{12}, red cell folate, antibodies against parietal cells or intrinsic factor.

*Pernicious anaemia is caused by autoimmune damage to gastric parietal cells causing atrophic gastritis and consequent reduced production of intrinsic factor needed for vitamin B_{12} absorption in terminal ileum.
†Subacute combined degeneration of the spinal cord is the degeneration of the dorsal and lateral columns of the spinal cord causing loss of joint and position sense, UMN weakness and spinocerebellar ataxia. Partially or completely relieved by restoring vitamin B_{12} levels.

Blood film: Abnormally large erythrocytes (macrocytes). May show cause.

Schilling's test: *Part I: Radiolabelled vitamin B_{12}* is given orally and non-radioactive B_{12} is given by IM injection to saturate vitamin B_{12}-binding proteins. Low levels of radiolabelled vitamin B_{12} in the urine (in the 24 h collection sample) indicates ↓ absorption.

Part II: Oral radiolabelled vitamin B_{12}, IM normal vitamin B_{12} (to saturate binding proteins) and oral intrinsic factor is given. If radiolabelled vitamin B_{12} is now detected in 24 h urine collection, the cause is likely to be intrinsic factor deficiency from pernicious anaemia or gastrectomy; otherwise, it suggests terminal ileal disease or bacterial overgrowth.

Bone marrow biopsy (rarely necessary): Megaloblasts (nucleated red cells) or myelodysplastic changes.

Investigations for suspected cause.

M: **Pernicious anaemia**: IM hydroxycobalamin (thrice weekly for 2 weeks, then every 3 months for life).

Folate deficiency: Oral folic acid.

Undetermined cause: Vitamin B_{12} and folate to avoid exacerbation of neuropathy caused by vitamin B_{12}.

C: In pernicious anaemia, ↑ risk of gastric cancer. In pregnancy, folate deficiency predisposes to spinal cord anomalies.

P: Majority are treatable if there are no complications.

Anaemia, microcytic

D: Anaemia associated with low MCV (< 80 fl).

A: **Iron-deficiency** (commonest cause):
blood loss: e.g. gastrointestinal tract, urogenital tract, Hookworm infection (*Ancylostoma duodenale*).
↓ *absorption:* small bowel disease, post-gastrectomy.
↑ *demands:* Growth, pregnancy.
↓ *intake:* Vegans.
Thalassaemia: See Thalassaemias.
Sideroblastic anaemia: Abnormality of haem synthesis. Can be inherited (X-linked), or secondary to alcohol, drugs (e.g. isoniazid, chloramphenicol), lead, myelodysplasia.
Anaemia of chronic disease*: Often normocytic but may be microcytic.
Lead poisoning (e.g. in scrap metal or smelting workers): Interferes with globin and haem synthesis.

A/R: Paterson–Brown–Kelly syndrome is anaemia associated with pharyngeal webs, dysphagia and glossitis.

E: Most common anaemia worldwide (particularly iron-deficiency anaemia).

H: **Non-specific:** Tiredness, lethargy, malaise, dyspnoea, pallor. Exacerbation of pre-existing angina or intermittent claudication. Family history of any causative diseases.
In lead poisoning: Anorexia, nausea, vomiting, abdominal pain, constipation, peripheral nerve lesions.

E: Signs of anaemia, e.g. pallor of skin and mucous membranes. Brittle nails and hair. If long-standing and severe, spoon-shaped nails (koilonychia).
Glossitis: Atrophy of tongue papillae.
Cheilitis: Angular stomatitis.
(Uncommon) Tachycardia, systolic flow murmurs.
Signs of thalassaemias (see Thalassaemias).
Lead poisoning: Blue line on the gums, peripheral nerve lesions (wrist or foot drop), encephalopathy, convulsions, ↓ consciousness.

P: **Microscopic:** (see Investigations).

I: **Blood:** FBC (↓ Hb,↓ MCV, reticulocytes), serum iron (↓ in iron deficiency), iron-binding capacity (↑ in iron deficiency), serum ferritin (↓ in iron deficiency), serum lead (if poisoning suspected).
Hb electrophoresis: For haemoglobin variants or thalassaemias.
Blood film:
Iron-deficiency anaemia: Microcytic (small), hypochromic (central pallor >one-third cell size), anisocytosis (variable cell size), poikilocytosis (variable cell shapes).
Sideroblastic anaemia: Dimorphic blood film with a population of hypochromic microcytic cells.
Lead poisoning: Basophilic stippling (coarse dots represent condensed RNA in the cytoplasm).

*Occurs in chronic inflammatory/autoimmune disease, chronic infections, e.g. TB/infective endocarditis, malignancy, chronic renal failure. Serum ferritin is normal/↑. It may be caused by ↓ RBC survival, ↓ erythropoietin response to the anaemia, ↓ iron release from bone marrow to erythroblasts. Treat the underlying condition.

Bone marrow (rarely needed): Erythroid hyperplasia and low iron levels.

Sideroblastic anaemia: Ring sideroblasts in the bone marrow (iron deposited in perinuclear mitochondria of erythroblasts, stain blue–green with Perls' stain).

If iron-deficiency anaemia in >40 years and postmenopausal women: Upper GI endoscopy, colonoscopy and investigations for haematuria should be considered if no obvious cause of blood loss.

M: **Iron deficiency:** Oral iron supplements (e.g. 200 mg ferrous sulphate tablets containing 65 mg of elemental iron, twice or three times daily taken with food). If oral iron intolerance or malabsorption, consider parenteral iron supplements (beware risk of anaphylaxis). Monitor Hb and MCV, aiming for Hb rise of 1 g/dL/week.

Thalassaemia: (see Thalassaemias).

Sideroblastic anaemia: Treat the cause (e.g. stop causative drugs). Pyridoxine can be used in inherited forms. If no response, consider blood transfusion and iron chelation.

Lead poisoning: Remove the source, dimercaprol, D-penicillamine, Ca^{2+} EDTA.

C: High output cardiac failure, complications of the cause.

P: Depends on the cause.

Anaphylaxis*

D: Life-threatening systemic hypersensitivity reaction to an allergen mediated by IgE antibodies.

A: Common allergens include drugs (e.g. penicillin), radiological contrast agents, latex, insect stings, eggs, fish, peanuts. Anaphylaxis may occur following repeated administration of blood products in patients with selective IgA deficiency (as a result of formation of anti-IgA antibodies).

A/R: Associated with other allergic hypersensitivity disorders (e.g. asthma, atopy, allergic rhinitis).

E: Relatively common. Anaphylaxis occurs in ~1 in 5000 exposures to parenteral penicillin or cephalosporin antibiotic.
1–2 % of patients receiving IV radiocontrast experience a hypersensitivity reaction (often minor).
0.5–1 % of children suffer from peanut allergy.
1 in 700 patients have selective IgA deficiency.

H: Acute onset of symptoms on exposure to allergen:
- wheeze;
- shortness of breath or sensation of choking;
- swelling of lips and face; and
- pruritus and rash.

E: **Bronchospasm:** Tachypnoea, wheeze, cyanosis.
Airway oedema: Swollen upper airways and eyes, rhinitis, conjunctival injection.
Skin: Urticarial rash (erythematous wheals) and angioedema.
Shock: Hypotension, tachycardia.

P: Type I hypersensitvity reaction occurs when a previously sensitized individual is exposed to an allergen. The allergen binds to preformed IgE attached to mast cells and basophils causing cross-linking. This results in degranulation and release of vasoactive compounds (e.g. histamine, prostaglandins and leukotrienes). These cause bronchospasm, ↑ capillary permeability and ↓ vascular tone, resulting in fluid loss into the extravascular space and tissue oedema. There is also further recruitment of inflammatory cells, which may cause a clinical deterioration several hours after the initial attack.

I: **Blood:** ABG. IgE levels (if measured) may be raised.
After the attack:
Allergen skin testing: Identifies allergen. Potentially dangerous as it may trigger anaphylactic attack.
RAST: Identifies specific IgE.

M: **Emergency management:**
- Stop any suspected drugs.
- *Resuscitation* according to principles of airway, breathing and circulation.
- *Secure airway* and give 100 % O_2. Intubation and transfer to ITU may be necessary so anaesthetist must be informed early.
- *Adrenaline* IM (0.5 mL of 1:1000). This can be repeated every 10 min according to response of pulse and BP.

*An anaphylactoid reaction is one that is clinically similar to anaphylaxis but antibodies are not responsible for the reaction, and may involve complement activation or non-immunological release of histamine.

- *Antihistamine* IV (10 mg chlorpheniramine) and *steroids* IV (100 mg hydrocortisone).
- *IV crystalloid or colloid* to maintain blood pressure. If hypotensive, lie patient flat with head tilted down.
- *Treat bronchospasm* with salbutamol ± ipratropium inhaler. Aminophylline IV infusion may be required.

Advice: Inform patient of allergen. Educate on use of adrenaline pen for IM administration. Provide Medicalert bracelet. Make note in patient's notes and drug charts.

C: Respiratory failure. Shock. Death.

P: Good if prompt treatment is given.

Angina pectoris

D: Acute central chest pain or tightness caused by cardiac ischaemia.

A: Angina results from coronary vessel narrowing, reducing myocardial blood supply and causing ischaemia. Most common cause is atherosclerosis. Other causes (spasm, e.g. from cocaine, arteritis, emboli) are rare.

A/R: **Risk factors:** Male, diabetes mellitus, family history, hypertension, hyperlipidaemia, smoking, previous history.

E: Common, prevalence is > 2 %. More common in males.

H: Chest pain or discomfort of acute onset. Central heavy tight 'gripping' pain that radiates to arms (usually left), neck, jaw or epigastrium. Exacerbated by cold weather, emotions and after meals.
Stable angina: Brought on by exertion (↑ myocardial demand for oxygen) and relieved by rest.
Unstable angina: Worsening or occurring at rest, with ↑ severity and frequency.
Decubitus angina occurs on lying down at night, possibly precipitated by cold sheets, ↑ heart rate in dreaming or left ventricular wall stress.

E: Signs of risk factors.

P: **Classical (stable or unstable):** Evidence of myocardial ischaemia secondary to atherosclerotic coronary arteries (see Myocardial infarction for pathology of atherosclerosis).
Prinzmetal's (variant): Caused by coronary vasospasm. Coronary arteries may be normal or atherosclerotic.
Syndrome X: Normal coronary arteries on angiograms despite angina and positive exercise ECG test. Possibly caused by functional or structural abnormalities of coronary microvasculature.

I: **Blood:** Cardiac enzymes (to exclude MI, troponin), lipid profile, glucose, amylase (exclude pancreatitis), FBC (anaemia can cause angina), TFT.
ECG: May be normal, ST depression, T wave inversion (Q waves show previous MIs), Prinzmetal's angina (ST elevation, which may be confused with MI).
ETT:* Positive in 75 % of patients with significant coronary artery disease, ST segment depression > 1 mm or a paradoxical ↓ in BP usually indicates severe coronary artery disease; normal test does not exclude the diagnosis. Dobutamine stress test is an alternative if patient is unable to exercise.
Cardiac angiogram: If symptoms not controlled with medical treatment or if ETT suggests poor prognosis.
Thallium-201 perfusion scan: ↓ Uptake in ischaemic myocardium. Not necessary in most cases.

M: **Acute unstable angina:**

- Admit, bed rest, high flow oxygen.
- Analgesia (diamorphine), antiemetic (metodopramide).
- Aspirin, clopidogrel if aspirin not tolerated.

*Contraindications: unstable angina, recent Q wave MI (< 5 days), severe aortic stenosis, uncontrolled arrhythmia, hypertension or heart failure. Stop if breathlessness or chest pain occurs, patient feels faint, arrhythmia, development of left bundle branch block or arteriovenous block, ST segment elevation or depression > 2 mm, fall in BP, excessive rise in BP (> 230 mmHg), failure of heart rate or BP to rise with effort, maximal or 90 % maximal heart rate for age is achieved.

- β-blocker (atenolol or metoprolol if not contra-indicated).
- Nitrate infusion.
- LMW heparin (e.g. enoxaparin)
- Monitor vital signs, O_2 Sats, ECG.
- If symptoms fail to improve, refer for urgent angiography ± angioplasty/CABG.
- Platelet glycoprotein IIb/IIIa antagonists (abciximab, tirofiban, eptifibatide) are of value in unstable angina (with aspirin and heparin) in:
  - patients at high risk of developing MI (tirofiban, eptifibatide)
  - reducing complications of percutaneous coronary intervention (abciximab, tirofiban, eptifibatide). These drugs should be used by specialists only.

Stable angina:

1 *Minimize cardiac risk factors:* Control BP (see Hypertension), hyperlipidaemia (see Hyperlipidaemia) and diabetes. Provide advice on smoking, exercise, weight loss and low-fat diet. All patients should receive aspirin (75 mg/day) unless contraindicated.

2 *Immediate symptom relief:* Glyceryl trinitrate can be given as a spray or sublingually.

3 *Long-term treatment:* The National Service Framework recommends β-blockers (e.g. atenolol, unless contraindicated), Ca^{2+} antagonists (e.g. verapamil, diltiazem) or nitrates (e.g. isosorbide nitrate). β-Blockers are the first choice. Dual therapy may be indicated if monotherapy is ineffective.

Percutaneous transluminal coronary angioplasty improves symptoms but does not improve survival. Re-stenosis rate ~20–30 % at 6 months. Coronary stenting ↓ risk of restenosis.

More severe cases (three-vessel or left main-stem coronary stenosis): Coronary artery bypass.

C: Patients are at risk of MI and other vascular diseases such as stroke and peripheral vascular disease.

P: Treatments and lifestyle changes ↓ risk of MI. The average annual mortality rate for patients with stable angina is 4 % per year. Unstable angina: The incidence of serious adverse outcomes (e.g. acute MI, death) in people taking aspirin, is 5–10% within the first week and about 15% at 30 days. 5–14% of patients with unstable angina die in the first year after diagnosis. Risk factors for an adverse event include: severity of presentation (e.g. duration of pain, evidence of heart failure), history (previous MI, left ventricular dysfunction, age, diabetes), ECG changes (e.g. severity of ST segment depression, deep T wave inversion), troponin concentration.

Ankylosing spondylitis

D: Seronegative inflammatory arthropathy affecting preferentially the axial skeleton and large proximal joints.

A: Unknown. Strong linkage with *HLA-B27* gene (> 90 % *HLA-B27*-positive, general population frequency ~8 %). Infective triggers, e.g. *Klebsiella* and antigen cross-reactivity with self-peptides have been suggested.

A/R: The *HLA-B27* allele, family history.

E: Common: affects ~0.25–1 % of UK population. Earlier presentation in ♂ (♂ : ♀ ~6:1 at 16 years and ~2:1 at 30 years), more common in white people.

H: Low back and sacroiliac pain disturbing sleep (worse in morning, improves on activity, returning with rest).
Progressive loss of spinal movement.
Symptoms of asymmetrical peripheral arthritis.
Pleuritic chest pain (caused by costovertebral joint involvement), heel pain (caused by plantar fasciitis).
Non-specific symptoms malaise, fatigue.

E: *Schober's test:* A mark is made on the skin of the back in the middle of a line drawn between the posterior iliac spines. A mark 10 cm above this is made. The patient is asked to bend forward and the distance between the two marks should ↑ by > 5 cm on forward flexion. This is reduced in ankylosing spondylitis. Reduced lateral spinal flexion and occiput–wall distance (with the patient standing next to the wall).
Tenderness over sacroiliac joints.
In later stages, thoracic kyphosis and spinal fusion, question-mark posture.
Signs of extra-articular disease: Anterior uveitis (red eye); apical lung fibrosis, ↓ chest expansion (fusion of costovertebral joints); aortic regurgitation (cardiac diastolic murmur).

P: **Spine:** Inflammation starts at the entheses (sites of attachment of ligaments to vertebral bodies). Persistent inflammatory enthesitis is followed by reactive new bone formation. Changes start in lumbar and progress to thoracic and cervical regions.

1 Squaring of the vertebral bodies.
2 Formation of syndesmophytes (vertical ossifications bridging the margins of the adjacent vertebrae).
3 Fusion of syndesmophytes and facet joints (bony ankylosis and spinal immobility).
4 Calcification of anterior and lateral spinal ligaments.

Sacroiliac joints: (see Investigations, radiograph).

I: **Blood:** FBC (anaemia of chronic disease), rheumatoid factor (negative), ↑ ESR/CRP, HLA-typing.
Radiography:
Anteroposterior and lateral view of spine: May show evidence of 'Bamboo spine' (see Pathology).
*Anteroposterior view of the sacroiliac joints:** Symmetrical blurring of joint margins. Later there are erosions, sclerosis and sacroiliac joint fusion.

*Sacroiliitis also occurs in other seronegative arthropathies: Reiter's syndrome (reactive arthritis), enteropathic arthropathy (inflammatory bowel disease), psoriatic arthropathy.

CXR: For evidence of apical fibrosis.
Lung function tests: Assesses mechanical ventilatory impairment from kyphosis.

M: **Medical:** NSAIDs can provide symptomatic relief. Sulfasalazine and other immunosuppressants may be useful as second-line treatment. Intra-articular injections of corticosteroids help acutely inflamed joints, especially with peripheral joint involvement. Recent trials with etanercept (TNF-α receptor fusion protein which inhibits TNF-α activity) are promising.
Physiotherapy: Educate on proper exercise and posture to maintain maximum range of back movements.

C: Respiratory impairment, lung fibrosis (typically apical), Achilles tendonitis, aortitis, aortic regurgitation, systemic amyloidosis (AA), cauda equina syndrome (rare).

P: Most may lead a normal life with intensive physiotherapy and surveillance for complications but 10 % progress to crippling disease.

Antiphospholipid syndrome

D: Characterized by antibodies against constituents of phospholipid membranes, arterial and venous thromboses, recurrent miscarriages and thrombocytopenia.

A: Unknown, but association with SLE suggests an autoimmune aetiology.

A/R: A small proportion have SLE or other autoimmune diseases, e.g. Sjögren's syndrome (secondary antiphospholipid syndrome).

E: More common in young ♀ (accounts for 20 % of strokes in $<$ 45-year-olds and 27 % of women with $>$ 2 miscarriages).

H: Recurrent miscarriages, history of arterial/venous thrombotic events (strokes, pulmonary embolism, DVT), headaches and migraine, chorea, epilepsy, history of autoimmune disease.

E: Livedo reticularis (network of cutaneous cyanotic vascularity).
Signs of systemic lupus (malar flush, discoid lesions, vasculitis, photosensitivity).
Signs of valvular heart disease.

P: Two main types of antibodies: lupus anticoagulant antibody and anticardiolipin antibodies. α_2-Glycoprotein 1 (phospholipid-binding protein) is the target of both antibodies.

Antiphospholipid antibodies may be involved in thrombosis by having an effect on vascular endothelial cells, platelet membranes and clotting components such as protein C, protein S and prothrombin.
Antiphospholipid antibodies ↓ annexin V, a placental and endothelial protein with anticoagulant activity.

I: **Blood:** FBC (↓ platelets), ESR (usually normal), clotting screen (↑ APTT).
Autoantibodies: Anticardiolipin antibodies and lupus anticoagulant antibodies, false-positive VDRL test for syphilis, ANA (usually negative).

M: **Medical:** Treat thrombotic episodes with SC heparin, followed by long-term anticoagulation with oral warfarin ± aspirin. Corticosteroids and cyclophosphamide may be beneficial in refractory cases. Future pregnancies should be closely monitored, and most should be given heparin as prophylaxis.
Advice: Avoid oral contraceptives and ↓ risk of vascular disease (smoking, hypertension, hyperlipidaemia). Warn patient about risk of miscarriage and thrombosis in pregnancies.

C: Fetal miscarriages. Thrombotic episodes causing Addison's disease (when adrenals are involved), or Budd–Chiari syndrome (when hepatic vein is involved), other sites for thrombosis include:
Arteries: cerebral, coronary, retinal and visceral;
Veins: deep or superficial leg, hepatic,.renal, portal or retinal.

P: Morbidity and mortality associated with antiphospholipid syndrome is high as effective treatment is not yet known. However, successful pregnancy rates are now much higher ($>$ 80 %).

D: A condition where a tear in the aortic intima allows blood to surge into the aortic wall, causing a split between the inner and outer tunica media, and creating a false lumen.

A: Degenerative changes in the smooth muscle of the aortic media are the predisposing event. Common causes and predisposing factors:

- Hypertension
- Aortic atherosclerosis
- Connective tissue disease (e.g. SLE, Marfan's, Ehlers–Danlos)
- Congenital cardiovascular abnormalities (e.g. aortic coarctation, bicuspid aortic valve)
- Aortitis (e.g. Takayasu's aortitis, tertiary syphilis)
- Iatrogenic (e.g. during angioplasty, insertion of intra-aortic balloon pump)
- Trauma

A/R: Hypertension is the biggest risk factor (> 90 % have hypertension).

E: Most common in ♂ between 40 and 60 years.

H: Sudden central 'tearing' pain, may radiate to the back.

Aortic dissection can lead to occlusion of the aorta and its branches:
Carotid obstruction: hemiparesis, dysphasia, blackout.
Coronary artery obstruction: chest pain (angina or MI).
Subclavian obstruction: ataxia, loss of consciousness.
Anterior spinal artery: paraplegia.
Coeliac obstruction: severe abdominal pain (ischaemic bowel).
Renal artery obstruction: anuria, renal failure.

E: Murmur on the back below left scapula, descending to abdomen.
Blood pressure: Hypertension (BP discrepancy between arms of > 20 mmHg), wide pulse pressure. If hypotensive may signify tamponade, check for pulsus paradoxus.
Aortic insufficiency: Collapsing pulse, early diastolic murmur above the aortic area.
Unequal arm pulses.
There may be a palpable abdominal mass.

P: **Macro:** Stanford classification divides dissection into type A (ascending aorta) and type B (descending aorta distal to the left subclavian artery). Expansion of the false aneurysm may obstruct the subclavian, carotid, coeliac and renal arteries.
Micro: Most have pre-existing cystic medial degeneration. This is elastic tissue fragmentation and separation of the elastic, fibrous and muscular elements of the tunica media.

I: **Blood:** FBC, cross-match 10 units of blood, U&E (renal function).
CXR: Widened mediastinum, localized bulge in the aortic arch.
ECG: Often normal. Signs of left ventricular hypertrophy or inferior MI if dissection compromises the ostia of the right coronary artery.
Echocardiography: Trans-oesophageal is highly specific.
CT/MRI scan: False lumen of dissection can be visualised.
Cardiac catherterization and aortography.

M: **Acute:** Resuscitate and restore blood volume with blood products. Best managed in ITU. Monitor pulse and BP in both arms, CVP, urinary catheter.

Surgical: *Type A dissection:* Emergency surgery because of the risk of cardiac tamponade. Affected aorta is replaced by a tube graft. Aortic valve may also be replaced.
Medical: *Type B dissection:* Control BP and prevent further dissection with IV nitroprusside and/or IV labetalol (use calcium-channel blocker if β-blocker contraindicated).

C: Aortic rupture, cardiac tamponade, pulmonary oedema, obstruction of the renal, carotid, subclavian, mesenteric and spinal arteries, MI.

P: Untreated mortality: 30 % at 24 h, 75 % at 2 weeks, operative mortality 10–25 %.
Prognosis for type B better than type A.

D: Reflux of blood from aorta into left ventricle during diastole.

A: **Aortic valve leaflet damage and abnormalities:**
- Infective endocarditis
- Rheumatic fever
- Trauma
- Bicuspid aortic valve

Aortic root dilation:
- Aortic dissection
- Aortitis, e.g. syphilis, Takayasu's arteritis
- Arthritides, e.g. rheumatoid arthritis, seronegative arthritides
- Severe hypertension

Others:
- Marfan's syndrome (see Marfan's syndrome)
- Pseudoxanthoma elasticum
- Ehlers–Danlos syndrome
- Osteogenesis imperfecta (see footnote to Mitral regurgitation)

A/R: (see Aetiology).

E: 75 % of cases are male, but most of those secondary to rheumatoid arthritis are female.

H: Initially asymptomatic. Later, symptoms of heart failure: exertional dyspnoea, orthopnoea, fatigue. Occasionally, angina.

E: Collapsing 'water-hammer' pulse and wide pulse pressure. Displaced thrusting heaving (volume-loaded) apex beat.
Early diastolic murmur at lower left sternal edge, better heard with the patient sitting forward with the breath held in expiration. An ejection systolic murmur is often heard because of ↑ flow across the valve.
Rare signs:
Austin Flint mid-diastolic murmur: over the apex, from turbulent reflux hitting anterior cusp of the mitral valve and causing a physiological mitral stenosis.
Quincke's sign: visible pulsations on nail-bed.
de Musset's sign: head nodding in time with pulse.
Becker's sign: visible pulsations of the pupils and retinal arteries.
Müller's sign: visible pulsation of the uvula.
Corrigan's sign: visible pulsations in neck.
Traube's sign: 'pistol shot' (systolic and diastolic beats) heard on auscultation of the femoral arteries.
Duroziez's sign: a systolic and diastolic bruit heard on compression of femoral artery with a stethoscope.
Hill's sign: popliteal cuff systolic pressure exceeding brachial pressure by $>$60 mmHg.

P: Reflux of blood into the left ventricle during diastole results in left ventricular dilation and ↑ end-diastolic volume and consequently ↑ stroke volume. The combination of ↑ stroke volume and low end-diastolic pressure in the aorta may explain the large volume, the collapsing pulse and the wide pulse pressure.

I: **CXR:** Cardiomegaly. Dilation of the ascending aorta. Signs of pulmonary oedema may be seen with left heart failure.
ECG: May show signs of left ventricular hypertrophy (deep S wave in V_{1-2}, tall R wave in V_{5-6}, inverted T waves in I, aVL, V_{5-6}, left axis deviation).

Echocardiogram: 2-D echo and M-mode may indicate the underlying cause (e.g. aortic root dilation, bicuspid aortic valve) or the effects of aortic regurgitation (left ventricular dilation/function, fluttering of the anterior mitral valve leaflet). Doppler echocardiography for detecting and assessing severity.

Cardiac catheterization: Visualization of regurgitating dye during diastole and to assess severity.

M: **Medical:** Vasodilators (e.g. nifedipine) and ACE-inhibitors reduce systemic vascular resistance and the afterload and the burden on the volume-loaded left ventricle. Treat the complications (e.g. heart failure).

Surgery: Aortic valve replacement in patients symptomatic of ventricular decompensation not controlled by medication and in asymptomatic patients with a left ventricular ejection fraction of $< 55\%$.

C: Left ventricular failure and pulmonary oedema.

P: Often well tolerated for many years without symptoms. Prognosis depends on the underlying aetiology. Aortic regurgitation caused by aortic dissection or infective endocarditis is fatal if not treated urgently.

Aortic stenosis

D: Narrowing of the left ventricular outflow at the aortic level.

A: **1** Stenosis secondary to rheumatic heart disease.
2 Calcification of a congenital bicuspid aortic valve.
3 Calcification/degeneration of a tricuspid aortic valve in the elderly.

A/R: Congenital bicuspid aortic valve may be associated with patent ductus arteriosus or coarctation of aorta.

E: Prevalence in ~3% of 75-year-olds. ♂ > ♀. Those with bicuspid aortic valve may present earlier (as young adults).

H: May be asymptomatic initially.
Angina (because of ↑ oxygen demand of the hypertrophied ventricles caused by aortic stenosis).
Syncope or dizziness on exercise, dyspnoea.

E: BP: narrow pulse pressure.
Slow-rising carotid pulse; forceful sustained thrusting undisplaced apex beat. Palpable thrill in the aortic area (if severe). Harsh ejection systolic murmur at aortic area, radiating to the carotid artery and apex. A_2 component of second heart sound may be softened or absent (because of calcification). Ejection click may be heard from a bicuspid valve.
Distinguish from aortic sclerosis.*

P: Depends on the cause. Results in hypertrophic ventricle (secondary to left ventricular outflow obstruction).

I: **ECG:** Signs of left ventricular hypertrophy (deep S wave in V_{1-2}, tall R wave in V_{5-6}, inverted T waves in I, aVL, V_{5-6}, left axis deviation), LBBB (caused by calcification of conducting tissues).
CXR: Post-stenotic enlargement of the ascending aorta, calcification of aortic valve.
Echocardiogram/Doppler: Visualizes structural changes of the valves and level of stenosis (valvar, supravalvar or subvalvar). Estimation of aortic valve area. Pressure gradient across the valve in systole and left ventricular function may be assessed.
Cardiac angiography: Differentiate from other causes of angina. Look for concomitant coronary artery disease (50% of patients with severe aortic stenosis have significant coronary artery disease).

M: **Medical:** Manage left ventricular failure (see Cardiac failure). Medical management of angina (see Angina pectoris). Antibiotic prophylaxis against infective endocarditis.
Surgical: Valve replacement is recommended if valve pressure difference is > 50 mmHg in a symptomatic patient. If unfit for surgery, balloon dilation (valvoplasty) may be performed but this is considered to be a palliative procedure and the rate of complications is high, e.g. MI, myocardial perforation, severe aortic regurgitation.

C: Arrhythmias, Stokes–Adams attacks, MI, left ventricular failure, sudden death.

P: Survival differs according to symptoms. In symptomatic patients with severe aortic stenosis causing left ventricular failure, average survival 50% at 18 months without surgery. Average survival with angina 5 years; syncope 3 years; dyspnoea 2 years.

*Aortic sclerosis is senile degeneration with no left ventricular outflow tract obstruction. The pulse character is normal, a thrill is not palpable and the ejection systolic murmur radiates only faintly. S_2 is normal.

Aspergillus lung disease

D: Lung disease associated with *Aspergillus* fungal infection.

A: Inhalation of the ubiquitous *Aspergillus fumigatus* spores. Disease presentation depends on the immune system of the host and the dose of the inhaled spores (particularly abundant in late autumn). It can produce three different clinical pictures:

1. *Aspergilloma:* growth of a *A. fumigatus* mycetoma ball in a pre-existing lung cavity (e.g. post-TB, old infarct or abscess).
2. *Allergic bronchopulmonary aspergillosis (ABPA):* caused by growth of *A. fumigatus* in bronchial walls causing recurrent respiratory symptoms (e.g. episodic eosinophilic pneumonia, progressing to lung fibrosis).
3. *Invasive aspergillosis:* causing necrotizing pneumonia and fungal dissemination (fungaemia).

A/R: Allergic aspergillosis more common in asthmatics.

Exposure to building work ↑ the risk of *Aspergillus* spore inhalation.
Invasive aspergillosis is most often seen in immunocompromised patients (e.g. HIV, leukaemia patients).

E: Uncommon. Most common in elderly and immunocompromised.

H: **Aspergilloma:** Asymptomatic, haemoptysis, which may be massive.
ABPA: Difficult to control asthma, recurrent episodes of pneumonia with wheeze, cough, fever and malaise.
Invasive aspergillosis: Dyspnoea, rapid deterioration, septic picture.

E: Tracheal deviation in large aspergillomas or in lobar collapse.
Cyanosis may develop in invasive aspergillosis.
There may be dullness in affected lung.
↓ Breath sounds, wheeze (ABPA).

P: **Aspergilloma:** Brown fungal balls within a pulmonary cavity with minimal invasion of surrounding tissue. Surrounding inflammation and fibrosis may be present.
ABPA: Type III (immune-complex-mediated) hypersensitivity reaction. Initially there is bronchoconstriction then, as inflammation persists, bronchiectasis develops. Mucous plugs can be shown to have fungal mycelium. With progressive disease, lung fibrosis develops, classically in the upper zones.
Invasive aspergillosis: Grey, sharply defined, necrotizing 'target lesions' spread throughout lung and may involve the heart and other organs. Often surrounded by haemorrhagic inflamed tissue.

I: **Blood:** FBC (eosinophilia), serology (↑ IgE, aspergillus preciptins present), ↑ ESR or CRP.
Sputum microscopy and culture: *A. fumigatus* may be visualized and cultured.
Lung function tests: *ABPA:* reversible airflow limitation, ↓ lung volumes/gas transfer in progressive cases.
CXR: *Aspergilloma:* Round opacity may be seen with a crescent of air around it.
ABPA: Transient patchy shadows, collapse, distended mucus-filled bronchi producing tubular shadows ('gloved fingers' appearance). Signs of complications: fibrosis in upper lobes (similar to tuberculosis), parallel-line shadows and rings (bronchiectasis).
CT scanning: *Invasive aspergillosis:* Nodules with surrounding 'ground glass' in filtrates (halo sign).

Allergen skin tests: Positive to *Aspergillus* antigens.

M: **Aspergilloma:** Surgical resection for large aspergillomas if uncontrolled or symptomatic.

ABPA: Bronchodilators (for symptomatic relief), steroids to reduce inflammation. Continuing low-dose steroids may be necessary.

Invasive aspergillosis: IV amphotericin B ± flucytosine. Amphotericin disrupts fungal membranes but is very nephrotoxic. Liposomal amphotericin is less toxic.

C: **Aspergilloma:** Secondary bacterial infection, massive haemoptysis or haemorrhage.

ABPA: Worsening of asthma, bronchiectasis, lobar collapse, lung fibrosis, respiratory failure.

Invasive aspergillosis: Septic shock, respiratory failure.

P: Grave prognosis for invasive aspergillosis. Good prognosis for allergic aspergillosis and aspergillomas but bronchospasm or haemoptysis can still lead to death.

Aspirin overdose

D: Excessive ingestion of aspirin causing toxicity.

A: Overdose can occur as a result of deliberate self-harm, suicidal intent or by accident (e.g. in children). Availability of aspirin is a major factor. Ingestion of 10–20 g can cause moderate–severe toxicity in adults.

A/R: In children < 4 years, even low doses of aspirin are associated with an increased risk of developing Reye's syndrome (metabolic acidosis, liver and CNS disturbances). Aspirin can also trigger an asthma attack in certain individuals.

E: One of the most common drug overdoses.

H: Ascertain the key facts:

- How much aspirin? • When? • Any other drugs? • Have you had any alcohol?

The patient may be asymptomatic initially.
Early symptoms: Flushed appearance, fever, sweating, hyperventilation, dizziness, tinnitus, deafness.
Late symptoms: Lethargy, confusion, convulsions, drowsiness, respiratory depression, coma.

E: Fever, tachycardia, hyperventilation, epigastric tenderness.

P: Aspirin (acetylsalicylate) ↑ respiratory rate and depth by stimulating the CNS respiratory centre. This hyperventilation produces respiratory alkalosis in the early phase. The body then compensates by increasing urinary bicarbonate and K^+ excretion, causing dehydration and hypokalaemia. Loss of bicarbonate together with the uncoupling of mitochondrial oxidative phosphorylation by salicylic acid and build up of lactic acid can lead to metabolic acidosis.

In severe overdoses, CNS depression and respiratory failure can occur.

I: **Blood:** Salicylate levels (for adults, 500–750 mg/L is a moderate overdose; >750 mg/L is a severe overdose), FBC, U&E (particularly ↓ K^+ if vomiting), LFT (↑ AST:ALT), clotting screen (↑ PT), glucose and other drug levels (e.g. paracetamol).
ABG: May show mixed metabolic acidosis and respiratory alkalosis.
ECG: May show signs of hypokalaemia: small T waves, U waves.

M: **Acute:** Resuscitate with attention to respiratory rate and blood gases. Treat hypovolaemia (rehydrate), hypokalaemia, hypoglycaemia; vitamin K for hypoprothrombinaemia (occasionally).
If <12 h after ingestion: Gastric lavage to empty the stomach, and oral activated charcoal to bind to and ↓ absorption of the drug.
Moderate cases (500–750 mg/L): Urine alkalinization with IV $NaHCO_3$ (with KCl) aims to ↑ salicylate excretion (aim for urine pH 7.5–8.5).
Severe cases (>750 mg/L) or in severe acidosis: Consider haemodialysis.
In all cases, monitor U&E, glucose (may ↑ or ↓), temperature, pulse, respiratory rate, BP, urine output.

C: Cerebral and pulmonary oedema (↑ capillary permeability).
Metabolic disturbances (↓ K^+, ↓ or ↑ Na^+, ↓ or ↑ glucose).
Acute renal failure.

P: If treated early, prognosis is good.

D: Chronic inflammatory airway disease characterized by variable reversible airway obstruction, airway hyper-responsiveness and bronchial inflammation.

A: **Genetic factors:** Positive family history, twin studies. Almost all asthmatic patients show some atopy (tendency of T lymphocyte (TH_2) cells to drive production of IgE on exposure to allergens). Linkages to multiple chromosomal locations point to 'genetic heterogeneity' for atopy and asthma.
Environmental factors: House dust mite, pollen, pets (e.g. urinary proteins, furs), cigarette smoke, viral respiratory tract infection, *Aspergillus fumigatus* spores. Breastfeeding may provide some protection.
Occupational: Exposure to isocyanates, epoxy resins.
Precipitating factors: Cold, viral infection, drugs (β-blockers, NSAIDs), exercise, emotions.

A/R: Allergic rhinitis, nasal polyps, urticaria, eczema, acid reflux and family history.

E: Affects 10% of children and 5% of adults. The prevalence of asthma appears to be increasing. Equal gender distribution. Acute asthma is a very common medical emergency and still responsible for 1000–2000 deaths/year in the UK.

H: Episodes of wheeze, breathlessness, cough; worse in the morning and at night. Ask about interference with exercise, sleeping, days off school and work. In an acute attack it is important to ask whether the patient has been admitted to hospital because of their asthma, or to ITU, as a gauge of potential severity.

E: Tachypnoea, use of accessory muscles, prolonged expiratory phase, polyphonic wheeze, hyperinflated chest.
Severe attack: PEFR $< 50\,\%$ predicted, pulse > 110/min, respiratory rate > 25/min, inability to complete sentences.
Life-threatening attack: PEFR $< 33\,\%$, silent chest, cyanosis, bradycardia, hypotension, confusion, coma.

P: **Micro:** Luminal mucus plugs, epithelial shedding, mixed cellular infiltrate of lymphocytes and eosinophils, oedema, submucosal mucous gland hyperplasia and smooth muscle hypertrophy.
Pathogenesis of inflammatory response in asthma:
Early phase (up to 1 h): Exposure to allergens in a presensitized individual results in cross-linking of IgE. IgE triggers mast cell degranulation releasing histamine and formation of other inflammatory mediators. These cause mucous hypersecretion, vasodilation, oedema, bronchoconstriction and airway obstruction.
Late phase (after 6–12 h): involves inflammatory cell, including lymphocyte, eosinophil and basophil, accumulation and perpetuation of the inflammation and bronchial hyper-responsiveness.

I: **Acute:** Peak flow, pulse oximetry, ABG, CXR (to exclude other diagnoses, e.g. pneumothorax, pneumonia), FBC (↑ WCC if infective exacerbation), CRP, U&E, blood and sputum cultures.
Chronic: *PEFR monitoring:* There is often a diurnal variation with a morning 'dip'.
Pulmonary function test: Obstructive defect, with improvement after a trial of a β_2-agonist.
Blood: Eosinophilia, *Aspergillus* antibody titres.
Skin prick tests: May help in the identification of allergens.

M: **Acute:** Resuscitate, monitor sat O_2, ABG and PEFR. Give high-flow oxygen, nebulized β_2-agonist bronchodilator salbutamol, ipratropium as required and steroid therapy (IV hydrocortisone or oral prednisolone). If not improving, start IV aminophylline. Monitor electrolytes closely (bronchodilators and aminophyline lower K^+). May need ventilation in severe attacks. If not improving or patient tiring, involve ITU early.

Discharge: When PEF >75% predicted or patient's best, diurnal variation <25%, inhaler technique checked, stable on discharge medication for 24 h, patient owns a PEF meter and has steroid and bronchodilator therapy. Arrange follow-up.

Chronic 'stepwise' therapy (British Thoracic Society guidelines): Start on the step appropriate to initial severity and step up or down to control symptoms. Treatment should be reviewed every 3–6 months.

Step 1 Short-acting inhaled β_2-agonist as needed. If used > 1/day, move to Step 2.

Step 2 As Step 1 plus regular low-dose inhaled steroids.

Step 3 As Step 1 plus either:

- regular high dose inhaled steroids, or
- regular low-dose steroid and long-acting β_2-agonist.

Step 4 As Step 1 plus high-dose inhaled steroids and long-acting β_2-agonist, plus trial of theophylline or cromoglycate.

Step 5 Addition of regular oral steroids.

Advice: Educate on proper inhaler technique. Patient education on disease and to develop an individualized management plan, with emphasis on avoidance of provoking factors.

C: Growth retardation, chest wall deformity (e.g. pigeon chest), recurrent infections, pneumothorax, respiratory failure, death.

P: Many children improve as they grow older. Adult-onset asthma is usually chronic.

Atrial fibrillation

D: Characterized by rapid, chaotic and ineffective atrial electrical conduction.

A: There may be no identifiable cause ('lone' atrial fibrillation). Secondary causes include thyrotoxicosis, pneumonia, alcohol, hypertension.
Heart: Mitral valve disease, ischaemic heart disease, rheumatic heart disease, cardiomyopathy, pericarditis, sick sinus syndrome,* atrial myxoma.
Lung: Bronchial carcinoma, pulmonary embolism.
Sarcoidosis, haemochromatosis.

A/R: Leading cause of strokes.

E: Very common in the elderly (~5 % of those >65 years). May be paroxysmal in young adults.

H: Palpitations, but often can be asymptomatic. Symptoms of the cause of the atrial fibrillation.

E: Irregularly irregular pulse, Apical–radial deficit. Signs of the underlying cause.

P: Depends on the cause (see Aetiology). Secondary causes lead to abnormal atrial electrical pathways which result in atrial fibrillation.

I: **ECG:** Uneven baseline (fibrillations) with absent P waves, irregular QRS complexes. Ventricular rate in untreated patients is often 150 beats/min (because AV node does not conduct all of the atrial impulses which may be as high as 600 beats/min).
Blood: Cardiac enzymes, TFT (free T_4, TSH), lipid profile, U&E, Mg^{2+}, Ca^{2+} (risk of digoxin toxicity ↑ with hypokalaemia, hypomagnesaemia, or hypercalcaemia).
Echocardiogram: To assess for mitral valve disease, left atrial dilation, left ventricular dysfunction or structural abnormalities.

M: Treat any reversible cause (e.g. thyrotoxicosis, chest infection).
For AF with <48 h from onset or anyone with haemodynamic compromise: Direct current cardioversion. Trans-oesophageal echocardiogram may be performed to exclude a left atrial thrombus.
For AF with >48 h from onset: Control the rate (digoxin or β-blockers) and anticoagulate for 3–4 weeks. Warfarin is the drug of choice.† Once appropriately anticoagulated (target INR: 2–3), chemical or direct current cardioversion (see below). Continue warfarin for 4 weeks after cardioversion.
DC cardioversion: Synchronized DC shock (2 × 100 J, 1 × 200 J) under general anaesthesia.

*Sick sinus (or tachy–brady) syndrome: caused by ischaemia, infarction or fibrosis of the sinus node (in the elderly), presenting with *bradycardia* (caused by intermittent failure of sinus node depolarization or impulse propagation to the atria), with ↑ P-P intervals (>2 s) and intermittent *tachycardia* (caused by ↑ ectopic pacemaker activity). Treated with pacemaker insertion for symptomatic bradycardia and antiarrhythmics for tachycardia, plus anticoagulation to reduce risk of thromboembolism.
†For young patients with no diabetes, hypertension or history of ischaemic heart disease or in cases where warfarin is contraindicated, aspirin is a reasonable but less effective alternative.
Note: **Atrial flutter** is characterized by atrial rate of 300/min and ventricular rate of 150/min (2: 1 heart block as AV node conducts every second beat). ECG shows a regular 'sawtooth' baseline (rate ~300/min). Treatment as for atrial fibrillation.

Chemical cardioversion: Flecainide (contraindicated in ischaemic heart disease), amiodarone.

(Note that the recent AFFIRM trial suggests that rhythm control by chemical or electrical cardioversion offers no survival advantage over rate control.)

Prophylaxis against AF: Sotalol, amiodarone or flecainide.

Chronic 'permanent' AF: Ventricular rate control with digoxin, verapamil or β-blockers. Anticoagulation.

Advice: Discuss the advantages and disadvantages of warfarin, lifestyle changes of cardiac risk factors.

C: Thromboembolism (e.g. embolic stroke ~4% risk per year, ↑ risk with left atrial enlargement or left ventricular dysfunction). Worsens any existing heart failure.

P: Chronic AF in a diseased heart does not usually return to sinus rhythm.

D: Characterized by proliferation of abnormal bacterial flora in the small intestine (upper intestinal bacterial counts $> 10^5$ colony forming units/mL). Also known as 'blind loop syndrome'.

A: **Motility disorders** (caused by stasis of intestinal contents): Diabetic autonomic neuropathy, amyloidosis, ileus.
Anatomical abnormalities (caused by stasis of intestinal contents or passage of colonic organisms into the small bowel): Jejunal diverticulosis, blind loop (side-to-end anastomosis), bowel obstruction, fistulae.
↓ **Gastric acid production** (caused by ↑ bacteria passing from mouth to the small intestine): gastric resection or vagotomy, chronic atrophic gastritis/pernicious anaemia, proton pump inhibitors.

A/R: (see Aetiology).

E: Uncommon. Children and elderly are more prone to bacterial overgrowth.

H: May be asymptomatic with no adverse consequences.
Diarrhoea, steatorrhoea (pale bulky offensive stool), malabsorption, weight loss, abdominal pain and nausea/vomiting.
Symptoms of vitamin B_{12} deficiency.
Rectal bleeding as a result of pouchitis (if bacterial overgrowth occurs in an ileo-anal anastomosis or ileal reservoir).

E: May be no signs or may be evidence of vitamin B_{12} deficiency and anaemia (see Anaemia, macrocytic).

P: *Escherichia coli*, *Klebsiella* and anaerobes (e.g. *Bacteroides*, *Clostridia* and *Enterococci*), replace the few Gram-positive aerobes derived from the mouth.
Pathogenesis of main features:
Diarrhoea: Enterocyte brush border damage leads to ↓ nutrient absorption and ↑ osmolality of intestinal contents.
Steatorrhoea: Deconjugation of bile acids by bacteria results in their premature absorption or precipitation as inert crystals, resulting in ↓ intraluminal bile acids and ↓ fat absorption and steatorrhoea.
Malabsorption: of nutrients as a result of bacterial metabolism and enterocyte damage.
Vitamin B_{12} deficiency: caused by increased uptake of the vitamin B_{12}–intrinsic factor complex by bacteria in the small bowel.

I: **Blood:** FBC (↓ Hb, ↑ MCV), serum vitamin B_{12}, red cell folate (normal or ↑ as a result of bacterial synthesis), Schilling's test (see Anaemia, macrocytic).
Breath test: Detection of exhaled $^{14}CO_2$ (after intake of ^{14}C-labelled bile salts by mouth) or hydrogen (after intake of glucose by mouth). Bacteria metabolize bile salts to $^{14}CO_2$, and glucose into hydrogen.
Proximal small intestinal aspiration: Microbiological culture, analysis of unconjugated bile acid proportion.
Small intestinal biopsy: To exclude coeliac disease, giardiasis and Whipple's disease (a small intestinal disease presenting with arthritis, neurological involvement, fever and lymphadenopathy that on biopsy shows PAS-positive macrophages containing the *Tropheryma whippeli* organism).
Barium follow-through: To detect structural abnormalities, e.g. jejunal diverticulosis, fistulae, strictures or altered intestinal motility.

M: **Treat the underlying cause:** e.g. surgical correction of the structural abnormality such as a stricture.

Antibiotics: e.g. amoxicillin–clavulanate (may cause diarrhoea) or cephalosporin and metronidazole. Rotating antibiotic regimens (e.g. ciprofloxacin, doxycycline and metronidazole) may be help to prevent the development of resistance.

Nutritional support: Correct deficiencies of vitamin B_{12}, vitamin K and calcium. More rarely, supplements of other fat-soluble vitamins (A, D, E) or oral iron may be needed.

C: Vitamin deficiencies, malnutrition.

P: Patients with an underlying motility disorder may have a poorer prognosis. If not responding to treatment, consider misdiagnosis, bacterial resistance or antibiotic-associated colitis.

D: Slow-growing malignancy of the basal keratinocytes in the epidermis of the skin.

A: Chronic sunlight exposure.

A/R: ↑ Incidence in immunosuppression and xeroderma pigmentosum (autosomal recessive condition associated with ↓ ability to repair DNA damage caused by ultraviolet light).
Gorlin's syndrome (a rare autosomal dominant mutation of gene signalling pathways associated with multiple BCCs in early adulthood, jaw cysts, bifid ribs and cutaneous palmar pits).

E: Most common cutaneous malignancy. Often occurring in the middle-aged and elderly.

H: (see Examination).

E: Occurs on exposed sites, primarily on nose and near the medial angle of the eye. Starts as a reddish dome-shaped papule with surrounding telangiectasia and may progress to central necrosis and ulceration, with classic 'rolled' pearl-like edge. There are several subtypes.
Nodular: Most common variety. Translucent dome-shaped nodules appearing over a period of months to years, mainly on head or neck.
Ulcerative: A nodular BCC that has ulcerated in the centre. There may be extensive local invasion (a 'rodent ulcer').
Cystic: Cystic lesion with overlying telangiectasia. Occurs predominantly on face.
Pigmented: A nodular BCC can become darkly pigmented, resembling a melanoma.
Morphoeic: Depressed firm pale plaques resembling a scar or localized scleroderma. Rare subtype.
Superficial: Thin, pink, scaling and crusted plaque with well-defined edge. There is a fine 'hair-like' margin. Usually occurs on trunk and limbs. Rare subtype.

P: **Microscopic:** Mass of basophilic keratinocytes push down into the dermis but retain contact with overlying epidermis. Lots of mitotic figures are visible. There is palisading of the small tumour cells at the periphery of the cellular islands.

I: Skin biopsy to establish diagnosis.

M: **Surgery:** For small lesions, curettage and cautery, but definitive treatment is wide excision. Micrographic surgery is important for tumours around eyes, nose, ears and for the morphoeic form.
Local radiotherapy or cryotherapy: If surgery is difficult or in the elderly. Contraindicated in morphoeic form.
Medical: Intralesional interferons useful if other options difficult. Follow-up should be arranged to check for recurrence.

C: Rarely metastatic, but can cause pressure or erode locally.

P: Good. 95 % cure rate.

Behçet's disease

D: Rare multisystem inflammatory disorder typically causing orogenital ulceration and uveitis.

A: Unknown. An immunogenic basis has been established. Viral (e.g. HSV) or streptococcal triggers, or exposure to toxic organic chemicals have been suggested.

A/R: Parents from Turkey, Greece or Japan. *HLA-B51*.

E: Rare, affecting young adults (third decade), ♂ > ♀ (also more severe in men). Higher prevalence in Japan (1 in 10 000), Turkey and Middle East. Prevalence in the UK, 1 in 170 000.

H: Recurrent painful ulcers in mouth and/or genital area.
Eye irritation or pain. Arthralgia (usually knees), arthritis (usually non-erosive, asymmetrical, involving the lower limb).
Neurological symptoms: headache, numbness in the extremities (peripheral neuropathy), and symptoms of other neurological complications.

E: International criteria for the diagnosis of Behçet's disease:
Required:
Recurrent painful oral ulceration: at least three times per year.
Plus two of the following four:
1 *Recurrent painful genital ulceration:* vulva, vagina or scrotum.
2 *Eye lesions:* anterior or posterior uveitis, retinal vasculitis, hypopyon.
3 *Skin lesions:* erythema nodosum, acne-like nodules, folliculitis.
4 *Positive pathergy test.*
Other clinical features: Signs of neurological complications mimicking meningitis, MS, malignancy or polyneuropathy.
Signs of GI ulcerations, abdominal pain, bloody diarrhoea.

P: **Micro:** There is typically inflammation around blood vessels with infiltration of polymorphs and mononuclear cells and giant cells. Thrombosis of large arteries and veins may occur or aneurysms, including pulmonary artery aneurysm, may occur. Affected joints show acute inflammatory infiltrate confined to superficial synovium only.

I: **Test for pathergy:** Following a needleprick, the puncture site becomes inflamed and a sterile pustule develops within 24–48 h.
Blood: Complement levels (C9 levels may be useful for monitoring progress); rheumatoid factor is negative.

M: **Medical:** Systemic immunosuppressants (systemic prednisolone, azathioprine) can be used. Topical corticosteroids can be used on localized oral or genital lesions.
Joint disease: NSAIDs for pain relief.
Mouth ulcers: Topical lidocaine corticosteroids or tetracycline.
Chronic uveitis: Ciclosporin A and chlorambucil.

C: Loss of vision, complications arising from the vasculitis affecting various major organ systems, CNS, skin, pulmonary (e.g. leading to thrombosis, aneurysm formation, bowel infarction, myocarditis).

P: Clinical course can be variable, with attacks lasting a few weeks, with young men having a poorer prognosis, life expectancy is normal unless complicated by severe vasculitis or CNS disease.

Bell's palsy

D: Idiopathic lower motor neurone facial (VII) nerve palsy.

A: Idiopathic. 60 % are preceded by an upper respiratory tract infection, suggesting a viral or postviral aetiology.

A/R: Pregnancy and diabetes are risk factors.

E: Annual incidence is 15–40 in 100 000. Most cases: 20–50 year. Equal gender distribution.

H: Prodrome of pre-auricular pain in some cases followed by acute (hours/days) onset unilateral facial weakness, droop, drooling and slurring of speech. Maximum severity within 1–2 days.
50 % experience facial, neck or ear pain or numbness.
Hypersensitivity to sound (hyperacusis caused by stapedius paralysis).
Loss of taste sense (uncommon).
Tearing or dry exposed eye.

E: Lower motor neurone weakness of facial muscles (affects all the ipsilateral muscles of facial expression and does not spare the muscles of the upper part of the face as seen in UMN facial nerve palsy).
Bell's phenomenon: Eyeball rolls up but eye remains open when trying to close the eyes. Although patient may report unilateral facial numbness, clinical testing of sensation is normal. The ear should be examined to exclude other causes (e.g. otitis media, herpes zoster infection).

P: Little is known as few pathology specimens are available.
Micro: Segmental demyelination in the facial canal may be seen. Axonal degeneration is rare but if present indicates delayed recovery.

I: Usually unnecessary except to exclude other causes, e.g. Lyme serology, herpes zoster serology.
EMG: May show local axonal conduction block in facial canal. Only useful $>$ 1 week after onset.

M: **Medical:** High-dose corticosteroids (prednisolone) is beneficial in the first few days of onset (given only if Ramsay Hunt's syndrome is excluded). Recent studies also show that aciclovir may shorten course of palsy.
Protection of cornea with protective glasses/patches and artificial tears.
Surgery: Lateral tarsorrhaphy (suturing the lateral parts of the eyelids together) if imminent or established corneal damage. Cosmetic surgery may be indicated in cases that fail to resolve.

C: Corneal ulcers, eye infection.
Aberrant reinnervation may occur, e.g. blinking may cause contraction of the angle of the mouth as a result of simultaneous innervation of obicularis oculi and ori.
Parasympathetic fibres may also aberrantly reinnervate causing 'crocodile tears' when salivating.

P: Most (85–90 %) recover function within 2–12 weeks with or without treatment.

D: Lung airway disease characterized by chronic bronchial dilation, impaired mucuociliary clearance and frequent bacterial infections.

A: Severe inflammation in the lung causes fibrosis and dilation of the bronchi. This is followed by pooling of mucus, predisposing to further cycles of infection, fibrosis, weakening and damage to bronchial walls.

A/R: Lung inflammation may be precipitated by:

- *Host defence defects:* e.g. Kartagener's syndrome,* cystic fibrosis, immunoglobulin deficiency.
- *Obstruction of bronchi:* foreign body, enlarged lymph nodes.
- *Severe pneumonia.*
- *Gastric reflux disease.*

E: Most often arises initially in childhood, incidence has ↓ with use of antibiotics, approximately 1 in 1000 per year.

H: Productive cough with purulent sputum or haemoptysis.
Breathlessness, chest pain, malaise, fever, weight loss.
Symptoms usually begin after an acute respiratory illness.

E: Finger clubbing. Coarse crackles (usually at the bases), wheeze.

P: **Macro:** Dilated bronchi with excess mucus collection.
Micro: Ulcerated epithelium with squamous metaplasia and infiltration by inflammatory cells.
Elastic and muscular component of the bronchi are replaced by fibrovascular granulation tissue and later collagen fibres. This weakens the walls.
Classified pathologically into follicular, saccular and atelectatic.

I: **Sputum:** Culture and sensitivity, common organisms in acute exacerbations: *Pseudomonas aeruginosa, Haemophilus influenzae, Staphylococcus aureus, Streptococcus pneumoniae, Klebsiella, Moraxella catarrhalis, Mycobacteria.*
CXR: Dilated bronchi may be seen as parallel lines radiating from hilum to the diaphragm ('tramline shadows'). It may also show fibrosis, atelectasis, pneumonic consolidations, or it may be normal.
High-resolution CT (1–2 mm slices): Dilated bronchi with thickened walls. Best diagnostic method.
Bronchography (rarely used): To determine extent of disease before surgery (radio-opaque contrast injected through the cricoid ligament or via a bronchoscope).
Other: Sweat electrolytes (see Cystic fibrosis), serum immunoglobulins (~10 % of adults have some immune deficiency), sinus X-ray (30 % have concomitant rhinosinusitis), mucociliary clearance study.

M: **Medical:** Appropriate antibiotics for acute infections and as prophylaxis for those with frequent exacerbations, bronchodilator therapy in patients with responsive disease.
Treat the cause of the bronchiectasis (e.g. IV immunoglobulins, proton pump inhibitors).
Physiotherapy: Cornerstone of management is sputum and mucus clearance techniques (e.g. postural drainage). Patient is taught to position themselves so the lobe to be drained is uppermost, ~20 min twice daily. These techniques reduce frequency of acute exacerbations and aids recovery during an infection.

*Kartagener's syndrome is caused by immotile cilia and is characterized by a combination of chronic sinusitis, infertility and situs inversus.

Surgical: Rarely used in UK except as a last resort. Various surgical options include localized resection, bronchial artery embolization, lung or heart–lung transplantation.

C: Life-threatening haemoptysis, persistent infections, empyema, respiratory failure, cor pulmonale, multiorgan abscesses (e.g. brain).

P: Most patients continue to have the symptoms after 10 years.

Budd–Chiari syndrome

D: Budd–Chiari syndrome is caused by obstruction to hepatic venous outflow.

A: Commonly caused by venous thrombosis (secondary to a hypercoagulable state) or malignancies. Occasionally, it may be caused by membranous venous webs in the inferior vena cava.

A/R: Associated with thrombosis of the inferior vena cava and portal vein.

E: Uncommon. Membranous venous webs are more common in Far East.

H: Presentation depends on the rapidity of onset, nature and anatomy of venous obstruction.
Acute: Rapid-onset abdominal pain and distension, jaundice and encephalopathy.
Chronic: Gradual development of the above symptoms or haematemesis/melaena as a result of variceal bleeding.

E: **Acute:** Abdominal tenderness, distension, signs of ascites. In severe cases, signs of hepatic failure.
Chronic: Jaundice, tender hepatomegaly, ascites, dependent oedema and dilated veins on the abdomen if inferior vena cava involvement.

P: **Macro:** Swollen purple-red liver with a tense capsule.
Micro: Thrombi in veins with centrilobular congestion and necrosis in affected regions. Within a few weeks of obstruction of the hepatic veins, fibrosis develops, with progression to nodular regeneration and cirrhosis within a few months. In many cases, there is enlargement of the caudal lobe (hypertrophy) as this often drains separately into the inferior vena cava.

I: **Blood:** LFT (raised transaminases), FBC, clotting and thrombophilia screen should be performed. In the chronic form, there may be evidence of renal impairment (hepatorenal syndrome).
Doppler ultrasound: ↓ Blood flow in hepatic vein,
Hepatic venogram and inferior venacavography: Enables visualization of the obstructed veins.
MRI: Can demonstrate the obstructed veins with a spider web pattern of vessels in the liver.

M: **Medical:** The underlying condition causing the thrombosis or obstruction should be treated. Anticoagulation therapy is usually necessary. In early stages, *in situ* thrombolytic therapy can be attempted. Management of complications (e.g. diuretics or paracentesis to control ascites, endoscopy to band varices).
Surgical or radiological: Procedures such as balloon dilation (angioplasty) with or without wall stents or TIPS may be performed. Surgical approaches include the creation of shunts from the portal system to the inferior vena cava. As a last resort, liver transplantation for fulminant hepatic failure, severe cirrhosis or following shunt thrombosis.

C: Liver failure, portal hypertension with ascites, GI haemorrhage, cirrhosis.

P: Depends on the speed and extent of hepatic vein thrombosis. Mortality is high in acute untreated cases. In chronic cases, 10-year survival rates are ~65 %. Factors associated with a better prognosis are younger age, better liver function as assessed by Child–Pugh score (see Liver failure).

Carcinoid syndrome

D: Syndrome caused by systemic release of hormones from carcinoid (neuroendocrine) tumours.

A: Carcinoid tumours are slow-growing neuroendocrine tumours and secrete hormones, often 5-HT (serotonin) but also substances such as histamine, prostaglandins, bradykinin and peptide hormones. Common sites include appendix and rectum, where they are often benign and non-secretory, but are also found in other parts of small or large gut, stomach, thymus, bronchus and other organs. Hormones released into the portal circulation are metabolized in the liver, and symptoms typically do not appear until there are hepatic metastases or release into the systemic circulation from bronchial or extensive retroperitoneal tumours.

A/R: 10 % of patients with MEN type 1 have carcinoid tumours.

E: Rare, annual UK incidence is 1 in 1 000 000. Asymptomatic carcinoid tumours are more common and may be an incidental finding after rectal biopsy or appendectomy.

H: Paroxysmal flushing, diarrhoea, crampy abdominal pain (↑ gut motility), wheeze, sweating, palpitations.

E: Facial flushing, telangiectasia, wheeze.
Right-sided heart murmurs: Tricuspid stenosis, regurgitation or pulmonary stenosis may be prominent if carcinoid tumour is secreting hormones into systemic circulation.
Nodular hepatomegaly in cases of metastatic disease.
Carcinoid crisis: tachycardia and hypotension in severe cases.

P: **Macro:** Solid and yellow-tan in appearance, may be classified into fore-, mid- or hindgut tumours, depending on their site of origin. There is often an area of fibrosis surrounding the primary. Classic sites include the appendix and the small bowel.
Micro: Carcinoid tumours are derived from enterochromaffin cells also known as APUD cells. Electron microscopy shows dense cytoplasmic granules containing hormonal peptides.

I: **24-h urine collection:** 5-HIAA levels (a metabolite of serotonin, false-positive with high intake of bananas and avocados).
Blood: Plasma concentrations of chromogranin B, fasting gut hormones.
CT or MRI scan: Localizes the tumour.
Radioisotope scan: Radiolabelled somatostatin analogue helps localize tumour.
Investigations for MEN-1: (see footnote to Hyperparathyroidism).

M: **Carcinoid crisis:** Octreotide infusion, also IV antihistamine and hydrocortisone.
Chronic: Multidisciplinary approach (gastroenterologists, oncologists, radiologists and surgeons). Octreotide (or other somatostatin analogues) inhibit hormone release and tumour growth. Radiolabelled octreotide may be beneficial (receptor-targeted therapy).
Supportive: Ondansetron and cyproheptadine (5-HT antagonists) can alleviate symptoms, rehydration (for diarrhoea), antiemetics and antidiarrhoeal treatment (codeine, loperamide).
Advice: Avoid precipitating factors (e.g. alcohol, spicy food, strenuous exercise).
Surgery: Surgical resection or debulking of the tumour.
Hepatic metastases: Hepatic artery embolization, chemotherapy (e.g. interferon-α).

C: Electrolyte imbalance (secondary to diarrhoea), metastases, fibrosis near a gut primary can result in bowel obstruction, hormones can cause tricuspid and pulmonary valve stenosis with consequent right heart failure.

P: As these tumours are generally slow-growing, mean survival is usually 5–10 years but can range up to 20 years. Earlier detection and treatment should improve quality of life and survival.

D: Acute cessation of cardiac function.

A: The classical reversible causes of cardiac arrest are the four H's and four T's:

Hypoxia	Tamponade, cardiac
Hypothermia	Tension pneumothorax
Hypovolaemia	Thromboembolism
Hypo- or Hyperkalaemia	Toxins

(+ other metabolic disorders)(sepsis, drugs, therapeutic agents)

A/R: –

E: –

H: Management precedes or occurs at same time as history (e.g. from witnesses).

E: Unconscious, patient is not breathing, absent pulses.

P: –

I: **Cardiac monitor:** Classification of the rhythm directs management (see below).
Blood ABG, U&E, FBC, cross-match, clotting, toxic screen.

M: **Safety:** Approach any arrest scene with caution as the cause of the arrest may still pose a threat. Defibrillators and oxygen are hazards. Help should be summoned as soon as possible.

Basic life support:*

1 If the arrest has just occurred, give a precordial thump.
2 Clear and maintain **A**irway with head-tilt (if no spinal injury), jaw-thrust and chin-lift.
3 Assess **B**reathing by look, listen and feel.
If not breathing, give two effective breaths immediately.
4 Assess **C**irculation at carotid pulse for 10 s.
If absent, give 15 chest compressions at rate of about 100/min.
5 Continue cycle of 15 chest compressions for every two breaths.
Check circulation every minute.
6 Proceed to advanced life support as soon as possible.

Advanced life support:* Attach cardiac monitor and defibrillator.

1 Assess the rhythm and check pulse.
2 If **VF** or pulseless **VT**,† defibrillate × 3 (First cycle at 200J, 200J, 360J. Further cycles at 360J) CPR for 1 min, return to **1**.
(Make sure no one is touching patient or bed when defibrillating.)
3 If EMD‡ or asystole, CPR for 3 min, return to **1**.
4 During CPR: check electrode, paddle positions and contacts. Attempt endotracheal intubation, high-flow oxygen, IV access, adrenaline (1 mg IV every 3 min). Consider amiodarone, atropine, pacing, buffers (e.g. bicarbonate).

*See latest UK Resuscitation Council guidelines.

†VT: > 3 successive ventricular extrasystoles (broad QRS complexes: > 120 ms) at a rate of > 120/min. Acute treatment of VT in patients with no haemodynamic compromise is with IV amiodarone. Patients at high risk of recurrent VT should be considered for implantable defibrillator which has been shown to be more effective than amiodarone. VF: irregular, rapid ventricular activation with no cardiac output.

‡EMD: Absence of cardiac output despite ECG showing electrical activity.

Treatment of reversible causes:
Hypothermia: Warm slowly.
Hypo- or Hyperkalaemia: Correction of electrolytes.
Hypovolaemia: IV colloids, crystalloids or blood products.
Tamponade: Pericardiocentesis under xiphisternum upwards and leftwards.
Tension pneumothorax: Needle into second intercostal space, mid-clavicular line.
Thromboembolism: (see Pulmonary embolism and Myocardial infarction).
Toxins: (see drug formulary for antidotes).

C: Irreversible brain damage, death.

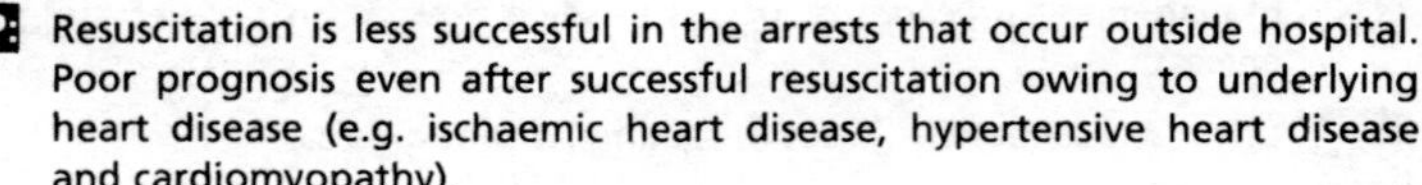

P: Resuscitation is less successful in the arrests that occur outside hospital. Poor prognosis even after successful resuscitation owing to underlying heart disease (e.g. ischaemic heart disease, hypertensive heart disease and cardiomyopathy).

D: Inability of the cardiac output to meet the body's demands despite normal venous pressures.

A: **Low output** (↓ cardiac output):
Left heart failure: Ischaemic heart disease, hypertension, cardiomyopathy, aortic valve disease, mitral regurgitation.
Right heart failure: Secondary to left heart failure, infarction, cardiomyopathy, pulmonary hypertension/embolus/chronic lung disease, pulmonary valve disease, tricuspid regurgitation, constrictive pericarditis/pericardial tamponade.
Biventricular failure: Arrhythmia, cardiomyopathy (dilated or restrictive), myocarditis, drug toxicity.
High output (↑ demand): Anaemia, beriberi, pregnancy, Paget's disease, hyperthyroidism, arteriovenous malformation.

A/R: (see Aetiology).

E: 10 % of > 65-year-olds.

H: **Left** (symptoms caused by pulmonary congestion): Dyspnoea (New York Heart Association classification):
1 no dyspnoea;
2 dyspnoea on ordinary activities;
3 dyspnoea on less than ordinary activities; and
4 dyspnoea at rest.
Orthopnoea, paroxysmal nocturnal dyspnoea, fatigue.
Acute LVF: Dyspnoea, wheeze, cough and pink frothy sputum.
Right: Swollen ankles, fatigue, ↑ weight (resulting from oedema), ↓ exercise tolerance, anorexia, nausea.

E: **Left:** Tachycardia, tachypnoea, displaced apex beat, bilateral basal crackles, third heart sound ('gallop' rhythm: rapid ventricular filling), pansystolic murmur (functional mitral regurgitation).
Acute LVF: Tachypnoea, cyanosis, tachycardia, peripheral shutdown, pulsus alternans, gallop rhythm, wheeze 'cardiac asthma', fine crackles throughout the lung.
Right: ↑ JVP, hepatomegaly, ascites, ankle/sacral pitting, oedema, signs of functional tricuspid regurgitation (see Tricuspid regurgitation).

P: **Macro:** Depends on cause. Dilated or hypertrophic ventricles, areas of fibrosis from old infarctions or fibrosed pericardium may be seen.

I: **Blood:** FBC, U&E, lipids, TFT. In acute LVF, ABG and cardiac enzymes.
CXR (in acute LVF): Cardiomegaly (heart > 50 % of thoracic width), prominent upper lobe vessels, pleural effusion, interstitial oedema ('Kerley B lines'), perihilar shadowing ('bat's wings'), fluid in the fissures.
ECG: Normal, ischaemic changes, arrhythmia, left ventricular hypertrophy (seen in hypertension).
Echocardiogram, technetium-99 scan: To assess ventricular contraction. If ejection fraction < 50 %: systolic dysfunction. Diastolic dysfunction: ↓ compliance leading to a restrictive filling defect.
Swan–Ganz catheter: Allows measurements of right atrial, right ventricular, pulmonary artery, pulmonary wedge and left ventricular end-diastolic pressures.

M: **Acute LVF:** *Cardiogenic shock:* Severe cardiac failure with low BP requires the use of inotropes (e.g. noradrenaline (norepinephrine), dobutamine) and should be managed in ITU.

Pulmonary oedema: Sit up patient, 60–100 % O_2 and consider CPAP or BiPAP. Other first-line therapies are diamorphine (venodilator and anxiolytic effect), GTN infusion (↓ preload), IV furosemide (frusemide) if fluid overloaded (venodilator and later diuretic effect). Monitor temperature, BP, respiratory rate, sat O_2, urine output, ECG.

Chronic LVF: Treat the cause (e.g. hypertension). Treat exacerbating factors (e.g. anaemia).

Medical: The following drug therapies are evidence-based.*

ACE-inhibitors: Inhibit Na^+ and water retention, vasoconstriction and improve symptoms and prognosis.

β-Blockers: Block the effects of chronically activated sympathetic system.

Spironolactone (aldosterone antagonist): Consider combination with furosemide (frusemide) to prevent hyperkalaemia.

Digoxin: Positive inotrope. Reduces hospital admissions, but does not improve survival.

Surgical: Heart transplantation (if < 65 years).

C: Respiratory failure, cardiogenic shock, death.

P: 50 % of patients with severe heart failure die within 2 years.

*Important trials include CIBIS-II and US-Carvedilol (role of β-blockers), SOLVD and CONSENSUS (role of ACE-inhibitors) and DIG study (role of digoxin).

D: A primary disease of the myocardium. Cardiomyopathy (CM) may be dilated (**DCM**), hypertrophic (**HCM**) or restrictive (**RCM**).

A: The majority are idiopathic.
DCM: Postviral myocarditis, alcohol, drugs (e.g. doxorubicin, cocaine), familial (~25 % of idiopathic cases, usually autosomal dominant), thyrotoxicosis, haemochromatosis, peripartum.
HCM: Up to 50 % of cases are genetic (autosomal dominant) with mutations in β-myosin, troponin T or α-tropomyosin (components of the contractile apparatus).
RCM: Amyloidosis, sarcoidosis, haemochromatosis, endomyocardial fibrosis.

A/R: (see Aetiology).

E: Prevalence of **DCM** and **HCM** is ~0.05–0.20 %. **RCM** is rare.

H: **DCM:** Symptoms of heart failure, arrhythmias, thromboembolism, sudden death.
HCM: Usually none. Syncope, angina, arrhythmias, sudden death (more common in young patients).
RCM: Dyspnoea, fatigue, arrhythmias, ankle or abdominal swelling.
Enquire about family history of sudden death.

E: **DCM:** ↑ JVP, displaced apex beat, functional mitral and tricuspid regurgitations, third heart sound.
HCM: Jerky carotid pulse, double apex beat, ejection systolic murmur.
RCM: ↑ JVP (Kussmaul's sign: further ↑ on inspiration), palpable apex beat, third heart sound, ascites, ankle oedema, hepatomegaly.

P: **DCM:** Dilation and impaired contraction of ventricles. Mural thrombi are common.
HCM: Asymmetrical left ventricle hypertrophy, septal bulge may partially obstruct outflow to aorta. Microscopy shows myocyte hypertrophy and disarray, interstitial fibrosis.
RCM: Myocardial thickening, fibrosis or amyloid deposition. Diastolic ventricular filling is restricted by the rigid ventricular walls.

I: **CXR:** May show cardiomegaly and signs of heart failure.
ECG: *All types:* Non-specific ST or T wave changes, conduction defects, arrhythmias, plus:
HCM: Left axis deviation, signs of left ventricular hypertrophy (see Aortic stenosis), Q waves in inferior and lateral leads.
RCM: Low voltage complexes.
Echocardiography: *DCM:* Dilated ventricles with 'global' hypokinesia.
HCM: Ventricular hypertrophy with disproportionate involvement of the septum.
RCM: Non-dilated non-hypertrophied ventricles. Atrial enlargement, preserved systolic function, diastolic dysfunction; granular or 'sparkling' appearance of myocardium in amyloidosis.
Cardiac catheterization, endomyocardial biopsy, histological examination: (? RCM).
Pedigree or genetic analysis.

M: **DCM:** Treat heart failure and arrhythmias. Consider implantable cardioverter defibrillator for recurrent ventricular tachycardias.

HCM: Treat arrhythmias with drugs, implantable cardioverter defibrillator for survivors of sudden death, reduce outflow tract gradients, dual-chamber pacing, surgery (e.g. septal myectomy, septal ablation with ethanol). Screen family members with ECG or echocardiography.
RCM: No specific treatment. Manage the underlying cause. Cardiac transplantation may be considered in end-stage heart failure (all cardiomyopathy types).

C: **All types:** Heart failure, arrhythmias (atrial and ventricular).
DCM and HCM: Sudden death and embolism.
HCM: Infective endocarditis.

P: **DCM:** Depends on the aetiology, New York Heart Association functional class and ejection fraction.
HCM: Ventricular tachyarrhythmias are the major cause of sudden death.
RCM: Poor prognosis, many die within the first year after diagnosis.

Carpal tunnel syndrome

D: Hand weakness and paraesthesia from compression of the median nerve in the carpal tunnel.

A: Narrowing of the carpal tunnel or enlargement of the contents compresses the median nerve which runs through it. Usually idiopathic but some common secondary causes include:

- fluid retention (e.g. in pregnancy, heart failure, liver failure, nephrotic syndrome);
- arthritis of the wrist (rheumatoid, osteoarthritis), previous wrist fractures, occupational misuse; and
- acromegaly, hypothyroidism, diabetes mellitus, obesity, amyloidosis.

A/R: Obesity and oral contraceptives are suggested risk factors.

E: Overall prevalence 2.7 %. Incidence in adults 0.1 % per year. Lifetime risk 10 %.

H: Tingling and pain in the hand and fingers (patients may be woken up at night). Weakness and clumsiness of hand.

E: Sensory impairment of median nerve (first 3 ½ fingers).
Tinel's sign: Tapping carpal tunnel triggers symptoms.
Phalen's test: Maximal flexion of the wrist for 1 min may cause symptoms.
Weakness and wasting of the thenar eminence (abductor pollicis brevis and opponens).
Signs of the underlying cause, e.g. hypothyroidism or acromegaly.

P: **Macro:** The carpal tunnel is made up of the flexor retinaculum anteriorly, the carpal bones posteriorly and laterally. It contains the median nerve, flexor pollicis longus, flexor digitorum profundus and superficialis tendons. There may be visible clues to the cause of compression: growths, oedema, inflammation or fibrosis.

I: **Blood:** TFT, ESR.
Nerve conduction study: Not always necessary. Shows conduction delay across wrist.

M: **Conservative:** Light wrist splint in a neutral position for a few weeks allows spontaneous resolution.
Medical: Local injection into carpal tunnel of long-acting steroid is effective. Worsens symptoms initially as a result of volume increase in carpal tunnel, diuretics are of uncertain benefit.
Surgical: Surgical decompression by division of the flexor retinaculum. Usually reserved for patients with intractable symptoms and motor involvement.

C: Permanent motor and sensory impairment of the hand.

P: Good. Majority of cases wax and wane over years. Secondary cases are more likely to progress further.

Cellulitis

D: Acute non-purulent spreading infection of the subcutaneous tissue, causing overlying skin inflammation.

A: Often results from penetrating injury (e.g. intravenous cannulation), local lesions (e.g. insect bites, sebaceous cysts, surgery) or fissuring (e.g. in anal fissures, toe web spaces), which allows pathogenic bacteria to enter the skin. In rare cases of septicaemia, it can arise spontaneously from blood-borne sources.

Most common organisms: *Streptococcus pyogenes* and *Staphylococcus aureus*. If occurring in the orbit, *Haemophilus influenzae* is the most common cause. The infection often arises from adjacent sinuses.

A/R: Main risk factors are poor hygiene and poor vascularization of tissue (e.g. diabetes mellitus).

E: Very common.

H: There may be history of a cut, scratch or injury.
Periorbital: Painful swollen red skin around eye.
Orbital cellulitis: Painful or limited eye movements, visual impairment.

E: **Lesion:** erythema, oedema, warm tender indistinct margins. Pyrexia may signify systemic spread.
Exclude abscess: Test for fluid thrill or fluctuation. Aspirate if pus suspected.
Periorbital: Swollen eyelids. Conjunctival injection.
Orbital cellulitis: Proptosis, impaired acuity and eye movement. Test for relative afferent pupillary defect, visual acuity and colour vision (to monitor optic nerve function).

P: **Micro:** Subdermal or subfascial bacterial growth. There is an acute inflammatory infiltrate composed mainly of polymorphs and macrophages. Localized vasodilation.

I: **Blood:** WCC, blood culture.
Discharge: Culture and sensitivity.
Aspiration: No pus. Not usually necessary unless abscess likely.
CT/MRI scan: When orbital cellulitis is suspected (to assess the posterior spread of infection).

M: **Medical:** Oral penicillins (e.g. flucloxacillin, benzylpenicillin, coamoxiclav) are effective in most community-acquired cases. In the hospital, treat empirically but change depending on sensitivity of any cultured organisms. IV use may be necessary.
Surgical: Orbital decompression may be necessary in orbital cellulitis. This is an emergency.
Abscess: Abscesses can be aspirated; incised and drained; or excised completely.

C: Sloughing of overlying skin. Localized tissue damage. In orbital cellulitis, there may be permanent vision loss and spread to brain, abscess formation, meningitis, cavernous sinus thrombosis.

P: Good with treatment.

D: Osteoarthritic degeneration of the lower cervical vertebral bodies causing compression of the spinal cord and/or nerve roots.

A: Degenerative change of vertebral bodies produces osteophytes, which protrude on to the exit foramina and spinal canal, and compress nerve roots (radiculopathy) or the anterior spinal cord (myelopathy).

A/R: Previous trauma, age and postmenopause.

E: Common in the elderly.

H: Neck pain or stiffness. Arm pain (stabbing or dull ache).
Paraesthesia, weakness, clumsiness in hands.
Weak and stiff legs.

E: **Arms:**

- Atrophy of forearm or hand muscles may be seen.
- Segmental muscle weakness in a nerve root distribution:
  C5: Shoulder abduction and elbow flexion weaknesses
  C6: Elbow flexion and wrist extension weaknesses
  C7: Elbow extension, wrist extension and finger extension weaknesses
  C8: Wrist flexion and finger flexion weaknesses.
- Hyporeflexia. In C5 and C6 lesions, 'inverted' reflexes (finger flexion seen on testing biceps or supinator tendon reflexes) may be seen as a result of LMN impairment at the level of compression and UMN impairment below the level.
- Sensory loss (mainly pain and temperature).
- Pseudoathetosis (writhing finger motions when hands are outstretched, fingers spread and eyes closed).

Legs (seen in those with cervical cord compressions):

- ↑ tone, weakness, hyper-reflexia and extensor plantars;
- ↓ Vibration and joint position sense (spinothalamic loss is less common) with a sensory level (few segments below the level of cord compression).

Lhermitte's sign: Neck flexion produces crepitus and/or paraesthesia down the spine.

P: **Macro:** Bony osteophytes and fibrocartilage protrude out into spinal canal and the exit foramina. The spinal vertebral bodies exhibit cystic changes subchondrally.

I: **Spinal X-ray (lateral):** Detects osteoarthritic change in the cervical spine, and excludes more serious causes. Poor sensitivity and specificity.
MRI: Assessment of root and cord compression and to exclude spinal cord tumour, many elderly people have some degree of cervical spondylosis and this may not be the cause of the symptoms.

M: **Conservative:** Physiotherapy. Soft neck collar to limit flexion–extension.
Medical: Supportive treatment with analgesia (e.g. NSAIDs, quinine sulphate).
Surgery: Spinal decompression, facetectomy, laminectomy (only about 50 % improve after surgery).

C: Acute spinal cord compression. Bladder and sphincter dysfunction.

P: If untreated, there can be a high quality of life impairment. Surgical treatment may only partially alleviate the impairment.

Chronic obstructive airway disease (COPD or COAD)

D: A chronic, slowly progressive lung disorder characterized by airflow obstruction, encompassing:
Chronic bronchitis: chronic cough and sputum production on most days for at least 3 months per year over 2 consecutive years; and
Emphysema: pathological diagnosis of permanent destructive enlargement of air spaces distal to the terminal bronchioles.

A: Bronchial and alveolar damage as a result of environmental toxins (e.g. cigarette smoke). A rare cause is α_1-antitrypsin deficiency (< 1 %) but should be considered in young patients or in those who have never smoked.

A/R: Risk factors are smoking (particularly if > 20 pack-years; 10–20 % of smokers will develop COPD), recurrent bronchopulmonary infections, occupational exposure in the mining and cotton industries. Overlaps and may often copresent with asthma.

E: Very common (prevalence up to 8 %). Presents in middle age or later. More common in males, but likely to change with ↑ female smokers. Responsible for large percentage of admissions. ~30 000 deaths/year.

H: Chronic cough and sputum production (see Definition). Breathlessness, wheeze, ↓ exercise tolerance.

E: **Inspection:** May have respiratory distress, use of accessory muscles, barrel-shaped overinflated chest, ↓ cricosternal distance, cyanosis. Note: clubbing is not normally a feature.
Percussion: Hyper-resonant chest, loss of liver and cardiac dullness.
Auscultation: Quiet breath sounds, prolonged expiration, wheeze, rhonchi and crepitations sometimes present.
Signs of CO_2 retention: Bounding pulse, warm peripheries, flapping tremor of the hands (asterixis). In late stages, signs of right heart failure (e.g. right ventricular heave, raised JVP, ankle oedema).

P: **Chronic bronchitis:** Narrowing of the airways resulting from inflammation of bronchioles (bronchiolitis) and bronchi with mucosal oedema, mucous gland hypertrophy, mucous hypersecretion and squamous metaplasia.
Emphysema: Destruction and enlargement of the alveoli distal to the terminal bronchioles, typically centriacinar in smokers and panacinar in α_1-antitrypsin deficiency. This results in loss of the elastic traction that keeps small airways open in expiration. Progressively larger emphyesematous spaces may develop, termed bullae when the diameter is > 1 cm.

I: **Blood:** FBC (↑ Hb and PCV as a result of secondary polycythemia, ↑ WCC in acute infective exacerbations).
ABG: May show hypoxia (↓ PaO_2), normal or ↑ $PaCO_2$.
Pulmonary function tests: Obstructive picture as reflected by ↓ PEFR, ↓ FEV_1: FVC ratio (mild, 60–80 %; moderate, 40–60 %; severe < 40 %), ↑ lung volumes and carbon monoxide gas transfer coefficient ↓ when significant alveolar destruction.
CXR: May appear normal or show hyperinflation (> 6 ribs visible anteriorly, flat hemi-diaphragms), ↓ peripheral lung markings, elongated cardiac silhouette.
ECG and echocardiogram: For cor pulmonale.
Sputum and blood cultures: In acute exacerbations for treatment.

M: Most important: stop smoking.

Medical:* *Bronchodilators:* β_2-*Agonists* (e.g. salbutamol) and anticholinergics (e.g. ipratropium), delivered by inhalers or nebulizers, provide symptomatic relief.

Steroids: Trial of inhaled beclometasone (6–8 weeks) and continue treatment if FEV_1 improves by $> 15\%$. In non-responders, long-term corticosteroid therapy is controversial. Oral corticosteroids are mainly reserved for acute exarcebations.

Oxygen therapy (only for those who stop smoking): Long-term home oxygen therapy has been shown to improve mortality. Indications are:

- $PaO_2 < 7.3$ kPa on air during a period of clinical stability.
- PaO_2 7.3–8.0 kPa and signs of secondary polycythaemia, nocturnal hypoxaemia, peripheral oedema or pulmonary hypertension.

Oxygen concentrators are more economical and useful in those requiring it for > 8 h/day.

Treatment of complications:

Acute infective exacerbations: 24 % O_2 via non-variable flow Venturi mask. Raise slowly if no improvement (measured by ABG) as there is a danger that a loss of hypoxic drive might cause respiratory arrest. Start empirical antibiotic therapy (first-line are amoxicillin or erythromycin). Corticosteroids (oral or inhaled) are of proven benefit. Vigorous chest physiotherapy is essential. Consider early ventilation in severe cases.

Prevention of infective exacerbations: Vaccination against pneumococcus and influenza.

C: Acute respiratory failure, infections (*Streptococcus pneumoniae*, *Haemophilus influenzae*), pulmonary hypertension and right heart failure, pneumothorax (resulting from bursting of emphysematous bullae), secondary polycythaemia.

P: High level of morbidity. 3-year survival rate of 90 % if age < 60 years and $FEV_1 > 50\%$ predicted; 75 % if > 60 years and FEV_1 40–49 % predicted.

*Refer to British Thoracic Society guidelines (*Thorax* 1997; **52**: S1–S28) and the UK Department of Health guidelines (available at http://www.prodigy.nhs.uk/) for complete information.

Cirrhosis

D: End-stage of chronic liver damage with replacement of normal liver architecture with diffuse fibrosis and nodules of regenerating hepatocytes. **Decompensated** when there are complications such as ascites, jaundice, encephalopathy or GI bleeding (see Liver failure).

A: **Chronic alcohol misuse:** Most common UK cause (see Alcoholic hepatitis and Alcohol dependence).
Chronic viral hepatitis: Hepatitis B or C are the most common causes worldwide.
Autoimmune hepatitis.
Inherited: α_1-Antitrypsin deficiency, haemochromatosis, Wilson's disease, galactosaemia, cystic fibrosis.
Drugs: e.g. methotrexate, hepatotoxic drugs.
Vascular: Budd–Chiari syndrome or hepatic venous congestion.
Chronic biliary diseases: Primary biliary cirrhosis, primary sclerosing cholangitis, biliary atresia.
Cryptogenic: In 5–10%.

A/R: NASH are at ↑ risk of developing cirrhosis (NASH is associated with obesity, diabetes, TPN, short bowel syndromes, hyperlipidaemia and drugs, e.g. amiodarone, tamoxifen).
Decompensation can be precipitated by infection, GI bleeding, constipation, high protein meal, electrolyte imbalances, alcohol and drugs, tumour development or portal vein thrombosis.

E: Among the top 10 leading cause of deaths worldwide.

H: Early non-specific symptoms: anorexia, nausea, fatigue, weakness, weight loss.
Symptoms caused by ↓ liver synthetic function: Easy bruising, abdominal swelling, ankle oedema.
Reduced detoxification function: Jaundice, personality change, altered sleep pattern, amenorrhoea.
Portal hypertension: Abdominal swelling, haematemesis, PR bleeding or melaena.

E: Stigmata of chronic liver disease:
Asterixis ('liver flap')
Bruises
Clubbing
Dupuytren's contracture
Erythema (palmar).
Jaundice, gynaecomastia, leuconychia, parotid enlargement, spider naevi, scratch marks, ascites ('shifting dullness' and fluid thrill), enlarged liver (shrunken and small in later stage), testicular atrophy, caput medusae (dilated superficial abdominal veins), splenomegaly (indicating portal hypertension).

P: **Micro:** Periportal fibrosis, loss of normal liver architecture and nodular appearance, either micronodular (< 3 mm, often caused by alcohol) or macronodular (> 3 mm). Grade refers to the assessment of degree of inflammation, whereas stage refers to the degree of architectural distortion, ranging from mild portal fibrosis to cirrhosis.
Macro: Enlarged liver or shrunken cirrhotic liver in later stages.

I: **Blood:** *FBC:* ↓ Hb, ↓ platelets as a result of hypersplenism.

LFT: May be normal or often ↑ transaminases, AlkPhos, γ-GT, bilirubin, ↓ albumin.
Clotting: Prolonged PT (↓ synthesis of clotting factors).
Serum AFP: ↑ In chronic liver disease, but high levels may suggest HCC.
Other investigations: To determine the cause, e.g. viral serology, α_1-antitrypsin, caeruloplasmin (Wilson's disease), iron studies (serum ferritin, iron, total iron binding capacity) for haemochromatosis, antimitochondrial antibody (primary biliary cirrhosis), ANA, SMA (autoimmune hepatitis).
Ascitic tap: Microscopy, culture and sensitivity, biochemistry (protein, albumin, glucose, amylase) and cytology. If neutrophils $>250/\text{mm}^3$, this indicates SBP.
Liver biopsy: Percutaneous or transjugular if clotting deranged or ascites present.
Imaging: Ultrasound, CT or MRI, MRCP.
Endoscopy: Examine for varices, portal hypertensive gastropathy.
Child–Pugh grading: Class A is score 5–6, Class B is score 7–9, Class C is score 10–15.

Score	1	2	3
Albumin (g/L)	>35	28–35	<28
Bilirubin (mg/dL)	<2	2–3	>3
Prothrombin time (s prolonged)	<4	4–6	>6
Ascites	None	Mild	Moderate or severe
Encephalopathy	None	Grade 1–2	Grade 3–4

M: **Medical:** Treat the cause if possible, avoid sedatives, opiates, NSAIDs and drugs that affect the liver. Nutrition is very important and if intake is poor, dietitian review and enteral supplements should be given; nasogastric feeding may be indicated.
Treat the complications:
Encephalopathy: Treat infections. Exclude a GI bleed. Lactulose, phosphate enemas and avoid sedation.
Ascites: Diuretics (spironolactone ± furosemide (frusemide)), salt restriction, therapeutic paracentesis (with human albumin replacement IV).
SBP: Antibiotic treatment (e.g. cefuroxime and metronidazole), prophylaxis against recurrent SBP with ciprofloxacin.
Surgical: Consider insertion of TIPS to relieve portal hypertension (if recurrent variceal bleeds or diuretic-resistant ascites) although it may precipitate encephalopathy. Liver transplantation is the only curative measure.

C: Portal hypertension with ascites, encephalopathy or variceal haemorrhage, SBP, hepatocellular carcinoma, renal failure (hepatorenal syndrome), pulmonary hypertension (hepatopulmonary syndrome).

P: Depends on the aetiology and complications. Generally poor; overall 5-year survival is ~50 %. In the presence of ascites, 2-year survival of ~50 %.

CNS tumours

D: Primary tumours arising from any of the brain tissue types.

A: In children, it probably reflects embryonic errors in development. In adults, the aetiology is unknown.

A/R: Neurofibromatosis type I is associated with gliomas. Previous brain trauma is a postulated risk factor.

E: Annual incidence of primary tumours 5–9 in 100 000. Two peaks of incidence (children and the elderly).

H: Headache or vomiting (↑ intracranial pressure), epilepsy (focal or generalized), focal neurological deficits (dysphagia, hemiparesis, ataxia, visual field defects, cognitive impairment), personality change.

E: Papilloedema/false localizing signs (↑ intracranial pressure), focal neurological deficits (visual field defects, dysphasia, agnosia, anopia, hemiparesis, ataxia, dysdiadochokinesis, hemispheric disconnection).

Specific localizing syndromes:

Olfactory groove tumours: Anosmia, frontal lobe dysfunction.

Cavernous sinus tumours: Opthalmoplegia (III, IV, VI nerve palsies), V_1 and V_2 sensory loss.

Foster Kennedy syndrome: Sphenoid wing meningioma compresses II nerve causing ipsilateral optic atrophy and contralateral papilloedema.

Pituitary adenomas: Endocrine signs, bitemporal hemianopia (suprasellar expansion and optic chiasm compression), hypopituitarism or hypersecretion of specific hormones from functioning tumours (e.g. acromegaly, hyperprolactinaemia, Cushing's disease).

Parinaud's syndrome: In pineal region impairing upgaze (because of proximity of the lesion to the superior midbrain) or obstructive hydrocephalus (at the level of third ventricle).

Parasagittal region tumours: Spastic paraparesis (mimicking cord compression).

Cerebellopontine tumours: Unilateral deafness, facial weakness, nystagmus.

P: **Meningioma:** Benign and most common primary CNS tumour.

Fibrilliary astrocytoma: Most common form, usually in cerebrum.

Pilocytic astrocytoma: Cystic, in cerebellum and brainstem.

Glioblastoma multiforme: High-grade invasive tumour.

Haemangioblastoma: Vascular tumours, often in the cerebellum.

Pituitary adenoma: Benign. Space-occupying and endocrine effects.

Oligodendroglioma: 10 % of gliomas. Epileptogenic.

Medulloblastoma: Invasive midline cerebellar tumour in children.

Ependymoma: Benign, in spinal cord and fourth ventricle.

Lymphoma: In immunosuppressed patients, highly malignant. 80 % occur in the posterior fossa in children, while in adults divided roughly equally between anterior and posterior fossa.

I: **CT/MRI:** To localize and characterize the lesion.

Blood: CRP, ESR, HIV screen.

Brain biopsy: Type and grading (degree of differentiation of tumour).

Caution: Lumbar puncture is contraindicated, may cause cerebral coning.

M: **Medical:** Anticonvulsants for epilepsy. Dexamethasone to reduce brain oedema. Chemotherapy and radiotherapy to reduce tumour size.

Surgery: Debulk or total resection of the tumour (especially for benign tumours). Not preferred if on dominant hemisphere or near speech centres. In pituitary adenomas, trans-sphenoidal resection is possible. Intraventricular shunts for hydrocephalus. Surgery may be inappropriate for low-grade glioma causing epilepsy only or for multiple metastases.

C: Pressure effect on surrounding tissue; herniation (falcine, tentorial, tonsillar); cerebrovascular accident (haemorrhage; see Stroke); focal or generalized fits (see Epilepsy).

P: Generally good for benign tumours, that are extra-axial (originate from meninges or cranial nerves). Malignant tumours that are intra-axial are generally incurable. Median survival is good in low-grade tumours (>5 year) but very poor in glioblastomas (about 9 months).

Coeliac disease

D: Inflammatory disease caused by intolerance to gluten, causing chronic intestinal malabsorption.

A: Sensitivity to the gliadin component of the cereal protein, gluten, triggers an immunological reaction in the small intestine leading to mucosal damage and loss of villi.

A/R: 10 % risk of first-degree relatives being affected. Strongly associated with dermatitis herpetiformis. There is a clear genetic susceptibility associated with *HLA-B8*, *DR3* and *DQW2* haplotypes.

E: Prevalence in UK is 1 in 2000. Very variable: 1 in 300 in the west of Ireland; very rare in East Asia.

H: May be asymptomatic.
Abdominal discomfort, pain and distention.
Steatorrhoea (pale bulky stool, with offensive smell and difficult to flush away), diarrhoea.
Tiredness, malaise, weight loss (despite normal diet).
Failure to 'thrive' in children, amenorrhoea in young adults.

E: **Signs of anaemia:** pallor.
Signs of malnutrition: Short stature, abdominal distension and wasted buttocks in children. Mid-arm muscle circumference or triceps skinfold thickness gives an indication of fat stores.
Signs of vitamin or mineral deficiencies (e.g. osteomalacia, easy brusing).
Intense, itchy blisters on elbows, knees or buttocks (dermatitis herpetiformis).

P: **Macro:** Villous atrophy in the small intestine (particularly the jejunum and ileum) giving the mucosa a flat smooth appearance.
Micro: Villous atrophy with crypt hyperplasia of the duodenum. The epithelium adopts a cuboidal appearance, and there is an inflammatory infiltrate of lymphocytes and plasma cells in the lamina propria.

I: **Blood:** FBC (↓ Hb), iron and folate, U&E, albumin, Ca^{2+} and phosphate.
Stool: Culture to exclude infection, faecal fat tests for steatorrhoea.
D-xylose test: Reduced urinary excretion after an oral xylose load indicates small bowel malabsorption.
Serology: Presence of IgA antigliadin, antiendomysial (against tissue trans-glutaminase) or antireticulin antibodies can be diagnostic. As IgA deficiency is common (1 in 50 with coeliac disease), immunoglobulin levels should also be measured.
Endoscopy: Visualization and biopsy of duodenum.

M: **Advice:** Withdrawal of gluten from the diet, with avoidance of all wheat, rye and barley products. Education and expert dietary advice is essential. The Coeliac Society offers patient support and advice.
Medical: Vitamin and mineral supplements. Oral corticosteroids may be used if the disease does not subside with gluten withdrawal.

C: Iron, folate and vitamin B_{12} deficiency, osteomalacia, ulcerative jejunoileitis, gastrointestinal lymphoma (particularly T cell), bacterial overgrowth.

P: With strict adherence to gluten-free diet, most patients make a full recovery. Symptoms usually resolve within weeks. Histological changes may take longer to resolve. A gluten-free diet needs to be followed for life.

D: A growth from the bowel wall that projects into the colonic lumen.

A: Classified into non-neoplastic and neoplastic polyps. Most are benign proliferations of mucosal epithelium (adenomas). Clinically significant because of malignant potential (see Colorectal carcinoma).

A/R: Multiple colonic polyps occur in some rare syndromes:
Peutz–Jeghers syndrome: Diffuse GI polyposis (most common in the small intestine) with mucocutaneous pigmentation of lips and gums. Autosomal dominant. Benign.
Inflammatory bowel disorder: Mucosal sloughing causes pseudopolyps. Colitis increases risk of malignancy.
Familial polyposis coli: Multiple colonic adenomas. Autosomal dominant. Caused by mutation in *APC* gene. Pre-malignant.
Gardner's syndrome: Osteomas, soft-tissue tumours, sebaceous cysts, congenital hypertrophy of retinal pigment epithelium and multiple colonic adenomas. Autosomal dominant. Pre-malignant.
Turcot's syndrome: Glioblastomas or medulloblastomas, with multiple colonic adenomas. Autosomal dominant. Pre-malignant.
Cronkhite–Canada syndrome: Alopecia, nail atrophy, pigmentation, watery diarrhoea and multiple stomach, small intestine and colonic adenomas. Pre-malignant.

E: Common. Prevalence is $>50\%$ of those over 60 years old.

H: Usually asymptomatic.
May cause a change in bowel habit.
Mucoid diarrhoea.
PR bleeding.
Symptoms of anaemia.

E: Usually no findings on examination.
May be palpable on PR examination if low in rectum.
Associated features of multiple polyposis syndromes.

P: **Macro:** It may be sessile or pedunculated and size ranges from millimetres to centimetres in diameter.
Micro: Non-neoplastic polyps include metaplastic (hyperplastic), inflammatory and hamartomatous polyps. Neoplastic polyps are adenomas, either tubular, tubulovillous or villous, the latter with a greater tendency to malignancy.

I: **Blood:** FBC (anaemia).
Stool: Occult or frank blood in stool.
Endoscopy: Colonoscopy is gold standard investigation. For multiple polyposis syndromes, an upper GI endoscopy is necessary to look for upper GI polyps. Polyps removed need to be histologically examined to determine their malignant potential.

M: **Endoscopy:** Colonoscopic polypectomy for small isolated polyps.
Surgical: Large polyps may have to be surgically resected. In multiple polyposis syndromes (particularly familial polyposis coli), early subtotal colectomy is recommended to reduce risk of malignancy.
Follow-up: Patients should be followed by colonoscopy every 2–4 years. Genetic screening of relatives may be necessary in multiple polyposis syndromes.

C: Malignant change, with highest risk in villous adenomas and in multiple polyposis syndromes. Risk of bowel obstruction.

P: Good if detected and treated before any malignant change.

Colorectal carcinoma

D: Malignant adenocarcinoma of the large bowel.

A: Environmental and genetic factors have been implicated. A sequence from epithelial dysplasia leading to adenoma and then carcinoma is thought to occur, involving accumulation of genetic changes in oncogenes (e.g. *APC, K-ras*) and tumour suppressor genes (e.g. *p53, DCC*).

A/R: Low-fibre diet (controversial), presence of colorectal polyps, previous colorectal cancer, family history,* inflammatory bowel disease (particularly long-standing ulcerative colitis). Inherited (autosomal dominant) disorders: Hereditary non-polyposis colorectal cancer (HNPCC) caused by mutations in mismatch repair genes (1–5% of colorectal cancers), familial adenomatous polyposis (FAP) caused by mutation in the APC gene.
NSAIDS and postmenopausal HRT may be protective.

E: Second most common cause of cancer death in the West. 20 000 deaths per year in the UK. Average age at diagnosis 60–65 years. Rectal carcinomas ♂ > ♀, colon carcinomas ♀ > ♂.

H: Symptoms will depend on the location of the tumour.
Left-sided colon and rectum: Change in bowel habit, rectal bleeding or blood/mucous mixed in with stools. Rectal masses may also present as tenesmus (sensation of incomplete emptying after defecation).
Right-sided colon: Later presentation, with symptoms of anaemia, weight loss and non-specific malaise or, more rarely, lower abdominal pain.
Up to 20 % of tumours will present as an emergency with pain and distension caused by large bowel obstruction, haemorrhage or peritonitis as a result of perforation.

E: Anaemia may be only sign, particularly in right-sided lesions, abdominal mass, with metastatic disease, hepatomegaly, 'shifting dullness' of ascites. Low-lying rectal tumours may be palpable on rectal examination.

P: **Macro:** 60 % rectum and sigmoid colon; 15–20 % in the ascending colon; and the remainder in the transverse and descending colon. Distal colon tumours tend to form an annular encircling ring around the bowel wall, causing 'napkin ring' constrictions, while proximal colon tumours tend to form polypoid exophytic masses.
Micro: Neoplastic change with deranged adenomatous or anaplastic cells and varying degrees of bowel wall penetration. Staging systems include Dukes' (see below) and the TNM system.

I: **Blood:** FBC (for anaemia), LFT, tumour markers (CEA to monitor treatment response or disease recurrence).
Stool: Occult or frank blood in stool (can be used as a screening test).
Endoscopy: Sigmoidoscopy, colonoscopy. Allows visualization and biopsy. Polypectomy can also be performed if isolated small carcinoma *in situ*.
Barium contrast studies: 'Apple core' stricture on barium enema.
Ultrasound scan for hepatic metastases.
Other staging investigations include CXR, CT or MRI, endorectal ultrasound.

*Risk of colorectal Cancer = 1:17 if one first degree relative affected, 1:10 if two affected, 1:50 if no close relative affected.

M: **Surgery:** Surgery is the only curative treatment. Operation depends on circumstances.

Caecum, ascending colon, proximal transverse colon: right hemicolectomy.

Distal transverse colon, descending colon: left hemicolectomy.

Sigmoid colon: sigmoid colectomy.

High rectum: anterior resection.

Low rectum: abdoperineal resection and end colostomy formation.

Emergency: Hartmann's procedure (proximal colostomy, resection of tumour and oversew of distal stump).

Survival in rectal tumours is improved if total mesorectal excision (removal of surrounding fascia). Isolated hepatic metastases may be successfully resected.

Radiotherapy: May be given in a neoadjuvent setting to downstage rectal tumours prior to resection or as adjuvant therapy to reduce risk of local recurrence.

Chemotherapy: Used as adjuvant therapy in Dukes' C, or sometimes B. 5-Fluorouracil (+folinic acid); many others are being assessed in clinical trials. Used to treat metastatic or recurrent disease, either systemically or regionally, e.g. liver infusion of chemotherapeutic drugs, often combined with embolization in hepatic metastases.

C: Bowel obstruction or perforation, fistula formation. Recurrence. Metastatic disease.

P: Prognosis varies depending on Dukes' staging.

Dukes'	Extent of spread	5-year survival (%)
A	Confined to bowel wall	80–90
B	Breached serosa but no lymph nodes	60
C	Breached serosa with lymph nodes	30
D	Distant metastases (usually liver)	<5

Congenital adrenal hyperplasia

D: Inherited disorders of adrenal steroid synthesis.

A: Autosomal recessive genetic defects in the steroid synthesis pathway result in ↓ cortisol (and, in some cases, ↓ aldosterone) synthesis. This produces a secondary rise in pituitary ACTH secretion causing enlargement of the adrenal glands and build-up of precursor steroids (e.g. androgenic steroids). Common defective enzymes include 21-hydroxylase (most common), 11β-hydroxylase and 17α-hydroxylase.

A/R: Associated with consanguinity.

E: Annual incidence of 21-hydroxylase deficiency and 11β-hydroxylase deficiency are 1 in 10 000 and 1 in 100 000, respectively. The rest are less common. 21-Hydroxylase deficiency is common among the Yupik Eskimos.

H & E: **21-Hydroxylase deficiency** (↓ aldosterone, ↑ androgens): Salt-losing crisis in infants (hypotension, hyponatraemia, hyperkalaemia).

Females: Virilization of fetuses, ambiguous genitalia (cliteromegaly, fused labia) or virilization, acne, hirsutism later in life, ↑ skeletal maturation.

Males: Precocious puberty (early pubic hair, penile and muscle enlargement, ↑ skeletal maturation).

11β-Hydroxylase deficiency (↑ 11-deoxycorticosterone (a mineralocorticoid), ↓ androgens): Hypertension, hypokalaemia.

Females: As 21-hydroxylase deficiency.

Males: As 21-hydroxylase deficiency.

17α-Hydroxylase deficiency (↑ 11-deoxycorticosterone (a mineralocorticoid), ↓ androgens): Hypertension, hypokalaemia.

Females: Failure to develop secondary sexual characteristics at puberty.

Males: Ambiguous or female genitalia.

P: **Macro:** Enlarged adrenal glands.

I: **Blood:** ^{17}OH-progesterone (↑ in 21-hydroxylase deficiency and 11β-hydroxylase deficiency), testosterone, ↑ basal ACTH, LH, FSH, U&E.

ACTH stimulation test: Inappropriately elevated ^{17}OH-progesterone levels after IM ACTH (should be performed in follicular phase of menstrual cycle).

Pelvic ultrasound: Excludes PCOS.

Karyotyping: Confirms gender of infant with ambiguous genitalia.

Molecular genetic testing: To confirm location of mutation.

M: **Acute salt-losing crisis:** IV saline, dextrose and hydrocortisone.

Medical: Glucocorticoid replacement with dexamethasone or hydrocortisone. Fludrocortisone in salt-losers. Treatment is monitored by measuring serum levels of ^{17}OH-progesterone and growth.

Advice: Genetic counselling. Antenatal screening occurs in UK.

C: Infertility. Short final adult height (because of premature epiphyseal closure without treatment).

P: Undiagnosed infants may die from salt-losing crisis. Otherwise, quality of life is usually good.

D: Chronic granulomatous inflammatory disease that can affect any part of the gastrointestinal tract. Grouped with ulcerative colitis and together they are known as inflammatory bowel disease.

A: Cause has not yet been elucidated, but thought to involve an interplay between genetic and environmental factors.

A/R: **Genetic:** *NOD2* gene (chromosome 16), *HLA-B27* in those with ankylosing spondylitis.
Environmental: Smoking (4–6 × risk), refined sugar intake. Infectious agents (e.g. *Mycobacterium*) proposed.
May be associated with autoimmune diseases (e.g. SLE, autoimmune thyroid disease).

E: Annual UK incidence is 5–8 in 100 000. Prevalence is 50–80 in 100 000. Affects any age but peak incidence is in the teens or twenties.

H: Crampy abdominal pain (caused by transmural and peritoneal inflammation, fibrosis or obstruction of bowel).
Diarrhoea (may be bloody or steatorrhoea).
Fever, malaise, weight loss.
Symptoms of complications.

E: Weight loss, clubbing, signs of anaemia.
Aphthous ulceration of the mouth.
Perianal skin tags, fistulae and abscesses.
Signs of complications.

P: **Macro:** Inflammation can occur anywhere along GI tract (40 % involving the terminal ileum), 'skip' lesions with inflamed segments of bowel interspersed with normal segments. Mucosal oedema and ulceration with 'rose-thorn' fissures (cobblestone mucosa), fistulae, abscesses.
Micro: Transmural chronic inflammation with infiltration of macrophages, lymphocytes and plasma cells. Granulomas with epithelioid giant cells may be seen in blood vessels or lymphatics.

I: **Blood:** FBC (↓ Hb, ↑ platelets, ↑ WCC), U&E, LFTs (↓ albumin), ↑ ESR, CRP (↑ or may be normal), haematinics to look for deficiency states: ferritin, vitamin B_{12} and red cell folate.
Stool microscopy and culture.
AXR for evidence toxic megacolon.
Erect CXR if risk of perforation.
Small bowel follow through: May reveal fibrosis/strictures (string sign of Kantor), deep ulceration (rose thorn), cobblestone mucosa.
Endoscopy (OGD, colonoscopy) and biopsy: May help to differentiate between ulcerative colitis and Crohn's disease, useful monitoring for malignancy and disease progression.
Radionuclide-labelled neutrophil scan: Localization of inflammation (when other tests are contraindicated).

M: **Acute exacerbation:** Fluid resuscitation, IV or oral corticosteroids, high dose 5-ASA analogues (e.g. mesalazine, sulfasalazine) may induce a remission in colonic Crohn's disease. Analgesia. Elemental diet may induce remission (more often used in children). Parenteral nutrition may be necessary.
Monitor: Temperature, pulse, respiratory rate, BP and markers of activity (ESR, CRP, platelets, stool frequency, Hb and albumin). Assess for complications.

Long-term: Steroids for acute exacerbations, regular 5-ASA analogues to ↓ number of relapses in Crohn's colitis. Alternatively, steroid-sparing agents (e.g. azathioprine, 6-mercaptopurine, methotrexate, infliximab).
Advice: Stop smoking, dietitian referral. Education and advice (e.g. from inflammatory bowel disease nurse specialists).
Surgery: Failure of medical treatment, failure to thrive in children, or the presence of complications.

C: **GI:** Haemorrhage, bowel strictures, perforation, fistulae (between bowel, bladder, vagina), perianal fistulae and abscess, GI carcinoma (5 % risk in 10 years), malabsorption.
Extraintestinal: Uveitis, episcleritis, gallstones, kidney stones, arthropathy, sacroiliitis, ankylosis spondylitis, erythema nodosum and pyoderma gangrenosum, amyloidosis.

P: Chronic relapsing condition. Two-thirds will require surgery at some stage and two-thirds of these >1 surgical procedure. Mortality rate twice that of general population.

Cryptogenic fibrosing alveolitis

D: Inflammatory condition of the lung resulting in fibrosis of alveoli and interstitium.

A: Unknown; proposed factors include environmental dusts, viral trigger or environmental injury potentiated by viral infection and immunological derangement. Certain drugs can produce a similar illness (e.g. bleomycin, methotrexate and amiodarone).

A/R: Occupational exposure to metal (steel, brass, lead) or wood (pine) in ~20 % cases; smoking (in 75 %); other associations reported are farming, hairdressing, stone cutting, animal and vegetable dusts.

E: Rare. Prevalence in UK is ~6 in 100 000. 2 × more ♂ affected. Mean age 67 years.

H: Gradual onset of progressive dyspnoea on exertion.
Dry irritating cough. No wheeze.
Symptoms may be preceded by a viral-type illness.
Fatigue and weight loss are common.
Full occupational and drug history important.

E: Finger clubbing (~50 %).
Bibasal fine late inspiratory ('velcro') crepitations.
Signs of right heart failure in advanced stages (e.g. right ventricular heave, raised JVP, peripheral oedema).

P: Varying areas of chronic inflammatory alveolitis with abundant lymphocytes, plasma cells and macrophages and fibrosis. Three histological patterns: usual interstitial pneumonia (UIP: patchy interstitial fibrosis, later: 'honeycomb' lung); desquamative interstitial pneumonia (DIP: Diffuse intra-alveolar accumulation of macrophages, mild thickening of alveolar septa, lymphoid aggregates); and non-specific interstitial pneumonia (NSIP).

I: **Blood:** ABG (normal in early disease, but ↓ PO_2 on exercise. Normal P_{CO_2} which rises in late disease).
Serology: One-third have rheumatoid factor or antinuclear antibodies.
CXR: Usually normal at presentation. Early disease may feature small lung fields and 'ground glass' shadowing. Later, there is reticulonodular shadowing (especially at bases), signs of cor pulmonale and eventually, in advanced disease, honeycombing.
High-resolution CT: More sensitive in early disease than CXR. Affecting mainly lower zones and subpleural areas, with reticular densities, honeycombing and traction bronchiectasis.
Pulmonary function tests: Restrictive ventilatory defect (↓ FEV_1, ↓ FVC with preserved or increased ratio), ↓ lung volumes, ↓ lung compliance and ↓ TLCO.
Bronchoalveolar lavage: To exclude infection and malignancy.
Lung biopsy: Gold standard for diagnosis but may not be appropriate.
Radionucleotide scans: Gallium scan is sensitive, but not specific. Raised clearance of inhaled radiolabelled-DPTA indicates ongoing inflammation.

M: **Medical:** No curative treatment available. Dual therapy trial with corticosteroids and azathioprine for 1 month is recommended. If responsive or disease stable (in up to 30 %), continue treatment. Corticosteroids should be stopped if there is deterioration. Cyclophosphamide can be used if azathioprine not tolerated.

Supportive care: Home oxygen may be necessary. Aggressive treatment of infections. Opiates in terminal stages for relieving distressing breathlessness. Psychosocial support is necessary because of poor long-term prognosis.
Surgical: Single lung transplantation is an option in selected patients.

C: Right heart failure, lung cancer (12 %), pulmonary embolus. Death from respiratory failure.

P: Poor; mean survival is only about 3 years. Good prognostic factors:
Clinical: young age, female, response to steroids.
Radiological: predominantly 'ground glass' shadowing.
Histology: DIP and NSIP better response to treatment than UIP.

D: Syndrome associated with chronic inappropriate elevation of free circulating cortisol.

A: **ACTH-dependent:** ACTH-releasing pituitary adenoma (Cushing's disease most common endogenous cause). Ectopic ACTH from oat cell bronchocarcinoma, carcinoid tumours, phaeochromocytoma.
Non-ACTH dependent: Adrenal adenoma/carcinoma/hyperplasia.
Iatrogenic: Steroids (most common overall cause).
(Rare) Meal dependent adrenal nodules.*

A/R: Associated with MEN-1. Rare associations in Carney's syndrome† and McCune–Albright syndrome.‡

E: ♂ : ♀ = 4:1. Peak incidence is 20–40 years; adrenal carcinomas more commonly present in childhood.

H: Increasing weight and fatigue.
Muscle weakness, myalgia, thin skin, easy bruising, poor wound healing, fractures (resulting from osteoporosis).
Polydipsia and polyuria.
Hirsutism, acne, frontal balding.
Oligo- or amenorrhoea, infertility, impotence.
Depression or psychosis.

E: Moon face (with plethoric complexion), buffalo hump.
Central obesity (because of altered fat distribution), pink/purple striae on abdomen, breast, thighs.
Proximal myopathy (difficulty rising from squat), thin skin, bruises.
Evidence of fractures (kyphosis in vertebral fracture).
Hirsutism, acne, frontal balding and poorly healing wounds.
Hypertension.
Ankle oedema (salt and water retention as a result of mineralocorticoid effect of excess cortisol).
Pigmentation in ACTH-dependent cases.

P: **ACTH dependent:** Excess ACTH causes bilateral diffuse or nodular hyperplasia of the adrenal glands and excess glucocorticoid synthesis and secretion.
ACTH independent: Hypersecretion of glucocorticoid by adrenal cortex, causing a negative feedback on ACTH production.

I: **Blood:** U&E (may show hypokalaemia), ↑ glucose, ↑ cortisol with loss of diurnal variation.
Screening test: ↑ 24-h Urinary free cortisol.
Confirmation tests: *Low-dose dexamethasone suppression test:* 0.5 mg orally every 6 h for 48 h. Normally, serum ACTH and cortisol are suppressed. In Cushing's syndrome, cortisol is not suppressed because the pituitary is less sensitive to negative feedback control.

*↑ Cortisol after meals, patients have ectopic overexpression of gastrointestinal peptide receptors in the adrenal cortex.
†Carney's syndrome: spotty skin pigmentation, atrial myxomas and peripheral nerve tumours.
‡McCune–Albright syndrome: fibrous dysplasia of bones with cysts, skin pigmentation and gonadal (precocious puberty), adrenal, pituitary and thyroid hyperfunction caused by a somatic mutation in α-subunit of the G protein and constitutive activation of hormone receptors in those tissues expressing the Gsα mutation.

To determine the underlying cause:
ACTH-independent (adrenal adenoma): ↓ ACTH.
- CT or MRI of adrenals shows structural lesions.

ACTH-dependent (pituitary adenoma): ↑ ACTH.
- *High-dose dexamethasone suppression test:* 2 mg orally every 6 h for 48 h. Serum cortisol is suppressed (> 50 %) in Cushing's disease.
- *Inferior petrosal sinus sampling:* Central:peripheral ratio of venous ACTH > 2:1.
- *CRH test:* Exaggerated ACTH and cortisol response to IV bolus CRH.

Pituitary MRI: Shows structural lesion.
ACTH-dependent (ectopic):
- If lung cancer is suspected: CXR, sputum cytology, bronchoscopy, CT scan.
- To find the ectopic cause: whole body venous sampling for ACTH.

M: **Medical:** Pre-operative or if unfit for surgery. Inhibition of cortisol synthesis with metyrapone or ketoconazole. Treat osteoporosis and provide physiotherapy for muscle weakness. In iatrogenic cases, discontinue administration, lower steroid dose, or use an alternative steroid-sparing agent.
Radiotherapy.
Surgical:
In pituitary adenomas: Trans-sphenoidal adenoma resection (hydrocortisone until pituitary function recovers).
In adrenal carcinoma: Surgical removal of tumour (> 5 cm) ± mitotane.
In ectopic ACTH production: Treatment is directed at the tumour.

C: Predisposition to infections (onychomycosis, dermatomycosis, pityriasis vesicolor), diabetes, osteoporosis.
Cardiovascular: Hypertension, IHD, thromboembolism.
Complications of surgery: CSF leakage, meningitis, sphenoid sinusitis, hypopituitarism.
Complications of radiotherapy: Hypopituitarism, radionecrosis, malignancy.

P: In the untreated, 5-year survival rate is 50 %.

D: Autosomal recessive inherited multisystem disease characterized by recurrent respiratory tract infections, pancreatic insufficiency, malabsorption and male infertility.

A: Caused by a defective *CFTR* gene on chromosome 7q, which encodes a cAMP-dependent Cl^- channel. This channel regulates Na^+ and Cl^- concentrations in exocrine secretions, especially in the lung and pancreas. Any loss of function mutations result in thick viscous secretions. >800 mutations reported, most common is ΔF508 phenylalanine deletion (75 % cases in UK).

A/R: Persons with obstructive azoospermia have an increased frequency of mutations in *CFTR* genes, but may be asymptomatic for cystic fibrosis.

E: Most common life-threatening autosomal inherited condition in white people. Incidence is 1 in 2500 live births. In UK, 1 in 25 are carriers.

H: **Lung:** Recurrent chest infections, chronic cough, wheeze, sputum, haemoptysis.
Gut: Meconium ileus (in neonates), steatorrhoea (caused by ↑ fat in the stool).
Other: Chronic sinusitis, nasal polyps, male infertility, arthritis.

E: **Chest:** Chest wall deformities, coarse crepitations and wheeze.
Signs of malnutrition: Anaemia, weight loss, signs of vitamin deficiencies, slow growth, failure to thrive in children, delayed puberty in adolescents.
Other: Clubbing, nasal polyps, signs of diabetes, hepatomegaly.

P: At birth, the lung is normal histologically but as the lung matures there is mucous gland hyperplasia, recurrent infection leads to fibrosis, consolidation and bronchiectasis. The pancreas shows fatty replacement, ductal obstruction from accumulation of thick secretions, reduced exocrine parenchyma and fibrosis.

I: **Sweat test:** Pilocarpine iontophoresis (low electrical current) stimulates sweat secretion which is collected and analysed for Na^+ and Cl^- (Cl^- levels >60 mmol is diagnostic of cystic fibrosis).
Neonatal screening: Standard day 6 Guthrie heal prick, blood is tested for immunoreactive trypsin (raised by 2–5 × in babies with cystic fibrosis).
CXR: May be normal in mild disease or show increased bronchial markings, ring shadows, fibrosis (often upper zone). Consolidation or bronchiectasis in more advanced cases.
Pancreatic assessment: Faecal elastase, faecal fat content, GTT, HbA1c.
Genetic analysis: For *CFTR* mutations.
Pulmonary function tests: To assess general lung function and to predict long-term prognosis.

M: Multidisciplinary specialist care is necessary.
Respiratory: Chest physiotherapy (postural drainage, regular exercise), positive expiratory pressure masks.
Bronchodilator therapy (if responsive).
Antibiotic prophylaxis and aggressive treatment of infections (especially *Pseudomonas*).
Influenza vaccination.

GI: Adequate nutritional intake is vital, using high-calorie oral supplements and oral pancreatic enzyme replacement, vitamin (especially fat-soluble) supplements.
Endocrine: Insulin replacement therapy if diabetes develops.
Surgical: Single lung or heart–lung transplants is an option in end-stage disease (5-year survival is 55 %).

C: Recurrent chest infections, bronchiectasis (particularly *Haemophilus*, *Staphylococcus* and *Pseudomonas*).
Malabsorption, meconium ileus, intussusception, rectal prolapse.
Diabetes mellitus Type I (30 % by late teens).
Male infertility (females are fertile but conception may be difficult).
Gallstones.

P: Life expectancy is in the third decade, but steadily improving. Those with pancreatic insufficiency and those colonized by *Pseudomonas* have poorer prognosis. Gene replacement therapy may be possible in the future.

D: The presence of thrombus in a deep vein, usually of the lower limb.

A: **Virchow's triad:**

1 Blood vessel wall injury.
2 Blood flow disturbance (stasis).
3 Blood hypercoagulability. These are risk factors for activation of coagulation and formation of venous thrombosis.

A/R: **Previous DVT.**

Stasis: Any surgery, trauma, immobility (e.g. long-haul flights), pregnancy, pelvic masses, obesity.

Thrombophilia: *Hereditary:* Protein C deficiency, protein S deficiency, antithrombin-III deficiency, 5′ prothrombin gene mutation and factor V Leiden (point mutation makes factor Va resistant to inactivation by protein C).

Acquired: Smoking, oestrogen contraceptive pill, malignancy, antiphospholipid syndrome, homocystinuria, polycythaemia, dehydration.

Other medical problems: Cardiac failure, recent MI, IBD, nephrotic syndrome.

E: Increasing incidence with increasing age. DVTs occur in many hospitalized patients, although the majority are asymptomatic and uncomplicated.

H: May be asymptomatic (25–50 %).

Presents with lower limb swelling or onset of deep pain, usually in the calf but may be above the knee.

There may be redness and warmth of the overlying skin or pain on weight bearing.

Mild fever.

Symptoms of pulmonary embolism (see Pulmonary embolism).

Enquire about risk factors above.

E: Unilateral lower limb swelling (usually calf), with diameter $\geq$1 cm compared with the other side. There may be overlying erythema, tenderness, heat, engorgement of the superficial veins. Occasionally, cyanotic discoloration of the limb (thrombosis involving the ileofemoral system).

Homan's sign: Resistance and pain on dorsiflexion of the foot, but the elicitation of Homan's sign is now discouraged because of the risk of precipitating embolism.

Low-grade pyrexia.

Signs of pulmonary embolism.

May be no signs on clinical examination ($\sim$50 %).

P: Thrombus formation is promoted by a component of Virchow's triad (see Aetiology), most commonly around the valves of the deep venous system of the calves. The thrombus may dissolve by fibrinolysis, or organize, with eventual recanalization (majority of cases). Before the latter occur, the thrombus may propagate proximally, or embolize to the pulmonary circulation.

I: **Blood:** D-dimers (degradation product of cross-linked fibrin) are sensitive but non-specific. Thrombophilia screen if indicated (e.g. multiple recurrent DVTs).

Prior to starting anticoagulation: FBC (platelets), U&E (renal function) and clotting screen.

Duplex ultrasonography: Positive predictive value in the proximal veins is 95 %, but sensitivity is only 50–75 % in calf veins.

Venography: Contrast medium is injected into a superficial vein of the foot but now rarely performed.

V/Q scan or CT pulmonary angiogram: If pulmonary embolism is suspected (see Pulmonary embolism).

M: **Prevention:** Treat avoidable risks, graded compression stockings, LMW heparin SC (e.g. enoxaparin), adequate hydration, early mobilization.

Medical: Anticoagulation with the following:

IV heparin: (binds to antithrombin III and ↑ rate of inactivation of thrombin and Xa). Given as a loading dose then constant infusion, monitoring the APTT to aim for 1.5–2.5 × normal.

LMW heparin: (inhibits factor Xa only) given SC is now commonly used, has longer duration of action than heparin and no APTT monitoring is required.

Warfarin: (inhibition of vitamin K dependent γ-carboxylation of factors II, VII, IX, X and protein C and S) is given for 3–6 months, monitoring INR with regular anticoagulant clinic appointments.

Avoid future risk factors for DVT (e.g. oral contraceptive pill).

Note: There is some evidence that DVT confined to the calf does not usually cause pulmonary embolism and anticoagulation is not indicated, this should be observed to ensure no proximal propagation.

Pulmonary embolism (see Pulmonary embolism).

C: Pulmonary embolism (5–20 % of symptomatic cases), deep venous insufficiency and postphlebitic syndrome. ↑ Risk of future DVT. Complications of treatment (e.g. bleeding, heparin-induced thrombocytopenia and thrombosis). Rarely, phlegmasia cerulea dolens (severe ileofemoral venous outflow obstruction).

P: Generally good, although there is risk of long-term sequelae of postphlebitic venous problems. If propagation and embolization occur, it can be fatal.

D: A disorder of inadequate secretion of or insensitivity to vasopressin (ADH) leading to hypotonic polyuria.

A: **Central or cranial diabetes insipidus:**

Acquired: Idiopathic, trauma (e.g. head injury, neurosurgery), tumours (e.g. craniopharyngiomas, pituitary tumours), infiltrative (e.g. sarcoidosis, tuberculosis), infection (e.g. meningitis, encephalitis), vascular (e.g. aneurysms, sickle cell disease, Sheehan's syndrome).

Familial: Autosomal dominant or recessive (see Associations).

Nephrogenic diabetes insipidus:

Acquired: Idiopathic, ↑ Ca^{2+}, ↓ K^+, drugs (e.g. lithium, demeclocycline), osmotic diuresis (diabetes mellitus), postobstructive uropathy, pyelonephritis, pregnancy.

Familial: Autosomal dominant (aquaporin-2 gene), X-linked recessive (VR_2 gene).

A/R: Cranial diabetes insipidus may be exacerbated during pregnancy because of vasopressinase produced by the placenta.

Diabetes insipidus may be part of the paraneoplastic syndrome associated with small cell bronchocarcinoma.

DIDMOAD (autosomal recessive syndrome of diabetes insipidus, diabetes mellitus, optic atrophy and deafness); Hand–Schüller–Christian disease (children 2–5 years, lytic lesions of skull, exopthalmos and diabetes insipidus).

E: Depends on aetiology, but median age of onset is 24 years. More common in males.

H: Polyuria, nocturia and polydipsia (excessive thirst). Enuresis and sleep disturbances in children.

Other symptoms depend on the aetiology.

E: Cranial diabetes insipidus has few signs if patients drink adequate fluids.

Urine output is often > 3 L/24 h.

If fluid intake <fluid output, signs of dehydration may be present (e.g. tachycardia, reduced tissue turgor, postural hypotension, dry mucous membranes).

Signs of the cause.

P: Failure of ADH secretion by the posterior pituitary (cranial) or insensitivity of the collecting duct (nephrogenic) to ADH. Water channels (aquaporins) fail to activate and the luminal membrane of the collecting duct remains impermeable to water. This results in large volume hypotonic urine and polydipsia.

I: **Blood:** U&E and Ca^{2+} (Na^+ may be rise secondary to dehydration, ↓ K^+ or ↑ Ca^{2+} as the aetiological factor). ↑ Plasma osmolality. ↓ Urine osmolality.

Water deprivation test:

Water is restricted for 8 h. Plasma and urine osmolality are measured every hour over the 8 h.

Weigh the patient (hourly) to monitor the level of dehydration; stop the test if the fall in body weight is > 3 %.

Desmopressin (2 μg IM) is given after 8 h and urine osmolality is measured.

Normal: Water restriction causes a rise in plasma osmolality and ↑ ADH secretion. This leads to ↑ water reabsorption in the collecting ducts. Urine is concentrated (urine osmolality > 600 mosmol/kg)

Diabetes insipidus: Lack of ADH activity means that urine is unable to be concentrated by the collecting ducts (urine osmolality < 400 mosmol/kg).
Cranial diabetes insipidus: Following administration of desmopressin, urine osmolality rises by > 50 %.
Nephrogenic diabetes insipidus: Following administration of desmopressin, urine osmolality rises by < 45 %.

M: Treat the identified cause if possible.
Cranial diabetes insipidus: Desmopressin (DDAVP), a vasopressin analogue, can be given 10 μg/day, intranasally. In mild disease, chlorpropamide or carbamazepine can be used to potentiate effects of residual vasopressin.
Nephrogenic diabetes insipidus: Sodium and/or protein restriction may help polyuria. Thiazide diuretics.

C: Hypernatraemic dehydration. Excess desmopressin therapy may cause hyponatraemia.

P: Variable depending on cause. Cranial diabetes insipidus may be transient following head trauma. Cure of cranial or nephrogenic diabetes insipidus may be possible on removal of cause, e.g. tumour resection, drug discontinuation.

D: Metabolic hyperglycaemic condition caused by insufficiency of pancreatic insulin production. Previously known as IDDM.

A: Results from insufficiency of pancreatic insulin production caused by damage to pancreatic islet β-cells. This can be due to:
1 autoimmune T-cell-mediated destruction (classically); or
2 damage to pancreas (e.g. chronic pancreatitis, trauma, haemochromatosis).

A/R: Associated with Addison's disease, autoimmune thyroid disease, pernicious anaemia, vitiligo and *HLA-DR3* and *4*.

E: Often of juvenile onset (< 30 years), affecting 3 in 1000 in UK, more common in white people.

H: May be incidental (routine blood tests).
Acute presentations (metabolic complications; see Examination).
Polyuria/nocturia (osmotic diuresis caused by glycosuria), polydypsia (thirst), tiredness, weight loss.
Symptoms of complications (see Complications).

E: **Acute presentations:**
Diabetic ketoacidosis: Nausea, vomiting, abdominal pain, polyuria, polydypsia, drowsiness, confusion, coma, Kussmaul breathing (deep and rapid), ketotic breath, signs of dehydration (e.g. dry mucous membranes, ↓ tissue turgor).
Hypoglycaemia: Neuroglycopenic and adrenergic signs: personality change, fits, confusion, coma, pale, sweating, tremor, tachycardia, palpitations, dizziness, hunger and focal neurological symptoms. (Note: hypoglycaemic symptoms may be masked by autonomic neuropathy, β-blockers and brain adapting to recurrent episodes.)
Others: (see Diabetes mellitus Type II).

P: The autoimmune aetiology is supported by autoantibodies directed to islet cell antigens such as GAD and insulin predate the clinical onset of IDDM, infiltration of the islets by lymphocytes, IDDM is associated with other autoimmune conditions (see Associations/Risk factors).
Diabetic ketoacidosis: ↓ ↓ Insulin and ↑ counter-regulatory hormones cause a catabolic state characterized by ↑ hepatic gluconeogenesis and ↓ peripheral utilization. Renal reabsorptive capacity of glucose is exceeded causing glycosuria, osmotic diuresis and dehydration. Increased lipolysis leads to ketogenesis and metabolic acidosis.

I: **Blood:** *Blood glucose:* Fasting blood glucose > 7 mmol/L or random blood glucose > 11 mmol/L. Two positive results are needed before diagnosis.
HbA1c: Estimates overall blood glucose levels in past month.
FBC: MCV, reticulocytes because increased erythrocyte turnover, causes misleading HbA1c levels.
U&E: Especially serum K^+ in diabetic ketoacidosis and when an ACE inhibitor is given.
Lipid profile.
Oral glucose tolerance test: (see Diabetes mellitus Type II).
Urine: MSU dipstick for protein, glucose and ketones.
Fundoscopy: Visualizes microvascular disease of diabetes.
Ultrasound or CT scan: Visualizes pancreatic inflammation or atrophy. Not usually necessary.

M: **Hypoglycaemia:** 50 mL of 50 % dextrose IV, or 1 mg IM glucagon.

Ketoacidosis:

Resuscitate: (A,B,C).

Tests: *Blood: FBC (↑ WCC even without infection), U&E (↑ urea and creatinine from dehydration), LFT, CRP, glucose (usually > 20 mmol/L), amylase (may ↑), blood cultures (for infection), ABG (metabolic acidosis with high anion gap), ketones.*

Urine: Glycosuria, ↑ ketones, MSU (microscopy, culture).

CXR: To exclude any infection.

ECG: To exclude MI.

IV fluid resuscitation: Rapid resuscitation using 0.9 % saline. (e.g. 1 L in 30 min, 1 L in 1 h, 1 L in 2 h, 1 L in 4 h, 1 L in 6 h). Use 5 % dextrose when blood glucose < 14 mmol/L.

Insulin (soluble): 8–10 units IV bolus (0.1 unit/kg), then 0.1 unit/kg/h IV infusion. Start an insulin sliding scale (hourly monitoring of blood glucose and adjusting insulin dose accordingly). Change to SC insulin when ketone levels normalize and patient is eating.

Potassium (if serum K^+ < 5 mmol/L, and patient is passing urine): Add 20 mmol/L K^+ to each litre of saline (30–40 mmol/L if serum K^+ < 3.5 mmol/L). Correction of ketoacidosis may cause hypokalaemia.

Monitoring: Temperature, pulse, respiratory rate, BP, sat O_2 and urine output hourly. Blood glucose, U&E, ABG and serum ketones also need regular monitoring.

Consider nasogastric tube (if unconscious, to prevent aspiration and gastric dilation), antibiotics, DVT prophylaxis, IV bicarbonate (if pH is < 7, controversial).

Chronic: (see Diabetes mellitus Type II). Many possible regimens of SC insulin, e.g.

1 mixed short- and long-acting insulin before breakfast and evening meal;

2 short-acting insulin three times daily before each meal and one long-acting insulin injection before bedtime.

Monitor: Control of symptoms (e.g. thirst, tiredness), regular finger prick tests by the patient, monitoring HbA1c levels (glycated haemoglobin should be < 7 %) every few months.*

Screening and management of complications and cardiovascular disease: (see Diabetes mellitus Type II).

Advice and patient education: (see Diabetes mellitus Type II).

C: **Emergencies:**

Diabetic ketoacidosis: May be precipitated by infection (30 %), errors in management (15 %), newly diagnosed diabetes (10 %), other medical disease (5 %), no cause identified (40 %).

Hypoglycaemia: Caused my missing a meal or overdosage of insulin.

Others: Neuropathy, nephropathy, retinopathy (see Diabetes mellitus Type II), peripheral vascular disease, ischaemic heart disease. Susceptible to infections (especially on feet). Fat hypertrophy at insulin injection sites.

P: Depends on early diagnosis, good glycaemic control and compliance with screening and treatment. Vascular disease and renal failure are major causes of increased morbidity and mortality.

*Diabetes Control and Complications Trial (DCCT) concluded that strict glycaemic control in Type I diabetes mellitus reduces the risk of development and progression of diabetic microvascular complications.

D: Metabolic hyperglycaemic condition caused by gradual relative insensitivity of body to insulin. Previously known as NIDDM.

A: Multifactorial (genetic and environmental). Linked to IGT* and obesity. In a tiny minority of patients, mutations in the insulin receptor, glucokinase, HNF-4α or HNF-1α have been identified. Mutations in glucokinase and HNF cause MODY (autosomally dominant inherited, age of onset < 25 years).

A/R: Obesity, family history, hypertension, hyperlipidaemia.

E: Often of adult onset, UK prevalence ~2 %, ↑ with age, six times more common in Asians.

H: May be incidental finding.
Polyuria, polydypsia, tiredness, infections (candidiasis, balanitis or pruritus vulvae).
Assess for other cardiovascular risk factors (e.g. hypertension, hyperlipidaemia, smoking).

E: Signs of chronic complications (see Complications and Diabetes mellitus Type I).
Diabetic foot: Both ischaemic and neuropathic signs. Dry skin, reduced subcutaneous tissue, corns and calluses, ulceration, gangrene. Charcot's arthropathy and signs of peripheral neuropathy, foot pulses may be ↓ in ischaemic foot.
Skin: Necrobiosis lipoidica diabeticorum (well-demarcated plaques on the shins or arms with shiny atrophic surface and red-brown edges), granuloma annulare (flesh-coloured papules coalescing in rings on the back of hands and fingers), diabetic dermopathy (depressed pigmented scars on shins).

P: ↓ Sensitivity of pancreatic β-islet cells to glucose and ↑ peripheral resistance to insulin. Impaired glucose tolerance is believed to precede diabetes mellitus Type II.
Microvascular: Best visualized in the retina (e.g. proliferative changes) and the kidneys (e.g. Kimmelstiel–Wilson changes in the basement membrane; see Complications).
Macrovascular: Hyalinization of arterioles, accelerated atherosclerosis.

I: **Blood and urine:** (see Diabetes mellitus Type I).
Oral glucose tolerance test: 75 g oral glucose load while fasting and measurement of blood glucose at 0, 1 and 2 h. Diabetes mellitus is diagnosed with a blood glucose of ≥ 11.1 mmol/L.
Exclude secondary causes, e.g. drugs, chronic pancreatitis, pancreatectomy, Cushing's syndrome, acromegaly.

M: **Hypoglycaemia:** (see Diabetes mellitus Type I).

HONK Coma†: Management similar to ketoacidosis, except use 0.45 % saline if serum Na^+ > 170 mmol/L, and a lower rate of insulin infusion (1–3 U/h). DVT prophylaxis with SC heparin.

*IGT (or insulin resistance) is a prediabetic condition. It is defined as an oral glucose tolerance test response of a 7.8–11.0 mmol/L at 2 h and a normal fasting blood glucose.
†Due to insulin deficiency, as diabetic ketoacidosis, but patient is usually old and may be presenting for the first time; history is longer (e.g. 1 week); there is marked dehydration, ↑ Na^+, ↑ Cl^-, ↑ glucose (> 35 mmol/L), ↑ osmolality (> 340 mosmol/kg), **no** acidosis.

Medical: Initially, controlling diet, encourage exercise and weight loss.
If not controlled and BMI < 25: Sulphonylureas (e.g. glibenclamide, gliclazide), which block ATP-sensitive K^+ channels in β-islet cells, stimulating insulin release.
If BMI is > 25: Metformin (inhibits hepatic gluconeogenesis). Replace metformin with a sulphonylurea if there are side-effects (e.g. diarrhoea, anorexia, lactic acidosis).
If not controlled: Combine metformin + sulphonylurea or try a thiazolidinedione (e.g. rosiglitazone, activates PPARγ and ↓ peripheral insulin resistance).
If not controlled: SC injections of intermediate-acting insulin at bed time. If still not controlled, add metformin (see Diabetes mellitus Type I for other regimens).
Other drugs: Acarbose (inhibits intestinal α-glucosidases to ↓ carbohydrate digestion); less used because of side-effects (bloating, flatulence).
Monitor: Control of symptoms (e.g. thirst, tiredness), finger prick tests by the patient (HbA1c: glycated haemoglobin should be < 7 %), ‡ regular follow-up by diabetic nurse specialist.
Screening for and management of complications:
Retinopathy: Regular examination for cataracts and retinopathy, laser photocoagulation if necessary.
Nephropathy: Monitor U&E and creatinine, urine dipstick testing for urine protein. BP check, ACE inhibitors, monitor changes in serum K^+.
Neuropathy: Regular examination and inspection of the feet for ulcers, joint vibration and pin prick testing, foot hygiene, gabapentin or amitriptyline for painful neuropathy.
Vascular disease: Regular cardiac and peripheral vascular examination. Monitor lipid profile.
Diabetic foot: Educate to examine feet regularly. Diabetic footwear. Podiatry assessment. Amitriptyline, gabapentin or opiates for painful neuropathy. For infections, clean and dress regularly. Swab for culture and sensitivity, IV antibiotics (e.g. flucloxacillin, cephalosporin and metronidazole). Look for osteomyelitis on X-ray. Surgical débridement or amputation.
Screen and reduce risk factors for cardiovascular disease: Lose weight, exercise, stop smoking, control blood pressure (with drugs), control lipid profile and treat hypercholesterolaemia or hypertriglyceridaemia.
Advice and patient education:
Information: Diabetic nurses, leaflets, websites, etc. explaining diabetes control, complications.
Nutrition: Optimizing meal plans, diet (complex carbohydrates as opposed to simple sugars, ↓ fat intake).
Foot care: Regular inspection, appropriate footwear, role of chiropodist.
Organizations: Local and national support groups.
Recognition of hypoglycaemia.
Monitoring with glucose and charting it. Monitoring for ketones during intercurrent illness.
Pregnancy: Strict glycaemic control and planning of conception.
Treatment: Action, duration and administration technique for insulin, change the site of injection, explain the need to plan exercise.

‡UK Prospective Diabetes Study (UK PDS) concluded that strict glycaemic control in patients with diabetes mellitus Type II ↓ the risk of development and progression of diabetic microvascular complications.

C: **Neuropathy:** Distal symmetrical sensory neuropathy, painful neuropathy, carpal tunnel syndrome, diabetic amyotrophy (asymmetrical wasting of proximal muscle), mononeuritis (e.g. III nerve palsy with preservation of pupillary response, VI nerve), autonomic neuropathy (e.g. postural hypotension), gastroparesis (abdominal pain, nausea, vomiting), impotence, urinary retention.

Nephropathy: Microalbuminuria, proteinuria and, eventually, renal failure. Prone to urinary tract infections and renal papillary necrosis.
Retinopathy: *Background:* Dot and blot haemorrhages, hard exudates.
Maculopathy: Macular oedema, exudates and haemorrhage of macula.
Preproliferative: Cotton wool spots, venous beading.
Proliferative: New vessels on the disc and elsewhere.
Also prone to glaucoma, cataracts, transient visual loss (sudden osmotic changes).
Vascular complications: Coronary, cerebrovascular, peripheral.

P: (see Diabetes mellitus Type I).

D: A disorder of the clotting cascade that can complicate a serious illness. DIC may occur in two forms.

1 Acute overt form where there is bleeding and depletion of platelets and clotting factors.

2 Chronic non-overt form where thromboembolism is accompanied by generalized activation of the coagulation system.

A: **Infection:** Particularly Gram-negative sepsis.

Obstetric complications: Missed miscarriage, severe pre-eclampsia, placental abruption, amniotic emboli.

Malignancy: *Acute DIC:* Acute promyelocytic leukaemia.

Chronic DIC: Lung, breast, GI malignancy.

Severe trauma or surgery.

Others: Haemolytic transfusion reaction, burns, severe liver disease, aortic aneurysms, haemangiomas.

A/R: (see Aetiology).

E: Seen in any severely ill patient.

H: The patient is severely unwell with symptoms of the underlying disease and confusion, fever, dyspnoea and evidence of bleeding.

E: Signs of the underlying aetiology, evidence of shock (hypotension, tachycardia, circulatory collapse).

Acute DIC: Petechiae, purpura, ecchymoses, epistaxis, mucosal bleeding, overt haemorrhage. Signs of end organ damage (e.g. local infarction or gangrene), respiratory distress, oliguria caused by renal failure.

Chronic DIC: Signs of deep venous or arterial thrombosis or embolism, superficial venous thrombosis, especially without varicose veins.

P: Aetiological agent (e.g. toxin) causes injury to endothelial cells leading to macrophage activation and activation of clotting cascade.

Acute DIC: Explosive thrombin generation depletes clotting factors and platelets, while simultaneously activating the fibrinolytic system. This leads to bleeding into the subcutaneous tissues, skin and mucous membranes, and occlusion of blood vessels by fibrin in the microcirculation. A vicious cycle develops.

Chronic DIC: The process is identical, but at a slower rate with time for compensatory responses, which diminish the likelihood of bleeding but give rise to a hypercoagulable state and thrombosis can occur.

I: **Blood:** There is no single diagnostic test.

Clotting: ↑ APTT, ↑ platelets, ↓ coagulation factors, ↓ fibrinogen, ↑ fibrin degradation products and D-dimers.

FBC: ↓ platelets, ↓ Hb.

Peripheral blood film: Red blood cell fragments (schistocytes).

Other investigations according to aetiology.

M: **Treat the underlying disease:** Avoid delay and treat vigorously in ITU setting with specialist input.

Acute DIC: With bleeding, blood components should be transfused as needed (e.g. fresh frozen plasma, cryoprecipitate and platelets). With ischaemia, anticoagulation can be considered after bleeding risk is corrected with blood products. Agents such as recombinant protein C are under trial.

Chronic DIC: If there is thromboembolism, anticoagulate.

C: Shock, acute renal failure, ARDS, life-threatening haemorrhage or thrombosis with organ ischaemia/infarction, death.

P: Mortality is high. Prognosis depends on the underlying disease and the severity of the coagulopathy.

Diverticular disease

D: The clinical condition resulting from the presence of diverticula (outpouchings) of the colonic mucosa and submucosa through the muscular wall of the large bowel. Diverticulitis is the inflammation of these diverticula as a result of impaction of faecalith within them and pooling of gut flora.

A: A low-fibre refined diet, common in the Western world, leads to loss of stool bulk. Consequently, high colonic intraluminal pressures must be generated to propel the stool, leading to herniation of the mucosa and submucosa through the muscularis.

A/R: Low-fibre refined diet, increasing age, connective tissue disorders.

E: Some form of diverticular disease is present in 30–50 % of the population > 50 years.

H: Often asymptomatic (80–90 %).
Recurrent left iliac fossa or suprapubic abdominal pain.
GI bleed: PR bleeding may be acute or chronic.
Diverticulitis: Pyrexia (from pooling of bacteria in diverticuli and inflammation).
Alternating constipation (pellet faeces) and diarrhoea.
Presentation with complications (e.g. pneumaturia, faecaluria, recurrent UTI caused by a vesicocolic fistula).

E: Usually normal.
Occasionally, lower abdominal tenderness and faecal loading.
Pain and an abdominal mass may be caused by a diverticular abscess.
Signs of anaemia may be present.

P: **Macro:** Diverticula are most common in the sigmoid and descending colon.
Micro: Diverticula consist of herniated mucosa and submucosa through the muscularis, particularly at sites of nutrient artery penetration with a peritoneal covering. There is an associated colonic smooth muscle hypertrophy resulting in luminal stenosis.

I: **Barium enema:** Can demonstrate the presence of diverticula with a saw-tooth appearance of lumen reflecting smooth muscle hypertrophy (should not be performed if there is a danger of perforation).
Sigmoidoscopy and colonoscopy: Diverticula are clearly visible.
Blood tests: FBC for anaemia, ↑ WCC and ↑ inflammatory markers in acute diverticulitis.

M: **GI bleed:** PR bleeding is often managed conservatively with IV rehydration, blood transfusion if necessary.
Diverticulitis: Antibiotics (cephalosporin and metronidazole).
Chronic: High-fibre diet with bulking agent (e.g. methylcellulose). Laxatives may be required if constipation is severe. Encourage high fluid intake.
Surgery: May be necessary with recurrent attacks or when complications develop. Sigmoid colectomy, fistulae resections or drainage of pericolic abscesses are some options.

C: Diverticulitis, pericolic abscess, perforation, colonic obstruction, fistula formation (bladder, small intestine, vagina), haemorrhage (caused by vessel erosion).

P: 10–25 % of patients will have one episode of diverticulitis. Of these, 30 % will have a second episode and 20 % of patients will have one or more complication after the first episode of diverticulitis.

D: A pruritic papulovesicular skin reaction to endogenous or exogenous agents.

A: Numerous varieties caused by a diversity of triggers.
Exogenous: Irritant, contact, phototoxic.
Endogenous: Atopic, seborrhoeic, pompholyx, varicose, lichen simplex.*

A/R: **Irritant:** Prolonged skin contact with a cell-damaging irritant (e.g. ammonia in nappy rash).
Contact: Non-naive exposure to allergen (commonly nickel, chromate, perfumes, latex and plants).
Atopic: Personal or family history of atopy (e.g. asthma, hay fever, rhinitis).
Varicose: Increased venous pressure in lower limbs.
Wiskott–Aldrich syndrome: Association of eczema, thrombocytopenia, immunological abnormalities and a predisposition to lymphoma and leukaemia.

E: **Contact:** Prevalence 4 %.
Atopic: Onset is commonly in the first year of life. Childhood incidence 10–20 %.

H: Itching (can be severe), heat, tenderness, redness, weeping, crusting.
Enquire into occupational exposures or irritants used at home (e.g. bleach).
Enquire into family/personal history of atopy.

E: **Acute:** Poorly demarcated erythematous oedematous dry scaling patches. Papules, vesicles with exudation and crusting, excoriation marks.
Chronic: Thickened epidermis, skin lichenification, fissures, change in pigmentation.
By type: *Contact and irritant:* Eczema reaction occurs where irritant/allergen comes into contact with the skin. In some cases, autosensitization (spread to other sites) can occur in contact eczema.
Atopic: Particularly affects face and flexures.
Seborrhoeic: Yellow greasy scales on erythematous plaques, particularly in the nasolabial folds, eyebrows, scalp and presternal area.
Pompholyx: Acute and often recurrent vesiculobullous eruption on palms and soles. Very painful.
Varicose: Eczema of lower legs, usually associated with marked varicose veins.
Nummular: coin shaped, on legs and trunk.
Asteatotic: dry, 'crazy paring' pattern.

P: **Irritant:** Physical damage to the skin.
Contact: Type IV delayed hypersensitivity to allergen.
Atopic: Believed to be caused by a dysregulation of immune system leading to proliferation of TH_2 cells in the skin. This, via IL-4, increases IgE receptors on antigen presenting cells and systemic production of IgE. Prevalence of IgE and IgE receptors facilitates antigen presentation, causing a vicious cycle.
Seborrhoeic: *Pityrosporum* yeast seems to have a central role.

*Lichen simplex is the thickening of skin secondary to a cycle of itch – scratch – itch, and is characterized by well-demarcated hyperpigmented lichenified plaques.

I: **Contact:** *Skin patch testing:* Disc containing postulated allergen is diluted and applied to back for 48 h. Positive if allergen induces a red raised lesion.
Atopic: *FBC:* ↑ Eosinophils and basophils.
Immunoglobulins: ↑ IgE (in 80 %).
Skin prick test: Rarely used because of anaphylactic risk.
RAST: Tests for allergen-specific IgE.
Swab for infected lesions: For bacteria, fungi and viruses.

M: **Irritant or contact:** Avoid precipitant. Barrier protection (e.g. gloves, barrier cream).
Atopic: Avoid precipitants. Topical steroids and tar ointment is useful in chronic eczema. Tacrolimus ointment for moderate to severe eczema not responding to potent steroids. Systemic immunosuppressants or phototherapy may be helpful in very severe cases.
Topical or systemic antibiotics for secondary infection. Medicated bandages (e.g. zinc paste for severe limb eczema). For pruritus, antihistamines (for children, mittens at night). Emollients (in bath water, as soap substitute or by direct application to affected area).
Seborrhoeic: Topical 1 % hydrocortisone and antifungal. Ketoconazole shampoo for scalp involvement.
Pompholyx: Potent topical steroids, potassium permanganate salts, systemic steroids in severe attacks.

C: Secondary infection, particularly from *Staphylococcus aureus* and HSV. HSV superinfection can be life-threatening. Molluscum contagiosum.†

P: Good prognosis for irritant eczema if the relevant agent is identified and avoided. Endogenous eczema may have a chronic relapsing course. 90 % of patients with atopic eczema have recovered by puberty.

†Molluscum contagiosum is a common childhood skin infection with multiple small translucent vesicle-like papules that have a central punctum. It is caused by a contact-transmissible pox virus. In adults, suspect HIV.

Encephalitis

D: Inflammation of the brain parenchyma.

A: In the majority of cases encephalitis is the result of a viral infection.
Virus: Most common in the UK is HSV. Other viruses are herpes zoster, mumps, adenovirus, coxsackie, echovirus, measles, EBV, HIV, rabies* (Asia), Nipah (Malaysia) and arboviruses transmitted by mosquitoes, e.g. Japanese B encephalitis (Asia), St. Louis and West Nile encephalitis (USA).
Non-viral: (rare) e.g. syphilis, *Staphylococcus aureus*.
Immunocompromised: CMV, toxoplasmosis, *Listeria*.

A/R: Travel to epidemic or endemic area. Seasonal (e.g. mumps, encephalitis in late winter or early spring). Immunocompromised.

E: Annual UK incidence is 7.4 in 100 000.

H: In many cases, encephalitis is a mild self-limiting illness.
Others: subacute onset (hours to days) headache, fever, vomiting, neck stiffness, photophobia, i.e. symptoms of meningism (meningoencephalitis) with behavioural changes, drowsiness and confusion. There is often a history of convulsions. Focal neurological symptoms, particularly dysphasia, hemiplegia and cranial nerve palsies may be present reflecting the site(s) of infection. Some patients report a recent viral infection.

E: ↓ level of consciousness with deteriorating GCS, seizures, pyrexia.
Signs of meningism: neck stiffness, photophobia, Kernig's test positive.
Signs of raised intracranial pressure: hypertension, bradycardia, papilloedema.
Focal neurological signs.
MSE may reveal cognitive or psychiatric disturbances.

P: May begin as an extra CNS primary viral infection. HSV encephalitis may be caused by reactivation of HSV-1 from the trigeminal ganglion, haematogenous spread or may reach the brain via the olfactory nerves. Lymphocytic infiltration and perivascular cuffing. Neuronal necrosis, cerebral oedema and glial proliferation may be seen.

I: **Blood:** FBC (↑ lymphocytes), U&E (SIADH may occur), glucose (compare with CSF glucose), viral serology, ABG.
MRI/CT: Excludes mass lesion. HSV produces characteristic oedema of the temporal lobe.
Lumbar puncture: ↑ Lymphocytes, ↑ monocytes, ↑ protein, glucose usually normal. CSF culture is difficult, PCR is now first line.
EEG: Characteristic pattern of abnormality, e.g. HSV slow waves in temporal lobes.
Brain biopsy: Now very rarely performed.

M: Resusitate and consider ITU. Start empirical IV aciclovir (± antibiotics) immediately, change as appropriate later. Mechanical ventilation if respiratory failure.
Monitor vital signs closely. Manage fluid balance closely (risk of cerebral oedema), consider dexamethasone.
Anticonvulsants. Antipyretics. Antiemetics. Analgesia for headache.

C: Postencephalitic neurological sequalae, particularly epilepsy and cognitive impairment in 10–30 % with variation according to viral aetiology.

P: Treated mortality is 20 %. Survivors may have epilepsy or cognitive impairment. Increased chance of sequelae in age > 30 years, GCS < 6 on initiation of treatment.

Epilepsy

D: More than two episodes of paroxysmal discharges of cortical grey matter resulting in a seizure.

A: The majority of cases are idiopathic.
CNS: Trauma, tumour, infection (meningitis; see Meningitis), encephalitis (see Encephalitis), abscess, toxoplasmosis), inflammation (vasculitis, MS), cerebrovascular disease.
Metabolic: Sodium imbalance, hyper- or hypoglycaemia, hypocalcaemia, hypoxia, porphyria, liver failure.
Drugs: Including withdrawal (e.g. alcohol, benzodiazepines).
Congenital anomalies: Particularly in hippocampi or temporal lobes.
Degenerative diseases: Alzheimer's disease or prion disease.
Hypertension: Malignant hypertension, eclampsia.

A/R: (see Aetiology).

E: Common. Prevalence is 1 % of general population. Peak age of onset is in early childhood or in the elderly.

H: Obtain history from a witness as well as the patient.
Partial (seizure localized to discrete area of cortex): Symptoms depend on region involved.
Precentral gyrus: Motor convulsions. In Jacksonian epilepsy, the spasm begins in corner of mouth or digit and spreads (Jacksonian march). There may be postictal flaccid paralysis (Todd's paralysis).
Temporal lobe: Aura (visceral and psychic symptoms: fear or déjà vu sensation), hallucinations (olfactory, gustatory or formed visual images), stereotyped automatisms (e.g. lip smacking).
Partial seizures may be *simple* (consciousness is retained) or *complex* (consciousness is impaired), partial seizures may spread to other areas of cerebrum (secondary generalized).
Generalized (seizure synchronously involving both hemispheres):
Tonic – clonic (grand mal): Vague symptoms before an attack (e.g. dizziness, irritability), loss of consciousness. Tonic phase characterized by generalized muscular spasms, followed by a clonic phase, characterized by repetitive jerks, faecal or urinary incontinence, tongue biting. After a seizure, there is often impaired consciousness, lethargy, confusion, headache, back pain, stiffness.
Absence (petit mal): Usual onset in childhood. Characterized by loss of consciousness but maintained posture (stops talking and stares into space for seconds), blinking or rolling up of eyes with other repetitive motor actions (e.g. chewing). No postictal phase.
Myoclonic: Adolescence onset. Involuntary jerking, particularly in the morning.

E: Depends on aetiology, usually normal between seizures.
Look for focal abnormalities indicative of brain lesions.

P: Columns (spindles) of cortical neurones generate bursts of action potentials. There is recruitment of surrounding neurones (hypersynchronization) and loss of surrounding inhibition, propagating about the neocortex. If both hemispheres are affected, loss of consciousness results.

I: **Blood:** FBC, U&E, LFT, glucose, Ca^{2+}, ABG prolactin (transient increase after a true seizure).
EEG: Characteristic waveforms (e.g. slow frequency, γ or δ waves, spindles). Note that 50 % of epilepsy patients have a normal EEG trace. Telemetry provides ambulatory measurements.

MRI or CT: Exclude structural brain lesion.
Other investigations: According to postulated aetiology.

M: **Status epilepticus** (seizure ≥30 min, failure to regain consciousness): Resuscitate and protect airway, breathing and circulation. IV or PR diazepam (repeat once after 15 min if needed), or IV lorazepam or clonazepam. If seizures recur or fail to respond after 30 min, IV phenobarbital bolus or phenytoin infusion under ECG monitoring. If these measures fail, consider anaesthesia using IV thiopental.

Treat the cause: e.g. correct hypoglycaemia or hyponatraemia.
Medical: Numerous anticonvulsant agents. Only start anticonvulsant therapy after second seizure.
Sodium valproate, lamotrigine (all seizure types), carbamazepine, phenytoin (generalized or partial), ethosuximide (absence), clonazepam (myoclonic).
Many new drugs are available: vigabatrine, gabapentin, topiramate.
Advice: Avoid triggers (e.g. alcohol, flickering light). Recommend supervision for swimming or climbing, driving is only permitted if seizure free for 1 year.
Surgery for refractory epilepsy: removal of definable epileptogenic focus.

C: Epilepsia partialis continua (partial seizure which continues for hours or days), muscular spasms and vertebral fractures in tonic – clonic seizures, depression.

P: 50 % remission at 1 year. Mortality 2 in 100 000/year, directly related to seizure or secondary to injury.

Erythema multiforme

D: An acute hypersensitivity reaction of the skin and mucous membranes.

A: Precipitating factor identified in only 50 % of cases.
Drugs: Sulphonamides, penicillin, phenytoin, barbiturates.
Infection: *Viral:* HSV, EBV, coxsackie, adenovirus, orf).
Bacterial: Mycoplasma pneumoniae, Chlamydiae.
Fungal: Histoplasmosis.
Inflammatory: Rheumatoid arthritis, SLE, sarcoidosis, ulcerative colitis.
Vasculitides: PAN, Wegener's granulomatosis.
Malignancy: Lymphomas, leukaemia, myeloma.
Radiotherapy.

A/R: (see Aetiology). Recipients of bone marrow transplants, HIV infection.

E: Can affect any age group, but most commonly children and young adults. ♂ : ♀ ~2 : 1.

H: Non-specific prodromal symptoms of upper respiratory tract infection.

Sudden appearance of itching/burning/painful skin lesions (see below), which may fade, leaving behind pigmentation.

E: Classic target ('bulls eye') lesions with a rim of erythema surrounding a paler area, vesicles/bullae, urticarial plaques. The lesions are often symmetrical, distributed over the arms and legs including the palms, soles and the extensor surfaces.

Stevens–Johnson syndrome is a severe form with bullous lesions and necrotic ulcers:

- *Affecting >2 mucous membranes:* conjunctiva, cornea, lips (haemorrhagic crusts), mouth, genitalia.
- *Systemic symptoms:* sore throat, cough, fever, headache, myalgia, arthralgia, diarrhoea and vomiting.
- *Shock:* hypotension, tachycardia.

P: Degeneration of basal epidermal cells and development of vesicles between the cells and the underlying basement membrane; lymphocytic infiltrate is seen around the blood vessels and at the dermal – epidermal junction. Immune complex deposition is variable and non-specific.
Stevens–Johnson syndrome is thought to be a form of TEN.*

I: Usually unnecessary as erythema multiforme and Stevens–Johnson syndrome are clinical diagnoses.
A skin biopsy for histology and direct immunofluorescence may be indicated in cases of diagnostic doubt.
Investigations may be necessary to determine the precipitating factor.
Blood: ↑ WCC, eosinophils, ESR, CRP, throat swab, serology, albumin (↓ in extensive exudation), ↑ urea (as a result of catabolic state and dehydration), autoantibodies.
Imaging: CXR (to exclude sarcoidosis and atypical pneumonias).

M: Symptomatic. Antihistamines (for itching) and NSAIDs (analgesia). Treat underlying cause, e.g. stop the implicated drug, treat the infection. Use of systemic corticosteroids is controversial. Oral aciclovir for recurrent episodes.

*TEN: widespread skin erythema leading to epidermal necrosis. Eventually, there is desquamation of epidermis in large sheets, leaving denuded shiny dermis underneath. High mortality (>30 %). Can be a reaction to drugs, e.g. penicillin, anticonvulsants, sulphonamides, NSAIDs, allopurinol.

Stevens–Johnson syndrome: Nurse in ITU. Close attention to fluid and electrolyes balance, heat loss, analgesia and the risk of secondary infections. Denuded areas are treated like burns. Mouth ulceration may be so severe that total parenteral nutrition is required. If the urethra is involved, catheterization is necessary.

C: Blindness in 3–10 % (if cornea affected), secondary infection of denuded areas, renal failure.

Stevens–Johnson syndrome: Lesions of respiratory tract can be complicated by pneumonia and respiratory failure.

P: Most cases of erythema multiforme resolve within 2–5 weeks. There may be recurrence in a small minority, usually triggered by HSV. Cases caused by drugs and *Mycoplasma* are more likely to progress to Stevens–Johnson syndrome. Mortality of Stevens–Johnson syndrome ~5–15 %.

Erythema nodosum

D: Skin lesion characterized by hypersensitivity reaction resulting in a characteristic vasculitis and panniculitis.

A: 25 % of cases have no underlying cause identified.

Infection: *Bacterial:* Streptococcus (especially β-haemolytic), TB, leprosy, *Yersinia*, rickettsia, *Chlamydia*.
Viral: EBV.
Fungal: Histoplasmosis, blastomycosis, coccidioidomycosis.
Protozoal: Toxoplasmosis.
Systemic disease: Sarcoidosis, IBD, Behçet's disease.
Malignancy: Leukaemia, Hodgkin's disease.
Drugs: Sulphonamides, penicillin, oral contraceptive pill, bromides, dapsone.
Pregnancy.

A/R: (see Aetiology).

E: Usually affects young adults. ♀ : ♂ ~3 : 1.

H: Multiple crops of tender blue-red nodules develop bilaterally on the shins and occasionally on the thighs and forearms. Fever, anorexia, weight loss, arthralgia and fatigue are often also present.

Symptoms of the underlying aetiology.

E: Crops of blue-red dome-shaped nodules usually present on both shins (occasionally involving thighs or forearms) which are tender to palpation. Low-grade pyrexia. Joints may be tender and painful on movement. Signs of the underlying aetiology.

P: **Pathogenesis:** Hypersensitivity reaction to foreign antigen leading to damage to the small blood vessels of the dermis and subcutaneous tissue. The shins are particularly affected because lymphatic drainage in this region is poor and hence removal of foreign antigens is slow.

Micro: Subcutaneous inflammatory changes which are vasculitic in origin with perivascular mixed cell infiltrate, oedema and giant cell formation. Septal panniculitis can also be seen.

I: To determine the underlying aetiology. Baseline tests include the following.

Blood tests: Anti-streptolysin O titre, FBC, CRP, ESR, serum ACE (↑ in sarcoidosis).
Throat swab and culture.
Mantoux/Heaf test: For TB.
CXR: To identify sarcoidosis, TB, disseminated fungal infections.

M: In most cases, manage conservatively. NSAIDs (as analgesia).
Treat the cause. Persistent cases may require corticosteroids, colchicine, azathioprine or dapsone.

C: None. Complications of the underlying cause.

P: The majority of cases resolve over 3–6 weeks leaving bruise marks. Occasionally, nodules may persist or recur over several months but they never ulcerate.

D: Non-specific intense widespread reddening of the skin often preceded by exfoliation.

A: **Pre-existing skin conditions:** Eczema, psoriasis.
Malignancy: Cutaneous T-cell lymphoma, lymphoma, leukaemia.
Adverse drug reaction.
Infection: HIV, toxic shock syndrome.
Idiopathic.

A/R: (see Aetiology).

E: Incidence: 1–2 in 100 000/year. 1 % of dermatological admissions. Age usually > 40 years. ♂ : ♀ = 2.5 : 1.

H: The skin feels hot and tight. Pruritus, erythema, scaling and shedding, fever and shivering. Symptoms of cardiac failure. The history should also be directed towards establishing aetiology.

E: The patient may be pyrexial or hypothermic. Erythema and scaling of ≥ 90 % of the skin. Evidence of skin shedding. The skin is hot and radiates warmth to the surroundings, can → hypothermia. Peripheral oedema, signs of volume depletion including ↓ BP and tachycardia. Signs of cardiac failure. Generalized lymphadenopathy. Signs of the underlying condition, e.g. psoriatic plaques.

P: **Pathogenesis:** Not fully known. Interaction of cytokines and cellular adhesion molecules → ↑ epidermal turnover rate → severe scaling and shedding → loss of fluid, electrolytes and albumin. There is increased blood flow through the skin which may cause temperature dysregulation and high-output cardiac failure.

I: **Skin biopsy:** in order to make a definitive diagnosis ± lymph node biopsy if significant lymphadenopathy.
Blood: *FBC: ↓ Hb, ↑ WBC* if secondary infection, may reveal underlying haematological dyscrasia.
ESR, U&E: May have ↓ Na^{+}, ↓ K^{+}, ↑ urea if lost through skin.
LFT: ↓ Albumin loss through the skin ± leakage to extracellular space from leaky capillaries.
Immunoglobulins: Hypergammaglobulinaemia, ↑ IgE.
Blood film: For Sezary cells in T-cell lymphomas.
ABGs: For renal failure (metabolic acidosis) and ARDS.
Imaging: ECG, CXR or echocardiogram may show signs of cardiac failure.

M: This is a dermatological emergency.

1. Nurse patient in a warm room.
2. Regular monitoring of vital signs.
3. Catheterize and insert a central venous line for monitoring of fluid balance if hypovolaemic.
4. Treat the underlying cause if identified.
5. Continue only vital medications.
6. Swab the skin for secondary infection.
7. Topical steroid and bandaging. Consider systemic steroid (controversial and never used in cases of psoriatic erythroderma).
8. Antihistamine for pruritus and sedative effect.
9. Management of complications.

C: Cardiac failure, renal failure, hypothermia, secondary infection, ARDS.

P: Mortality ~ 20–40 %.

Essential thrombocythaemia

D: A myeloproliferative disorder characterized by persistently elevated platelet count, not attributable to secondary causes: iron deficiency, infection, inflammation, haemorrhage, hyposplenism, trauma or malignancy.

A: Disorder of bone marrow stem cells of unknown aetiology causing proliferation of megakaryocytes and overproduction of platelets. Very rare familial variants, some associated with mutations in thrombopoietin gene.

A/R: Other myeloproliferative disorders, polycythaemia rubra vera, chronic myeloid leukaemia or myelofibrosis.

E: Rare. UK annual incidence ~1 in 100 000. Mean age is 50–60 years but 20 % are < 40 years.

H: May be asymptomatic and diagnosed on routine blood count (20 %).
Venous or arterial thrombosis (e.g. MI, stroke, superficial thrombophlebitis, DVT): Present in 20–50 % at presentation.
Spontaneous haemorrhage (e.g. GI bleeding, epistaxis, bruising): A patient may complain of headaches or visual disturbance; rarely, pruritus.
Erythromelalgia: Characteristic burning sensation felt in the hands or feet, promptly relieved by aspirin.

E: Splenomegaly is present in 30 %, but often the spleen has atrophied because of repeated thrombosis and infarction.

P: Bone marrow is hypercellular (similar to polycythaemia rubra vera) but with ↑ megakaryocytes.

I: Diagnosis based on exclusion of secondary causes and other myeloproliferative disorders.
Blood: FBC (persistently ↑ platelets, often $> 1000 \times 10^9$/L. About one-third have ↑ red cell count and ↑ WCC). Urate levels and LDH levels normally ↑.
Blood film: Platelet anisocytosis (variation in size) with circulating megakaryocyte fragments. There may be signs of hyposplenism (e.g. Howell–Jolly bodies, target cells).
Bone marrow biopsy: (see Pathology).
Tests of platelet function: Aggregation in response to adenosine diphosphate, is consistently abnormal and may help distinguish between primary and secondary causes.
Cytogenetics (for Philadelphia chromosome or *BCR-ABL* fusion gene): To exclude myeloid leukaemia.

M: **Medical:** Low-dose aspirin daily reduces risk of thrombosis. Goal is to control the platelet count ($< 600 \times 10^9$/L), thereby reducing risk of thrombosis. Hydroxyurea is the most widely used agent. Interferon-α and anagrelide (reduces megakaryocyte hyperproliferation and differentiation) can also be used. Platelet-pheresis can be used to rapidly but transiently lower counts.

C: Thrombosis, haemorrhage, development of another myeloproliferative disease or transformation to acute leukaemia. For women, ↑ risk of miscarriage and intrauterine growth retardation during pregnancy.

P: A chronic disease which is often stable for 10–20 years. There is a risk (< 5 %) of transformation to myelofibrosis or acute leukaemia.

D: Interstitial inflammatory disease of the distal gas-exchanging parts of the lung caused by inhalation of organic dusts. Also known as hypersensitivity pneumonitis.

A: Inhalation of antigenic organic dusts containing microbes (bacteria, fungi or amoebae) or animal proteins induce a hypersensitivity response in susceptible individuals. Examples are as follows:
Farmer's lung: mouldy hay containing thermophilic actinomycetes.
Pigeon/budgerigar fancier's lung: bloom on bird feathers and excreta.
Mushroom worker's lung: compost containing thermophilic actinomycetes.
Humidifier lung: water-containing bacteria and *Naegleria* (amoeba).
Maltworker's lung: barley or maltings containing *Aspergillus clavatus*.

A/R: Associated with certain occupations as above. Less common in smokers.

E: Uncommon, 2% of occupational lung diseases, 50% of reported cases affect farm workers (incidence is about 4–10 in 100 000/year), marked geographical variation reflecting dependence on occupational causes.

H: **Acute:** Presents 4–12 h postexposure. Reversible episodes of dry cough, dyspnoea, malaise, fever, myalgia. Wheeze and productive cough may develop on repeat high-level exposures.
Chronic: Poorly reversible manifestation in some, slowly ↑ breathlessness and ↓ exercise tolerance, weight loss. Exposure is usually chronic, low level and there may be no history of previous acute episodes.
Full occupational history and enquiry into hobbies and pets important.

E: **Acute:** Rapid shallow breathing, pyrexia, inspiratory crepitations.
Chronic: Fine inspiratory crepitations (see Cryptogenic fibrosing alveolitis). Finger clubbing is rare.

P: Antigenic organic particles (0.5–5.0 μm), deposited in alveoli and small airways, incite an inflammatory response (a combination of type III antigen – antibody complex hypersensitivity reaction and a type IV granulomatous lymphocytic inflammation).
Acute: Inflammatory cellular infiltration into alveoli and small bronchioles, with development of non-caseating granulomas.
Chronic: Increased foamy macrophages in alveoli. Development of interstitial fibrosis. In the late stage, there is 'honeycombing' of the lung, creating a more restrictive lung disease picture.

I: **Blood:** FBC (neutrophilia, lymphopenia), ABG (↓ Po_2, ↓ Pco_2).
Serology: Precipitating IgG to fungal or avian antigens in serum; however, these are not diagnostic as are often found in asymptomatic individuals.
CXR: Often normal in acute episodes, may show 'ground glass' appearance with alveolar shadowing or nodular opacities in the middle and lower zones. In chronic cases, fibrosis is prominent in the upper zones.
High-resolution CT: Detects early changes before CXR. Patchy 'ground glass' shadowing and nodules.
Pulmonary function tests: Restrictive ventilatory defect (↓ FEV_1, ↓ FVC with preserved or increased ratio), ↓ TLCO.
Bronchoalveolar lavage: Increased cellularity with ↑ $CD8^+$ suppressor T cells. Lung biopsy (transbronchial or thoracopic).

M: **Advice:** Complete avoidance of exposure to the antigen (e.g. change of work practice or hobby), if this is problematic, then minimize exposure and encourage use of respiratory protection masks.

Medical: *Acute flare:* Spontaneous recovery is usually within 1–2 days, corticosteroids may accelerate recovery but do not appear to affect long-term outcome.

Chronic disease: Trial of high-dose oral prednisolone for 1 month may be carried out, this is gradually reduced, or stopped if no objective response demonstrated.

General: Regular follow-up to monitor lung function. Environmental assessment is necessary for risk posed to others. In UK, farmer's lung patients are entitled to compensation, depending on the degree of disability.

C: Progressive lung fibrosis, pulmonary hypertension, right heart failure.

P: The acute form generally resolves if further exposure is prevented, with chronic disease some patients will improve while a minority progress to lung fibrosis.

D: A hereditary neurodegenerative disease primarily affecting the spinocerebellar and corticospinal tracts, the dorsal columns and peripheral nerves.

A: Autosomal recessive inheritance. There is expansion of the triplet repeats (*GAA*) in the *FRDA* gene (on chromosome 9q), leading to reduced levels or altered function of the protein product, frataxin which may be involved in mitochondrial iron transport and antioxidation.

A/R: Family history, parental consanguinity.

E: Uncommon; prevalence is 1 in 50 000. Most common inherited ataxia.

H: Age of presentation is usually 8–16 years, progressing over years.

Gait abnormality: Staggering or swaying with frequent falls. Clumsy hands and feet. Dysarthria, titubation (head tremor).
Lower limb weakness, ascending to upper limbs and eventually paralysis.
Cardiac: Angina, palpitations, dyspnoea.

Other systems: Reduced visual acuity (30 %), diabetes mellitus Type I (20 %), deafness (10 %).

E: **Cerebellar signs:** Ataxia of all four limbs, dysarthria, nystagmus, intention tremor, dysdiadochokinesis and titubation. Clumsy, swaying and broad-based gait.

UMN signs: Spastic limb paralysis, extensor plantar reflexes. Reflexes are reduced because of simultaneous damage to peripheral nerves.
Dorsal column signs: Absent joint position and vibration sense, particularly in the lower limbs.
Musculoskeletal deformity: Kyphoscoliosis, pes cavus (high arched foot) and pes equinovarus (heel turned inward, foot plantar flexed with a raised medial border).
Optic atrophy (less commonly): ↓ Visual acuity and pale optic discs.
Sensorineural deafness

P: Multisystem disease not just affecting the central nervous system. Degeneration of the spinocerebellar tracts, corticospinal tracts, peripheral nerves and dorsal columns. Cardiac myocyte hypertrophy and fibrosis. Optic atrophy. The reason for the ↑ incidence of diabetes is unclear.

I: **Genetic testing:** Karyotype analysis of patient. Should be offered to family members.

MRI brain and spinal cord
Electrophysiology: Electromyography and nerve conduction studies. Large myelinated fibres are predominantly affected.
Cardiac assessment: ECG and echocardiogram.
Blood: Fasting blood glucose.

M: **Medical:** Supportive care is best provided by a multidisciplinary team. Physiotherapy, occupational and orthopaedic therapy is needed because of physical disability. DVT prophylaxis and care of pressure areas caused by long-term immobility. Speech and language therapy. Genetic counselling of patient and family. Management of diabetes and cardiomyopathy.

C: Diabetes mellitus. Cardiomyopathy.

P: Poor. Most patients are wheelchair-bound by age 20. Life expectancy is ~40–50 years, and death is usually a result of cardiac complications.

Gallstones

D: Presence of gallstones in the gallbladder or the biliary tree.

A: **Mixed stones** (80 %): Contain cholesterol, calcium bilirubinate, phosphate and protein, occurring because of imbalance between bile salt and cholesterol components, nucleation factors or gallbladder stasis.

Pure cholesterol stones (10 %).

Pigment stones (10 %): Black crystalline stones caused by hyperbilirubinaemia secondary to haemolytic disorders or cirrhosis. Brown pigment stones may be caused by liver fluke *Clonorchis sinensis* infestation.

A/R: **Mixed or pure cholesterol stones:** ↑ Age, female, obesity, diabetes mellitus, parenteral nutrition, drugs (contraceptive pill, octreotide), family history, interruption of the enterohepatic recirculation of bile salts.

Pigment stones: Haemolytic disorders (e.g. sickle cell, thalassaemia, hereditary spherocytosis), residence in the Far East where liver flukes are more common.

E: Very common. UK prevalence is about 10 %. Increases with age, ♀ : ♂ ~3 : 1 but equal sex ratio ≥65 years. 50 000 cholecystectomies are performed annually in UK.

H: **Asymptomatic** (90 %).

Biliary colic: Sudden onset, severe RUQ or epigastric pain, may radiate to right scapula. Often lasts several hours and worsened by a fatty meal or alcohol. Often associated with nausea and vomiting.

Acute cholecystitis: Patient systemically unwell, fever, prolonged upper abdominal pain.

Ascending cholangitis: RUQ pain, fever and rigors, jaundice (Charcot's triad).

E: **Biliary colic:** RUQ or epigastric tenderness.

Acute cholecystitis: Tachycardia, pyrexia, RUQ or epigastric tenderness. Murphy's sign (pain on inspiration on palpation of the RUQ as the inflamed gallbladder descends and contacts the palpating fingers).

Ascending cholangitis: Pyrexia, rigors, RUQ tenderness, jaundice.

P: **Biliary colic:** Caused by impaction of a gallstone in the cystic duct. Resolves when stone falls back into gallbladder. If stone remains impacted this leads to inflammation and acute cholecystitis.

Ascending cholangitis: Occurs when a stone passes into common bile duct and becomes impacted causing pain, bile stasis, bacterial proliferation and inflammation with risk of Gram-negative septicaemia.

I: **Blood:** FBC (↑ WCC in acute cholecystitis and ascending cholangitis), LFT (↑ alkaline phosophatase and bilirubin in ascending cholangitis), blood cultures (if pyrexia), amylase (risk of pancreatitis).

Ultrasound: Demonstrates gallstones, gallbladder wall thickness and the presence of dilation of biliary ducts.

AXR: Gallstones radio-opaque in 10 % of cases. Mainly to exclude other causes of an acute abdomen.

CT abdomen: May visualize other causes of biliary tree pain.

ERCP: Identifies and allows intervention for stones stuck in biliary tree.

Technetium-labelled HIDA scintigraphy: Allows assessment of gallbladder function (contractility) and detects non-gallstone obstructions.

M: **Acute:** On acute presentation, all patients need analgesia, antiemetics, IV fluids and should be nil by mouth. Morphine analgesia is not preferred as it can cause spasm of the sphincter of Oddi.
Biliary colic: No specific treatment. Usually self-resolving.
Acute cholecystitis: IV antibiotics (e.g. cephalosporin).
Ascending cholangitis: IV antibiotics (e.g. cefuroxime and metronidazole). Urgent biliary drainage if obstruction is present by ERCP or by percutaneous route (percutaneous transhepatic cholangiography).
Surgery: Laparoscopic or open cholecystectomy are usually performed after a delayed interval (8–12 weeks) from the acute event (either of the above three presentations). This is the standard treatment.
Medical: Dissolution therapy (e.g. with oral bile acid ursodeoxycholate) is slow and poorly effective, with stones often recurring). Lithotripsy (sonic shockwaves) is another option of limited effectiveness.

C: Chronic cholecystitis, mucocoele, gallbladder empyema, obstructive jaundice, pancreatitis, stricturing of the biliary tree, cholecystenteric fistula (causing gallstone ileus), cholecystocholedochal fistula (Mirrizzi's syndrome), porcelain gallbladder (thick-walled fibrotic premalignant gallbladder).

P: 2% with gallstones develop symptoms each year. Gallstone-induced acute cholecystitis, obstructive jaundice and cholangitis are indications for definitive treatment by cholecystectomy.

Gastric carcinoma

D: Gastric malignancy, most commonly adenocarcinoma, more rarely lymphoma, leiomyosarcoma.

A: Most cases are probably caused by environmental insults in genetically predisposed individuals that lead to mutation and subsequent unregulated cell growth.

A/R: Diet high in smoked and processed foods, nitrosamines, smoking, alcohol, *Helicobacter pylori* infection and atrophic gastritis. Blood group A (1.2 relative risk). Pernicious anaemia. Partial gastrectomy. Gastric polyps.

E: Common cause of cancer death worldwide, with highest incidence in Asia, especially Japan. Sixth most common cancer in UK (annual incidence is 15 in 100 000). ♂ ♀ ~2 : 1. Age > 50 years. Cancer of the antrum/body is becoming less common, while that of the cardia and gastro-oesophageal junction is increasing.

H: Early often asymptomatic.
Early satiety or epigastric discomfort.
Weight loss, anorexia, nausea and vomiting.
Haematemesis, melaena, symptoms of anaemia.
Dysphagia (tumours of the cardia).
Symptoms of metastases, particularly abdominal swelling (ascites) or jaundice (liver involvement).

E: May be none. Epigastric mass. Abdominal tenderness. Ascites.
Signs of anaemia.
Many eponymous signs:
Virchow's node/Troisier's sign: palpable lymph nodes in left supraclavicular fossa.
Sister Mary Joseph node: metastatic nodule on umbilicus.
Krukenberg's tumour: ovarian metastases.

P: **Micro:** Adenocarcinoma, intestinal or diffuse subtypes (Lauren classification).
Macro: Polypoid, ulcerating or infiltrative (Borrmann classification), if widespread may cause linitis plastica (leatherbottle stomach). Gastric carcinomas can spread directly through stomach wall, via lymph nodes, transcoelomic with peritoneal deposits or haematogenous to liver, lungs, brain, ovaries.

I: **Upper GI endoscopy:** With multiquadrant biopsy of all gastric ulcers.
Blood: FBC (for anaemia), LFT.
CT/MRI: Staging of tumour and planning of surgery.
Ultrasound of liver: Staging of tumour.
Bone scan: Staging of tumour.
Endoscopic ultrasound: Assess depth of gastric invasion and local lymph node involvement.
Laparoscopy may be needed to determine if tumour is resectable.

M: **Surgery:** Various surgical techniques, depending on size and location of the tumour.
Bilroth I partial gastrectomy: Excision of tumour and distal stomach. Duodenal stump is anastomosed with remainder of stomach. Suitable for antral tumours.
Bilroth II partial gastrectomy: Excision of tumour and distal stomach. Duodenal stump is oversewn and remainder of the stomach is anastomosed to jejunum (gastrojejunostomy). Suitable for antral tumours.

Total gastrectomy: Removal of stomach and spleen. Oesophagojejunostomy. Suitable for large tumours.
Ivor–Lewis gastrectomy: Proximal gastrectomy and distal oesophagectomy, with oesophagoantrostomy and pyloroplasty. Suitable for cardial or fundal tumours.
Roux-en-Y reconstruction: Duodenal stump oversewn. Distal duodenum anastomosed to jejunum.
Palliative: Debulking surgery. Gastrojejunostomy or intubation to bypass and maintain enteral nutrition.
Medical: Chemotherapy (e.g. 5-fluorouracil, platinum agents) prolongs survival by a few months.

C: Dysphagia, gastric outlet obstruction, upper GI haemorrhage, iron-deficiency anaemia. Early and late complications of gastrectomy (e.g. dumping syndrome, diarrhoea, deficiencies of vitamin B_{12}).

P: Generally poor with $< 10\%$ overall 5-year survival. About 50 % in those with early disease undergoing resection.

Gastroenteritis

D: Acute inflammation of the lining of the GI tract, manifested by nausea, vomiting, diarrhoea and abdominal discomfort.

A: Can be caused by viruses, bacteria, protozoa or toxins contained in contaminated food or water.

Viral: Rotavirus, adenovirus, astrovirus, calcivirus, Norwalk virus, small round structured viruses.

Bacterial: *Campylobacter jejuni*, *Escherichia coli* (particularly 0157), *Salmonella*, *Shigella*, *Vibrio cholerae*, *Listeria*, *Yersinia enterocolitica*.

Protozoal: *Entamoeba histolytica*, *Cryptosporidium parvum*, *Giardia lamblia*.

Toxins: From *Staphylococcus aureus*, *Clostridium botulinum*, *Clostridium perfringens*, *Bacillus cereus*, mushrooms, heavy metals, seafood.

Commonly contaminated foods: Improperly cooked meat (*Staphylococcus aureus*, *Clostridium perfringens*), old rice (*Bacillus cereus*, *Staphylococcus aureus*), eggs and poultry (*Salmonella*), milk and cheeses (*Listeria*, *Campylobacter*), canned food (botulism).

A/R: Risk groups include travellers, patients in large institutions.

Haemolytic – uraemic syndrome is associated with toxins from *E. coli* 0157.

Guillian–Barré syndrome may occur weeks after recovery, e.g. *Campylobacter* gastroenteritis.

E: Common, and often under-reported, a serious cause of morbidity and mortality in the developing world.

H: Sudden onset nausea, vomiting, anorexia.

Diarrhoea (bloody or watery), abdominal pain or discomfort, fever and malaise.

Enquire about recent travel, antibiotic use and recent food intake (how cooked, source and whether anyone else ill).

Time of onset: Toxins (early; 1–24 h), bacterial/viral/protozoal (12 h or later).

Effect of toxin: Botulinum causes paralysis; mushrooms can cause fits, renal or liver failure.

E: Diffuse abdominal tenderness, abdominal distension and bowel sounds are often increased.

If severe, pyrexia, dehydration, hypotension, peripheral shutdown.

P: Depending on the organism or toxin, there are different pathogenic mechanisms.

Non-inflammatory mechanisms: e.g. *Vibrio cholerae*, enterotoxigenic *E. coli* produce enterotoxins that cause enterocytes to secrete water and electrolytes.

Inflammatory mechanisms: e.g. *Shigella*, enteroinvasive *E. coli* release cytotoxins and invade and damage the epithelium, with greater invasion and bacteraemia in the case of *Salmonella typhi*.

I: **Blood:** FBC, blood culture (helps identification if bacteriaemia present), U&E (dehydration).

Stool: Faecal microscopy for polymorphs, parasites, oocysts, culture, electron microscopy (used to diagnose viral infections). Analysis for toxins, particularly for pseudomembranous colitis (*Clostridium difficile* toxin).

AXR or ultrasound: To exclude other causes of abdominal pain.

Sigmoidoscopy: Often unnecessary unless IBD needs to be excluded.

M: **Medical:** Bed rest, fluid and electrolyte replacement with oral rehydration solution (containing glucose and salt). IV rehydration may be necessary in those with severe vomiting. Most infections are self-limiting. Antibiotic treatment is only warranted if severe or the infective agent has been identified (e.g. ciprofloxacin against *Salmonella, Shigella, Campylobacter*).

Typhoid fever: (see Typhoid and paratyphoid fever).
Botulinism: Botulinum antitoxin IM and manage in ITU.
Public health: Often a notifiable disease. Educate on basic hygiene and cooking.

C: Dehydration, electrolyte imbalance, prerenal failure, secondary lactose intolerance (particularly in infants). Sepsis and shock (particularly *Salmonella* and *Shigella*).

Botulinism: Respiratory muscle weakness or paralysis.

P: Generally good, as the majority of cases are self-limiting.

Gastro-oesophageal reflux disease (GORD)

D: Inflammation of the oesophagus caused by reflux of gastric acid and/or bile.

A: Disruption of mechanisms that prevent reflux (physiological lower oesophageal sphincter, mucosal rosette, acute angle of junction, intra-abdominal portion of oesophagus). Prolonged oesophageal clearance contributes to 50 % of cases.

A/R: Associated with the development of Barrett's oesophagus.* Risk factors include hiatus hernia, obesity, pregnancy, intake of caffeine, fat or alcohol, smoking, drugs (e.g. tricyclic antidepressants), increased gastric volume (large meal, delayed gastric emptying), systemic sclerosis.

E: Common, prevalence 5–10 % adults.

H: Substernal burning discomfort or 'heartburn' aggravated by lying supine, bending or large meals and drinking alcohol. Pain relieved by antacids. Waterbrash. Regurgitation of gastric contents.
Aspiration may result in voice hoarseness, laryngitis, nocturnal cough and wheeze ± pneumonia (rare).
Dysphagia (caused by formation of peptic stricture after long-standing reflux).

E: Usually normal. Occasionally, epigastric tenderness, wheeze on chest auscultation, dysphonia.

P: **Pathogenesis:** Prolonged reflux of acidic stomach contents causes oesophageal mucosal erosions, ulceration and an inflammatory (neutrophils and eosinophils) infiltrate. Chronic reflux may result in a fibrotic reaction and stricture formation.

I: **Upper GI endoscopy, biopsy** and cytological brushings to confirm the presence of oesophagitis, exclude the possibility of malignancy (all patients >45 years).
Barium swallow: Hiatus hernia, peptic stricture, extrinsic compression of the oesophagus can be visualised.
CXR: Not specifically for GORD. Incidental finding of hiatus hernia (gastric bubble behind cardiac shadow).
24-h oesophageal pH monitoring: pH probe placed in lower oesophagus determines the temporal relationship between symptoms and oesophageal pH.

M: **Advice:** Lifestyle changes, weight loss, elevating head of bed, avoid provoking factors, stopping smoking, lower fat meals, avoiding large meals late in the evening.
Medical: Antacids and alginates, H_2 antagonists (e.g. ranitidine) or proton pump inhibitors (e.g. lansoprazole) is sufficient for most patients.
Endoscopy: Yearly endoscopic surveillance of Barrett's oesophagus, stricture dilation.
Surgery: Antireflux surgery for those with symptoms despite optimal medical management or in those intolerant of medication.
Nissen fundoplication (fundus of the stomach is wrapped around the lower oesophagus and held with seromuscular sutures) helps reduces any hiatus hernia and reduce reflux.

*Barrett's oesophagus is characterized by metaplasia of oesophageal squamous epithelium and replacement with columnar epithelium. This is a premalignant condition with an increased risk of dysplasia and adenocarcinoma.

C: Oesophageal ulceration, peptic stricture, anaemia, Barrett's oesophagus and oesophageal adenocarcinoma.

P: 50 % respond to lifestyle measures alone. In patients who require drug therapy withdrawal is often associated with relapse. 20 % of patients undergoing endoscopy for GORD have Barrett's oesophagus.

Giant cell arteritis (temporal arteritis)

D: Granulomatous inflammation of large arteries, particularly branches of the external carotid artery, most commonly the temporal artery.

A: Unknown. Associated with *HLA-DR4* and *HLA-DRB1*.

A/R: 40–60 % of cases are associated with PMR, while only 15 % of cases of PMR are associated with giant cell arteritis.

E: Annual incidence is 18 in 100 000. ♀ : ♂ = 2–4 :1. Peak age onset 65–70 years.

H: Subacute onset, usually over a few weeks.
Headache: Scalp and temporal tenderness (pain on combing hair). Jaw and tongue claudication.
Visual disturbances: Blurred vision. Sudden blindness in one eye (amaurosis fugax*).
Systemic features: Malaise, low-grade fever, lethargy, weight loss, depression.
Symptoms of PMR: Early morning pain and stiffness of the muscles of the shoulder and pelvic girdle.

E: Swelling and erythema overlying the temporal artery. Scalp and temporal tenderness.

Thickened non-pulsatile temporal artery.
Visual disturbances.

P: Granulomatous inflammation of all layers of the arterial wall with giant cell formation in the internal elastic lamina. Replacement of the vessel by a fibrous cord. Thrombosis may occur followed by recanalization or embolism to the ophthalmic artery leading to visual disturbances, amaurosis fugax or sudden monocular blindness.

I: **Blood:** ↑ ESR typically, FBC (anaemia of chronic disease).
Temporal artery biopsy: Within 36 h of starting corticosteroids. Note that a negative biopsy does not exclude the diagnosis, because skip lesions occur.

M: **Medical:** Start on high dose oral prednisolone (40–60 mg/day in divided doses) immediately to prevent visual loss. The majority of patients experience immense symptomatic relief within 48 h of commencing steroid therapy. ↓ Dose of prednisolone gradually (according to symptoms and ESR) to a maintenance dose of 7.5–10 mg/day. Many patients require prednisolone for at least 2 years.

C: Permanent monocular blindness.

P: In most cases the condition lasts for ~2 years before complete remission.

*Amaurosis fugax is a gradual descending mono-ocular ‘curtain’ of vision loss.

D: Optic neuropathy with typical field defect usually associated with raised IOP.

A: **Primary:** Acute closed-angle glaucoma (ACAG), primary opened-angle glaucoma (POAG), chronic closed-angle glaucoma.
Secondary: Trauma, uveitis, steroids, rubeosis iridis (diabetes, central retinal vein occlusion).
Congenital: Buphthalmos, other inherited ocular disorders.
It is believed that ↑ IOP is caused by ↓ outflow of aqueous humour which can be caused by:

- obstruction to outflow by approximation of iris to cornea closing iridocorneal angle and trabecular meshwork/canal of Schlemm causing a rapid and severe rise in IOP (ACAG);
- resistance to outflow through trabecular meshwork (POAG); or
- blockage of trabecular meshwork by blood, inflammatory cells, etc. (secondary causes).

A/R: **ACAG:** Hypermetropia.

POAG: Genetics, age, diabetes, myopia, race (Afro-Carribean).

E: Prevalence 1 % over 40 years, 10 % over 80 years (POAG). Third most common cause of blindness worldwide

H: **ACAG:** Severely painful red eye, vomiting, impaired vision, haloes around lights.
POAG: Usually asymptomatic, peripheral visual field loss may be noticed.
Congenital: Buphthalmos (ox eye), watering, cloudy cornea.

E: **ACAG:** Red eye, hazy cornea, loss of red reflex, fixed and dilated pupil, eye tender and hard on palpation, cupped optic disc, visual field defect (arcuate scotoma), moderately raised IOP.

POAG: Optic disc may be cupped. Usually no signs.

P: Two theories for the mechanism by which elevated IOP damages nerve fibres:

1 by causing mechanical damage to the optic nerve axons; or
2 by causing ischaemia of the axons by decreasing blood flow at the optic nerve head.

I: **Slit-lamp examination:** (see Examination).

Tonometry: To measure ocular pressure (normal 15 mmHg, POAG 22–40 mmHg, ACAG > 60 mmHg).
Gonioscopy: To assess the iridocorneal angle.
Fundoscopy: To detect pathologically cupped optic disc (cup : disc ratio > 0.6 or an asymmetry of 0.2).
Visual field testing: Arcuate scotoma (early), tunnel vision (late).

M: **ACAG (medical emergency):** IV acetazolamide (500 mg), 4 % pilocarpine topically, analgesics, antiemetics.
Long-term: *Topical:* Timolol (β-blockers ↓ secretion of aqueous humour).
Carbonic anhydrase inhibitor: Dorzolamide (↓ secretion of aqueous humour).
Parasympathomimetics: Pilocarpine (constricts pupil and opens up trabecular meshwork).
Sympathomimetics: Brimonidine (α_2-agonist).
Prostaglandin analogues: Latanoprost (↑ flow via alternative uveoscleral drainage pathway).
Laser treatment: Trabeculoplasty for POAG; iridotomy for ACAG.

Surgery: Drainage surgery (trabeculectomy) ±5-fluorouracil to prevent postoperative scarring.

C: **Congenital:** Amblyopia and visual loss.
POAG: Visual loss.
ACAG: Visual loss and anterior synechiae.

P: Poor prognosis for congenital glaucoma caused by amblyopia. Prognosis in acquired glaucoma depends on early diagnosis and treatment.

D: Glomerulonephritis is immunologically mediated inflammation of renal glomeruli.

A: There are many different types of glomerulonephritis with differing aetiologies (see Pathology).
Some types of glomerulonephritis are ascribed to deposition of antigen–antibody immune complexes in the glomeruli that lead to inflammation and the activation of complement and coagulation cascades. The immune complexes may either form within the glomerulus (probably more commonly) or be deposited from the circulation. The antigens in the immune complexes are often unknown but may occasionally be associated with the following.
Infection: *Bacterial: Streptococcus viridans*, group A β-haemolytic streptococci, staphylococci, gonococci, *Salmonella*, syphilis.
Viral: Hepatitis B/C, HIV, measles, mumps, EBV, VZV, coxsackie.
Protozoal: Plasmodium malariae, schistosomiasis, filariasis.
Inflammatory/systemic diseases: SLE, systemic vasculitis, cryoglobulinaemia.*
Drugs: gold, penicillamine.
Tumours.
Other types of glomerulonephritis are ascribed to complement abnormalities or T cell dysfunction.

A/R: May be associated with tubulointerstitial lesions, abnormalities of complement activation.

E: Makes up to 25 % of cases of chronic renal failure.

H: Haematuria, subcutaneous oedema, polyuria or oliguria, proteinuria. History of recent infection.
Symptoms of uraemia or renal failure (acute and chronic).

E: May present with the signs of the following:
- hypertension;
- proteinuria (< 3 g/24 h);
- haematuria (microscopic or macroscopic, especially IgA nephropathy);
- nephrotic syndrome (usually for minimal-change glomerulonephritis in children and membranous glomerulonephritis in adults; see Nephrotic syndrome);
- nephritic syndrome (haematuria, proteinuria, subcutaneous oedema, oliguria, hypertension, uraemia);
- renal failure (acute or chronic); and
- partial lipodystrophy (loss of subcutaneous fat in MPGN type II).

P: Classified based on the site of nephron pathology and its distribution.
Minimal-change glomerulonephritis: Normal appearance on light microscopy. Electron microscopy: loss of epithelial foot processes.
Membranous glomerulonephritis: Thickening of GBM from immune complex deposition. Associated with Goodpasture's syndrome.†

*Cryoglobulins are immunoglobulins that precipitate in cold, and may be monoclonal or polyclonal. They can cause cutaneous vasculitis.
†Goodpasture's syndrome occurs resulting from anti-GBM antibody that binds to an antigen in the basement membrane. The antibody also reacts with pulmonary capillary basement membrane and can cause pulmonary haemorrhage.

Membranoproliferative glomerulonephritis (MPGN): Thickening of GBM, mesangial cell proliferation and interposition.

Type 1: Subendothelial immune complex deposits and reduplication of GBM.

Type 2: Dense intramembranous deposits (stain only for C3).

Focal segmental glomerulosclerosis: Glomerular scarring. Associated with HIV.

Focal segmental proliferative glomerulonephritis: Mesangial and endothelial cell proliferation. 'Focal' refers to involvement of some of the glomeruli, 'segmental' refers to involvement of parts of individual glomeruli.

Diffuse proliferative glomerulonephritis: Same as above but affects all glomeruli.

IgA nephropathy: Mesangial cell proliferation and mesangial IgA and C3 deposits.

Crescentric glomerulonephritis: Crescent formation by macrophages and epithelial cells, which fills up Bowman's space.

Focal segmental necrotizing glomerulonephritis: Peripheral capillary loop necrosis (e.g. in Wegener's granulomatosis, microscopic polyarteritis and other vasculitides). Often evolves into crescentric glomerulonephritis.

I: **Blood:** FBC, U&E and creatinine, LFT (albumin), lipid profile, complement studies (C3, C4, C3 nephritic factor in MPGN), ANA, anti-double stranded DNA, ANCA, anti-GBM antibody, cryoglobulins if appropriate.

Urine: Microscopy (dysmorphic RBCs, red-cell casts), 24-h collection: creatinine clearance, protein.

Imaging: AXR, ultrasound, IVU (to exclude other pathology).

Renal biopsy: Light microscopy, electron microscopy, immunofluorescence microscopy.

Investigations for associated infections.

M: **Fluid balance:** Monitor input/output and weight changes, avoid added salt and restrict fluid if there are signs of fluid overload or ↑ BP.

Treatment of complications: (see Hypertension; Renal failure, acute; Renal failure, chronic, Nephrotic syndrome).

Focal necrotizing glomerulonephritis, rapidly progressive crescentric glomerulonephritis, glomerulonephritis associated with SLE, primary vasculitides: steroids, azathioprine, ciclosporin A, cyclophosphamide.

Consider plasma exchange, especially for severe disease affecting the basement membrane.

C: Pulmonary oedema, increased risk of hypertension, hypertensive encephalopathy, uraemia, renal failure complications of nephrotic syndrome, pre-eclampsia in pregnancy.

P: Minimal-change glomerulonephritis and postinfective diffuse proliferative glomerulonephritis mostly resolve.

Risk of CRF: Focal segmental sclerosis 50–75 %; focal proliferative glomerulonephritis 25 %; membranous glomerulonephritis ~30 %; MPGN >75 %.

Poor prognostic factors: ↑ Creatinine when first seen, ↑ BP, persistent proteinuria.

D: A disorder of uric acid metabolism causing recurrent bouts of acute arthritis caused by deposition of monosodium urate crystals in joints, and also soft tissues and kidneys.

A: The underlying metabolic disturbance is hyperuricaemia which may be caused by the following.
Increased urate intake or production: ↑ Dietary intake, ↑ nucleic acid (purine) turnover (e.g. lymphoma, leukaemia, polycythaemia vera, psoriasis) or, rarely, caused by ↑ synthesis (e.g. Lesch–Nyhan syndrome*).
Decreased renal excretion: Idiopathic, drugs (e.g. 'CANT LEAP': ciclosporin, alcohol, nicotinic acid, thiazides, loop diuretics, ethambutol, aspirin (low-dose), pyrizinamide), renal dysfunction.

A/R: Male, ↑ age, postmenopausal women, high alcohol intake, obesity, hyperlipidaemia, hypertension, diabetes mellitus, family history, ischaemic heart disease.

E: Prevalence 0.2 %. ♂ : ♀ ~10:1. Very rare in prepuberty and in premenopausal women. More common in higher social classes. Common in certain ethnic groups, e.g. Polynesian and Maori.

H: **Acute attack:** May be precipitated by trauma, infection, alcohol, starvation, introduction or withdrawal of hypouricaemic agents. Sudden excruciating monoarticular pain, usually the metatarsophalangeal joint of the great toe. The symptoms peak at 24 h and resolve in 7–10 days. Occasionally, acute attacks present with cellulitis, polyarticular or periarticular involvement. Attacks are often recurrent, but the patient is symptom free between attacks.
Intercritical gout: Asymptomatic period between acute attacks.
Chronic tophaceous gout: Follows repeated acute attacks. Persistent low-grade fever, polyarticular pain with painful tophi (urate deposits), best seen on tendons and the pinna of the ear.
Symptoms of urate urolithiasis: (see Renal calculi).

E: **Acute attack:** Erythematous warm tender swollen joint with ↓ range of movement and inability to bear weight. Low-grade pyrexia.
Chronic tophaceous gout: Yellow-ivory painful urate crystals called tophi may be seen through the skin (e.g. on the pinna of the ear, elbow, hands, tendons).

P: Excess monosodium urate crystals are deposited in joints, soft tissues and the urinary tract. Neutrophils phagocytose the crystals. This causes disruption of the lysosomal membrane and release of enzymes and oxygen free radicals into the tissues causing tissue damage.

I: **Synovial fluid aspirate:** Diagnosis depends on the presence of monosodium urate crystals which are needle-shaped and negatively birefingent under polarized light. Microscopy and culture (to exclude septic arthritis).
Blood: FBC (↑ WCC), U&E, ↑ urate (but may be normal in acute gout), ↑ ESR.
AXR/KUB film: Uric acid renal stones are often radiolucent.

M: **Acute attack:** NSAIDs. Colchicine if NSAIDs contraindicated. Intra-articular corticosteroids. Intramuscular ACTH for difficult cases.
Surgery: May be necessary for large or ulcerating tophus.

*Lesch–Nyhan syndrome is a result of hypoxanthine–guanine phosphoribosyl transferase deficiency, and presents with chorea, ↓ IQ and self-mutilation.

Prevention: Treat associated features (e.g. obesity) with lifestyle changes and drugs.

Medical prophylaxis: Allopurinol (xanthine oxidase inhibitor) provides prophylaxis against acute attacks. Alternative prophylaxis agents include long-term colchicine (risk of neuromyopathy), probenecid or sulfinpyrazone (uricosurics). Encourage ↑ fluid intake to lower risk of renal calculi.

C: Renal failure, urate urolithiasis, urate nephropathy. Secondary infection or ulceration of tophi.

P: 75 % have a second attack within 2 years. Treatment often necessary in long term.

Guillain–Barré syndrome

D: Acute ascending inflammatory demyelinating polyneuropathy.

A: Precise aetiology unknown:

- Idiopathic in about 40 %.
- Postinfection (1–3 week): herpes viruses (e.g. zoster, CMV), bacterial (e.g. *Campylobacter jejuni*), HIV.
- Malignancy (lymphoma, Hodgkin's disease).
- SLE.
- Postoperative.

A/R: None.

E: Annual UK incidence is 1–2 in 100 000. Affects all age groups.

H: Progressive symptoms of ≤ 1 month duration of ascending symmetrical limb weakness (lower>upper).
Paraesthesia may be present.
Cranial nerve involvement (e.g. dysphagia, dysarthria, facial weakness and diplopia).
In severe cases, the respiratory muscles may be affected.
Miller–Fisher variant (rare): Opthalmoplegia, ataxia and arreflexia, with little if any limb weakness.

E: Hypotonia, flaccid paralysis, arreflexia (ascending upwards from feet to head).
Cranial nerve palsies: facial nerve weakness (lower motor neurone pattern), abnormality of eye movements, binocular diplopia, signs of bulbar palsy.
Type II respiratory failure is important to identify early (e.g. CO_2 flap, bounding pulse, drowsiness).
Autonomic function may be impaired.

P: Incompletely understood. Believed to be an immune (cell-mediated) demyelination of peripheral nerves and/or spinal nerve roots. Autoallergic perivascular infiltration of macrophages and lymphocytes, as part of a peripheral inflammatory demyelinating process with axonal sparing.

I: **Lumbar puncture:** ↑ CSF protein, cell count and glucose normal.
EMG: ↓ Conduction velocity.
Blood: Antiganglioside antibodies positive in Miller–Fisher variant and 25 % of Guillain–Barré syndrome cases.
Arterial blood gases: Type II respiratory failure (hypoxia, hypocapnia) indicates a need for intubation.
Spirometry: ↓ Full vital capacity.
ECG: Arrhythmias may develop.

M: **Acute:** Supportive treatment is the core. Monitor vital capacity, ABG and ECG. DVT prophylaxis, regular physiotherapy with care of pressure areas. Dysphagia may warrant nasogastric feeding. Respiratory muscle compromise or inability to protect airway requires artificial ventilation. High-dose IV immunoglobulin or plasmapheresis may reduce duration or severity of disease.

C: Respiratory failure, cardiac arrhythmias, sepsis, pulmonary embolus, incomplete recovery, relapse, death.

P: 85 % complete recovery, usually within 3–6 months. 10 % have residual neurological disability. Minority have future relapses. Mortality rate of 5 %.

Haemochromatosis

D: Body iron overload resulting from excessive intestinal iron absorption which may lead to organ damage (particularly liver, joints, pancreas, pituitary and heart).

A: Inherited form is caused by a mutation in the *HFE* gene on chromosome 6p. Most common mutation (90 %) is C282Y, less common is H63D. *HFE* codes for a protein involved in iron transport; however, the exact mechanism leading to increased iron uptake is not yet clear.

A/R: Can be exacerbated by high alcohol intake.

E: Carrier frequency is up to 1 in 10 but not all express disease, prevalence of those affected are ~1 in 400 (in white people). Typical age of presentation 40–60 years. Females have a later onset and less severe presentation as a result of iron loss through menstruation.

H: May be asymptomatic.
Non-specific symptoms of weakness, fatigue, lethargy, abdominal pain.
Later features include joint pains (small or large joints), symptoms of liver disease, diabetes mellitus, hypogonadism, cardiac failure.
Exclude causes of secondary iron overload (e.g. multiple transfusions).

E: May be normal, but with severe iron overload:
Skin: Pigmentation ('slate-grey') resulting from ↑ melanin deposits.
Liver: Hepatosplenomegaly.
Heart: Signs of heart failure (unusual), arrhythmias.
Hypogonadism: Testicular atrophy, loss of hair, gynaecomastia.

P: **Macro:** The enlarged liver is dark brown because of deposition of excess iron as haemosiderin (iron-rich protein).
Micro: Liver cells accumulate iron, visualized using Perls' stain. Iron is initially deposited in periportal hepatocytes (pericanalicular lysosomes), later in Kupffer cells, bile duct epithelial cells and portal tract connective tissue, later leading to fibrosis and cirrhosis.

I: **Blood:** ↑ Iron, ↓ TIBC, ↑ ferritin and transferrin saturation (false-positives in alcoholic liver disease or in any inflammation).
Gene typing of *HFE*
Tests for complications in various organs:
Liver: LFT may be normal or deranged. Liver biopsy to assess tissue damage. MRI may be used to estimate the degree of iron loading.
Pancreas: Fasting or random blood glucose to test for diabetes mellitus.
Pituitary function test: Early morning cortisol, LH, FSH, testosterone.
Heart: ECG, echocardiography.
Joint X-ray: Linear calcification (chondrocalcinosis).

M: **Regular venesection:** One unit of blood (~450 mL with 200 mg iron) once or twice weekly until serum iron and ferritin are in normal ranges. Maintenance venesection of 1 unit every 3 months, aiming for a serum ferritin < 50 μg/L, transferrin saturation < 50 %.
Screening of relatives: Serum ferritin and genotyping.

C: Arthritis, cirrhosis, diabetes, dilated cardiomyopathy and cardiac failure and arrhythmias, hypogonadism, ↑ risk of hepatocellular carcinoma.

P: Reducing iron overload decreases mortality from cardiac and liver failure and returns the life expectancy of non-cirrhotic non-diabetic patients to normal. Hypogonadism and arthritis may not be reversed by venesection.

D: Triad of microangiopathic haemolytic anaemia, acute renal failure and thrombocytopenia. There are two forms: D^+ (diarrhoea-associated form); and D^- (no prodromal illness identified).

A: **Infection:** Verotoxin-producing *Escherichia coli* 0157 (from contaminated water, meat, dairy products), *Shigella*, neuraminidase-producing infections (e.g. pneumococcal respiratory tract infection), HIV.
Drugs: Oral contraceptive pill, ciclosporin, mitomycin, 5-fluorouracil.
Familial: Autosomal dominant or recessive inheritance.
Others: Malignant hypertension, malignancy, pregnancy, SLE, scleroderma.

A/R: Haemolytic uraemic syndrome overlaps with **thrombotic thrombocytopenic purpura (TTP)** which has the additional features of fever and fluctuating CNS signs.

E: Uncommon, D^+ haemolytic uraemic syndrome often affects young children, occurs more often in summer in epidemics and is the most common cause of acute renal failure in children. **TTP** mainly affects adult females.

H: **GI:** Severe abdominal colic, watery diarrhoea that becomes blood-stained.
General: Malaise, fatigue, nausea, fever $< 38\,°C$ (D^+ form).
Renal: Oligo- or anuria, haematuria.

E: **General:** Pallor (from anaemia), slight jaundice (from haemolysis), bruising (severe thrombocytopenia), generalized oedema, hypertension and retinopathy.
GI: Abdominal tenderness.
CNS signs: Especially in TTP (weakness, ↓ vision, fits, ↓ consciousness).

P: An aetiological factor causing endothelial injury results in platelet aggregation, release of unusually large vWF multimers and activation of platelets and the clotting cascade. This results in small vessel thrombosis, particularly the glomerular afferent arteriole and capillaries, which undergo fibrinoid necrosis. This is followed by renal ischaemia and acute renal failure. The thrombi also promote intravascular haemolysis. In **TTP** systemic microvascular platelet aggregation causes ischaemia of brain and other organs. Dysfunction/loss of the vWF-cleaving protease (ADAMTS 13) contributes to the pathogenesis.

I: **Blood:** *FBC:* Normocytic anaemia, ↑ neutrophils, ↓↓ platelets.
U&E: ↑ Urea, creatinine, urate, K^+, ↓ Na^+.
Clotting: Normal platelets, APTT and fibrinogen levels, abnormality may indicate DIC.
LFT: ↑ Unconjugated bilirubin, ↑ LDH from haemolysis.
Blood cultures.
ABG: ↓ pH, ↓ bicarbonate, ↓ $Paco_2$, normal anion gap.
Blood film: Fragmented red blood cells, ↑ reticulocytes, spherocytes.
Urine: > 1 g protein/24 h, haematuria, fractional excretion $Na^+ > 1\%$.
Stool samples: Light and electron microscopy, culture.
ECG: Risk of arrhythmia and cardiac arrest resulting from hyperkalaemia.
Renal biopsy: Contraindicated in severe thrombocytopenia. In cases of diagnostic doubt:
D^+ form: arteriolar necrosis, glomerular capillary thrombosis;
D^- form: intimal proliferation in arterioles.

M: Requires specialist supportive management.

Medical: Treat hypovolaemia (from diarrhoea, vomiting, capillary leak), control hypertension, IV fluids and furosemide (frusemide) may establish diuresis and prevent the need for dialysis. Haemodialysis if severe uraemia, hyperkalaemia, acidosis. Blood transfusion for anaemia. Plasma exchange and FFP infusions may be required.

TTP: plasma exchange and FFP infusions; refractory cases: steroids, vincristine, splenectomy and antiplatelet agents.

C: Neurological complications, hyperkalaemia.

D$^+$ form: GI infarction, rectal prolapse, acute tubular necrosis, acute or chronic renal failure.

D$^-$ form: Cardiomyopathy, malignant hypertension.

P: Most children with D$^+$ form recover. Adults have a poorer outcome with 70 % having complete recovery. ~17 % remain dialysis-dependent. 7 % overall mortality (often with CNS involvement). Mortality is higher in **TTP**.

D: Bleeding diatheses resulting from an inherited deficiency of clotting factor. Three subtypes:
Haemophilia A: (most common). Caused by a deficiency in factor VIII.
Haemophilia B: caused by a deficiency in factor IX (Christmas disease).
Haemophilia C: (rare). Caused by a deficiency in factor XI.

A: Haemophilia A and B exhibit X-linked recessive inheritance. A variety of genetic changes have been described. 30 % of cases are new mutations.

A/R: Family history, consanguinity.

E: Incidence of haemophilia A is ~1 in 10 000 males and for haemophilia B is 1 in 50 000 males. Haemophilia C is more common in Ashkenazi Jews.

H: Symptoms usually begin from early childhood.
Swollen painful joints occurring spontaneously or with minimal trauma (haemarthroses). Painful bleeding into muscles.
Haematuria. Excessive bruising or bleeding after surgery or trauma.
Female carriers usually asymptomatic, but may have low enough levels to cause excess bleeding after trauma.

E: Multiple bruises.
Muscle haematomas. Haemarthroses. Joint deformity.
Nerve palsies (nerve compression by haematoma).
Signs of iron-deficiency anaemia.

P: **Haemophilia A:** Factor VIII is a vital co-factor in the intrinsic pathway of the coagulation cascade, when activated by thrombin it accelerates the activity of the clotting cascade 200 000-fold.
Haemophilia B: Activated factor IX converts factor X → Xa.
Both prolong the APTT which reflects the activity of the intrinsic and the common pathway.

I: **Blood:** Clotting (↑ APTT), coagulation factor assays (↓ factor VIII, IX or XI depending on condition; see Definition).
Genetic studies: Karyotype analysis of patient and family.
Other investigations according to complications (e.g. arthroscopy).

M: Specialist management and follow-up at a haemophilia centre.
Mild haemophilia A (factor VIII ≥ 10 % of normal): Intranasal or IV DDAVP (vasopressin analogue) mobilizes factor VIII from stores. Alternatively, oral transexamic acid (a fibrinolytic inhibitor) can be used.
Moderate to severe haemophilia: Transfusion with factor VIII or IX concentrate (depending on haemophilia subtype) is needed to maintain levels at 20–50 % of normal. In severe bleeding or preoperatively, more rigorous transfusion to 70–100 % of normal is necessary.
Advice: Avoid antiplatelet drugs (e.g. aspirin) and IM injections. Hepatitis A and B vaccination. Specialist referral for complications.
Lifestyle: Avoid contact sports. Medicalert card or bracelet. Genetic counselling for patient and family.

C: Severe and fatal haemorrhage. Crippling joint deformity.
10–15 % of patients develop antibodies to the clotting factor (particularly recipients of factor VIII).
Hepatitis C and HIV infection in patients who received clotting concentrates before 1985 in developed countries.

P: The availability of safer blood products and home treatment programmes mean that most people with haemophilia can lead a relatively normal life.

Heart block

D: Impairment of the atrioventricular (AV) node impulse conduction, as represented by the interval between P wave and QRS complex.

First-degree AV block: Prolonged conduction through the AV node.

Second-degree AV block: *Mobitz type I (Wenckebach):* Progressive prolongation of AV node conduction culminating in one atrial impulse failing to be conducted through the AV node. The cycle then begins again.

Mobitz type II: Intermittent or regular failure of conduction through AV node. Also called by the number of normal conductions per abnormal one (e.g. 2 : 1 or 3 : 1).

Third-degree (complete) AV block: No relationship between atrial and ventricular contraction. Failure of conduction through the AV node leads to a ventricular contraction generated by a focus of depolarization within the ventricle (ventricular escape).

A: MI or ischaemia (most common cause).
Infection (e.g. rheumatic fever, infective endocarditis).
Drugs (e.g. digoxin, β-blockers, Ca^{2+} channel antagonists).
Metabolic (e.g. hyperkalaemia, cholestatic jaundice, hypothermia).
Infiltration of conducting system (e.g. sarcoidosis, cardiac neoplasms, amyloidosis).
Degeneration of the conducting system.

A/R: None.

E: Majority of the 250 000 pacemakers implanted each year (worldwide) are for heart block.

H: **First-degree:** Asymptomatic.

Wenckebach: Usually asymptomatic.

Mobitz type II and third-degree block: May cause Stokes–Adams attacks (syncope caused by ventricular asystole). Other presentations include dizziness, palpitations, chest pain and heart failure.

E: Often normal. Examine for signs of the cause.

Complete heart block: Slow large volume pulse and JVP may show 'cannon waves'.

Mobitz type II and third-degree block: Signs of a reduced cardiac output (e.g. hypotension, heart failure).

P: Anatomical or functional impairment of the conducting system (AV node, bundle of His or Purkinje system).

I: **ECG (consider ambulatory or 24-h Holter):**

First-degree: Prolonged PR interval (> 0.2 s).

Mobitz I (Wenckebach): Progressively prolonged PR interval, culminating in a P wave that is not followed by a QRS. The pattern then begins again.

Mobitz II: Intermittently a P wave is not followed by a QRS. There may be a regular pattern of P waves not followed by a QRS (e.g. two P-waves per QRS, indicating 2 : 1 block).

Third-degree (complete): No relationship between P waves and QRS complexes. If QRS initiated by focus in the bundle of His, the QRS is narrow. QRS initiated more distally are wide and slow rate (~ 30 beats/min).

Look for other signs of cause, e.g. ischaemia.

CXR: Cardiac enlargement, pulmonary oedema.

Blood: TFT, digoxin level, cardiac enzymes, troponin.

Echocardiogram: Wall motion abnormalities, aortic valve disease, vegetations.

M: **Chronic block:** Permanent pacemaker insertion is recommended in patients with third-degree heart block, advanced Mobitz type II and symptomatic Mobitz type I.
Acute block (e.g. secondary to MI): If associated with clinical deterioration, IV atropine and consider temporary (external) pacemaker.

C: Asystole. Cardiac arrest. Heart failure. Complications of any pacemaker inserted.

P: Mobitz type II and third-degree block usually indicate serious underlying cardiac disease.

Hepatitis, autoimmune

D: Liver inflammation associated with autoantibodies.

A: Unknown, although genetic predisposition and autoimmune pathogenesis likely. Four subtypes classified according to autoantibodies.
Type I: High titres of antinuclear (ANA) and antismooth muscle (ASM) antibodies.
Type II: High titres of antiliver/kidney microsomal antibodies (anti-LKM).
Type III: Antisoluble liver antigen.
Type IV: No autoantibodies described.

A/R: Associated with *HLA-DR3* and *HLA-DR4*, other autoimmune conditions or family history of autoimmune disease (e.g. diabetes mellitus Type I, vitiligo). Also associated with keratoconjuctivitis sicca, renal tubular acidosis, peripheral neuropathy.

E: Eight times more common in females. Age is 20–40 years, with type II more common in children.

H: May be asymptomatic and discovered incidentally by abnormal LFT.
Insidious onset: Malaise, fatigue, anorexia, weight loss, nausea, jaundice, ammenorrhoea, epistaxis.
Acute hepatitis (25 %): Fever, jaundice, nausea, vomiting, diarrhoea, RUQ pain, anorexia. Some may also present with serum sickness (e.g. arthralgia, polyarthritis, maculopapular rash).
It is important to take a full history to rule out other potential causes of liver disease (e.g. alcohol, drugs).

E: Stigmata of chronic liver disease, e.g. spider naevi (see Cirrhosis).
Ascites, oedema and encephalopathy are late features.
Cushingoid features (e.g. rounded face, cutaneous striae, acne, hirsuitism) may be present even before the administration of steroids.

P: Uncertain. It is thought that an environmental trigger (e.g. viral infection) leads to hepatocyte expression of HLA antigens which then become the focus of a principally T-cell-mediated autoimmune attack. The raised titres of ANA, ASM and anti-LKM are not thought to directly injure the liver. The chronic inflammatory changes are similar to those seen in chronic viral hepatitis with lymphoid infiltration of the portal tracts and hepatocyte necrosis, leading to fibrosis and, eventually, cirrhosis.

I: **Blood:** *LFT:* ↑↑ AST and ALT, ↑↑ γ-GT, ↑ AlkPhos, ↑ bilirubin, ↓ albumin in severe disease.
Clotting: ↑ PT in severe disease.
FBC: Mild ↓ Hb, also ↓ platelets and WCC from hypersplenism if portal hypertension present.
Auto-antibodies: Hypergammaglobulinaemia is typical (polyclonal gammopathy) with the presence of ANA, ASM or anti-LKM autoantibodies.
Liver biopsy: Needed to establish the diagnosis. Shows interface hepatitis or cirrhosis.
Other investigations: To rule out other causes of liver disease, e.g. viral serology (hepatitis B and C) caeruloplasmin and urinary copper (Wilson's disease), ferritin and transferrin saturation (haemochromatosis), α_1-antitrypsin (α_1-antitrypsin deficiency) and antimitochondrial antibodies (primary biliary cirrhosis).
Ultrasound, CT or MRI of liver and abdomen: To visualize structural lesions.
ERCP: To rule out primary sclerosing cholangitis.

M: **Medical:** Immunosuppression with steroids (e.g. prednisolone), followed by maintenance treatment with gradual reduction in dose (treatment is often long term). Azathioprine may be used in the maintenance phase as a steroid-sparing agent with frequent monitoring of LFT and FBC.
Surgical: For those with end-stage disease, liver transplant may be indicated.

C: Fulminant hepatic failure. Cirrhosis and complications of portal hypertension (e.g. varices, ascites). Hepatocellular carcinoma. Side-effects of corticosteroid treatment.

P: 35–50 % remain in remission when immunosuppression is withdrawn. 50 % require lifelong maintenance. 5-year survival rate is 85 % if treated and 50 % if untreated. 5-year survival after liver transplantation is > 80 %.

Hepatitis, viral: A and E

D: Hepatitis caused by infection with the RNA viruses, hepatitis A (HAV) or hepatitis E virus (HEV), that follow an acute course without progression to chronic carriage.

A: HAV is a picornavirus and HEV is a calicivirus. Both are small non-enveloped single-stranded linear RNA viruses of ~7500 nucleotides, with transmission by the faecal–oral route.

A/R: Poor sanitation, contaminated water, poor food hygiene with contaminated shellfish a cause of food-borne HAV, travel to endemic countries, sewage workers, outbreaks in families, institutions (e.g. schools). Hepatitis E can be very severe in pregnant women (fatality rate ~20 %).

E: HAV is endemic in most of the developing world, infection often occurs subclinically, especially in children. In the developed world, better sanitation means that seroprevalence is lower, age of exposure ↑ and hence is more likely to be symptomatic. Annual UK incidence is 5000 cases (seroprevalence ~5 %). HEV is endemic in Asia, Africa and Central America, tending to occur in epidemics.

H: Incubation period for HAV or HEV is 3–6 weeks.
Prodromal period: Malaise, anorexia (distaste for cigarettes in smokers), fever, nausea and vomiting.
Hepatitis: Prodrome followed by dark urine, pale stools and jaundice lasting ~3 weeks. Occasionally, itching and jaundice last several weeks in HAV infection (owing to cholestatic hepatitis).

E: Pyrexia, jaundice, tender hepatomegaly, spleen may be palpable (20 %). Absence of stigmata of chronic liver disease, although a few spider naevi may appear, transiently.

P: Both viruses replicate in hepatocytes and are secreted into bile. Liver inflammation and hepatocyte necrosis is caused by the immune response, with targeting of infected cells by $CD8^+$ T cells and natural killer cells. Histology shows inflammatory cell infiltratation (neutrophils, macrophages, eosinophils and lymphocytes) of the portal tracts, zone 3 necrosis and bile duct proliferation.

I: **Blood:** LFT (↑↑ AST and ALT, ↑ bilirubin, ↑ AlkPhos), ↑ ESR. In severe cases, ↓ albumin and ↑ platelets.
Viral serology:
Hepatitis A: Anti-HAV IgM (during acute illness, disappearing after 3–5 months), anti-HAV IgG (recovery phase and lifelong persistence).
Hepatitis E: Anti-HEV IgM (↑ 1–4 weeks after onset of illness), anti-HEV IgG. Hepatitis B and C viral serology is also necessary to rule out these infections.
Urinalysis: ↑ Urobilinogen, ↑ bilinogen.

M: **Medical:** No specific management. Bed rest and symptomatic treatment (e.g. antipyretics, antiemetics). Colestyramine for severe pruritus. Corticosteroids may help resolve prolonged cholestatic symptoms.
Prevention and control:
Public health: Safe water, sanitation, food hygiene standards. Both are notifiable diseases. Personal hygiene and sensible dietary precautions when travelling.

Immunization (HAV): Passive immunization with IM human immunoglobulin is only effective for a short period. Active immunization with killed HAV vaccine offers safe and effective immunity for those travelling to endemic areas, high-risk individuals (e.g. residents of institutions).
At present, there is no effective vaccine for HEV.

C: Fulminant hepatic failure develops in 0.1 % cases of HAV, 1–2 % of HEV but up to 20 % in pregnant women. Cholestatic hepatitis with prolonged jaundice and pruritus may develop after HAV infection.
Posthepatitis syndrome: Continued malaise for weeks to months after LFT returning to normal.

P: Recovery is usual within 3–6 weeks. Occasionally, a relapse during recovery. There are no chronic sequelae. Fulminant hepatic failure carries an 80 % mortality.

Hepatitis, viral: B and D

D: Hepatitis caused by infection with hepatitis B virus (HBV) which may follow an acute or chronic (defined as viraemia and hepatic inflammation continuing > 6 months) course.
Hepatitis D virus (HDV), a defective virus, may only co-infect with HBV or superinfect persons who are already carriers of HBV.

A: HBV is an enveloped, partially double-stranded DNA virus. Transmission is by sexual contact, blood and vertical transmission. Various viral proteins are produced including core antigen (HBcAg), surface antigen (HBsAg) and *e* antigen (HBeAg). HBeAg is a marker of increased infectivity.
HDV is a single-stranded RNA virus coated with HBsAg, resembling satellite viruses found in plants.

A/R: Hepatitis B infection is associated with IV drug abuse, unscreened blood and blood products, infants of HBeAg positive mothers and sexual contact with HBV carriers. Risk of persistant HBV infection varies with age, with younger individuals—especially babies—more likely to develop chronic carriage. Genetic factors are associated with increased rates of viral clearance.

E: Common. 350 million worldwide infected with HBV, 1–2 million deaths annually. Common in South East Asia, Africa and Mediterranean countries. HDV also found worldwide. HBV is relatively uncommon in the UK.

H: Incubation period 3–6 months.
1–2 week *prodrome* of malaise, headache, anorexia, nausea, vomiting, diarrhoea, RUQ pain.
May experience serum-sickness-type illness (e.g. fever, arthralgia, polyarthritis, urticaria, maculopapular rash).
Jaundice then develops with dark urine and pale stools.
Recovery is usual within 4–8 weeks. 1 % may develop fulminant liver failure.
Chronic carriage may be diagnosed after routine LFT testing or if cirrhosis or decompensation develops.

E: **Acute:** Jaundice, pyrexia, tender hepatomegaly, splenomegaly, cervical lymphadenopathy in 10–20 %. Occasionally, urticaria/maculopapular rash.
Chronic: May have no findings, signs of chronic liver disease or decompensation.

P: Liver inflammation and hepatocyte necrosis caused by antibody and cell-mediated immune responses to viral replication. Histology can be variable, from mild to severe inflammation and changes of cirrhosis. HBsAg may give a 'ground glass' appearance to hepatocytes using certain tissue stains.

I: **Blood:** *Viral serology:*
Acute HBV: HbsAg positive, IgM vs. HbcAg.
Chronic HBV: HbsAg positive, IgG vs. HBcAg, HbeAg positive or negative (latter in precore mutant variant).
HBV cleared or immunity: anti-HBsAg positive, IgG vs. HBcAg.
HDV infection: detected by IgM or IgG vs. HDV.
PCR: Detection of HBV DNA is the most sensitive measure of ongoing viral replication.
LFT: ↑↑ AST and ALT. ↑ Bilirubin. ↑ AlkPhos.
Clotting: ↑ PT in severe disease.

Liver biopsy: Percutaneous, or transjugular if clotting is deranged or ascites is present.

M: **Prevention:** Blood screening, instrument sterilization, safe sex practices. *Passive immunization:* Hepatitis B immunoglobulin (HBIG) following acute exposure and to neonates born to HbeAg positive mothers (in addition to active immunization).

Active immunization: Recombinant HbsAg vaccine for individuals at risk and neonates born to HBV positive mothers. Immunization against HBV protects against HDV.

Medical: *Acute HBV hepatitis:* Symptomatic with bed rest, antiemetics, antipyretics, colestyramine for pruritus. Notification to the consultant in communicable disease control.

Chronic hepatitis: SC interferon-α (cytokine produced in response to viral infection which augments natural antiviral mechanisms). Side-effects include 'flu-like symptoms, fever, chills, myalgia, headaches, also bone marrow suppression, depression, necessitating discontinuation in 5–10 % of patients. Alternatively, oral lamivudine (nucleoside analogue). Others, e.g. adefovir, are under clinical trials.

C: Fulminant hepatic failure (1 %), chronic HBV infection (~10 % adults, much higher in neonates), cirrhosis and hepatocellular carcinoma, extra-hepatic immune complex disorders including glomerulonephritis, polyarteritis nodosa. Superinfection with HDV may lead to acute liver failure or more rapidly progressive disease.

P: In adults, 10 % infections become chronic and of these, 20–30 % will develop cirrhosis. Factors predictive of a good response to interferon include high serum transaminases, low HBV DNA, active histological changes and the absence of complicating diseases.

Hepatitis, viral: C

D: Hepatitis caused by infection with hepatitis C virus (HCV), often following a chronic course (~80 % cases).

A: HCV is a small enveloped single-stranded RNA virus of the flavivirus family. As it is an RNA virus, fidelity of replication is poor and mutation rates high, resulting in different HCV genotypes, and even in a single patient many viral quasi-species may be present. Transmission occurs via the parenteral route.

A/R: Recipients of blood and blood products prior to virus identification and screening in the early 1990s. IV drug users, non-sterile acupuncture and tattooing, those on haemodialysis and health care workers. Sexual and vertical transmission are uncommon (1–5 %, ↑ risk in those co-infected with HIV).

E: Common. Prevalence is 0.5–2 % in developed countries, with higher rates in certain areas (e.g. Middle East) because of poor sterilization practices. Different HCV genotypes have different geographical prevalence.

H: 90 % of acute infections are asymptomatic with < 10 % becoming jaundiced with a mild 'flu-like illness.
May be diagnosed after incidental abnormal LFT or in older individuals with complications of cirrhosis.
Occasional extrahepatic manifestations include:
- skin rash, caused by mixed cryoglobulinaemia causing a small vessel vasculitis; and
- renal dysfunction, caused by glomerulonephritis.

E: May be no signs or may be signs of chronic liver disease in long-standing infection.

P: Although HCV is hepatotrophic, it is not thought that the virus is directly hepatotoxic, rather that the humoral and cell-mediated response leads to hepatic inflammation and necrosis. On liver biopsy, chronic hepatitis is seen and a characteristic feature is lymphoid follicles in the portal tracts. Fatty change is also common and features of cirrhosis may be present. Transaminase levels bear little correlation to histological changes, hence biopsy is needed to assess the degree of liver damage and prognosis.

I: **Blood:** *HCV serology:* Anti-HCV antibodies, either IgM (acute) or IgG (past exposure or chronic).
Reverse-transcriptase PCR: Detection and genotyping of HCV RNA.
LFT: Acute infection causes ↑ AST and ALT, mild ↑ bilirubin. Chronic infection causes 2–8 times elevation of AST and ALT, often fluctuating over time. Sometimes normal.
Liver biopsy: To assess degree of inflammation and liver damage.

M: **Prevention:** Screening of blood, blood products and organ donors, needle exchange schemes for IV drug abusers, instrument sterilization. No vaccine available at present.
Medical: *Acute:* No specific management and mainly supportive (e.g. antipyretics, antiemetics, colestyramine). Notification of the consultant in communicable disease control.
Chronic: Recombinant SC interferon-α (a natural cytokine produced by the body in response to viral infection which augments natural antiviral mechanisms), either standard or pegylated formulations (prolongs $t_{1/2}$). Dose and duration of treatment depends on viral genotype. Side-effects (see Hepatitis, viral: B and D). Combination therapy with ribavarin (guanosine nucleotide analogue) results in a greater response rate.

C: Fulminant hepatic failure in acute phase (0.5 %), chronic HCV carriage, cirrhosis and hepatocellular carcinoma. Less common are porphyria cutanea tarda, cryoglobulinaemia, glomerulonephritis.

P: ~80 % exposed progress to chronic HCV infection and of these 20–30 % develop cirrhosis over 10–20 years.

Hepatocellular carcinoma

D: Primary malignancy of hepatocytes, usually occurring in a cirrhotic liver.

A: Gene mutation resulting in unregulated cell proliferation, probably because of chronic liver damage as a result of ↑ mitotic rate or toxins. In the case of chronic HBV, it is caused by incorporation of the viral genome into hepatocyte nuclear DNA. Mutations in the tumour suppressor gene *p53* are common.

A/R: Chronic HBV or HCV infection, cirrhosis (particularly that associated with alcohol), male gender, aflatoxin (*Aspergillus flavus* fungal toxin found on stored grains), anabolic and sex steroids.

E: 30 times less common than secondaries. Rare in West (1–2 in 100 000/year). One of most common malignancies of Asia and sub-Saharan Africa (up to 500 in 100 000/year). ♂ : ♀ = 4 : 1. Mean age is 50–60 years (in West), 30–40 years (in areas of high incidence). In rare fibrolamellar subtype, ♂ = ♀ and mean age 35 years.

H: Weight loss, anorexia, malaise, fever, RUQ pain.
Abdominal distention (ascites) usually in a patient with known chronic HBV, HCV or cirrhosis.
May present with complications or with symptoms caused by paraneoplastic effects.

E: Tender, irregular hepatomegaly.
Hepatic friction rub or bruit.
Signs of decompensated liver disease may be present (e.g. jaundice, encephalopathy; see Liver failure).
Signs of paraneoplastic manifestations.

P: Single or multiple nodules or diffusely infiltrative tumour within a (usually cirrhotic) liver parenchyma. If well-differentiated, carcinoma cells form a trabecular arrangement similar to that of normal liver but often tumour cells are poorly differenciated and anaplastic. The tumour may undergo haemorrhage and necrosis as a result of poor stromal support. Invasion, vascular and lymphatic, is common.

I: **Blood:** ↑ AFP (tumour marker that is often raised in up to 90 %), vitamin B_{12}-binding protein is a marker of fibrolamellar hepatocellular carcinoma. Biochemical evidence of paraneoplastic syndromes (e.g. ↓ glucose, ↑ Ca^{2+})
Abdominal ultrasound: Not sensitive for tumours < 1 cm.
Duplex scan of liver: May be used to demonstrate large vessel invasion (e.g. into hepatic or portal veins).
CT or MRI: Shows structural lesion.
Hepatic angiography: With lipiodol (an iodized oil taken up by the tumour).
Liver biopsy: Confirms histology of tumour but there is small risk of tumour seeding along biopsy tract.
Staging: CXR, CT thorax, radionuclide bone scan.
Screening: AFP and 6-monthly abdominal ultrasound in at-risk individuals.

M: **Surgery:** Surgical resection possible in < 10 % (40–50 % of fibrolamellar hepatocellular carcinoma), tumours must be small and localized. Liver transplantation if disease is small and localized to the liver. Tumour embolization may be carried out in the period prior to transplantation to reduce tumour growth.

Medical or interventional radiography: Usually palliative.
Systemic chemotherapy: (e.g. doxorubicin, cisplatin, carboplatin) in fibrolamellar hepatocellular carcinoma.
Local therapy: Percutaneous ethanol injection, microwave or radiofrequency ablation are approaches used. Tumour embolization with particles, chemotherapy agents or radiolabelled ^{131}I in lipiodol.

C: Liver decompensation, cachexia, tumour necrosis and pain; more rarely, rupture and intraperitoneal bleeding, paraneoplastic syndromes.

P: Poor (mean survival is months from diagnosis). After liver transplantation, 5-year survival rate is ~20 %.

Herpes simplex

D: Disease resulting from HSV1 or HSV2 infection.

A: HSV is an α herpes virus (dsDNA). Transmitted via close contact with an individual shedding the virus (e.g. kissing, sexual intercourse).

A/R: Close contact. Multiple sexual partners. Immunosuppression.

E: 90 % adults seropositive for HSV1 by 30 years. 35 % adults >60 years seropositive for HSV2. Over one-third of world population have recurrent HSV infections and are therefore capable of transmitting the disease.

H: **HSV1:** Primary infection is often asymptomatic. If symptomatic, can present with:

1 pharyngitis;
2 gingivostomatis, may make eating very painful; and
3 herpetic whitlow, inoculation of virus into a finger.

Recurrent infection/reactivation (herpes labialis/'cold sore'): prodrome (6 h) peri-oral tingling and burning. Vesicles appear (48 h duration), ulcerate and crust over. Complete healing 8–10 days.

HSV2: Very painful blisters and rash in genital, perigenital and anal area. Dysuria. Fever and malaise.

HSV encephalitis: Usually HSV1 (see Encephalitis).

HSV keratoconjunctivitis: Epiphoria (watering eyes), photophobia.

E: **HSV1 primary infection:** Tender cervical lymphadenopathy. Erythematous, oedematous pharynx. Oral ulcers filled with yellow slough (gingivostomatitis). Digital blisters/pustules (herpetic whitlow).

Herpes labialis: Perioral vesicles/ulcers/crusting.

HSV2: Maculopapular rash, vesicles and ulcers (external genitalia, anal margin, upper thighs), inguinal lymphadenopathy, pyrexia.

HSV encephalitis: (see Encephalitis).

HSV keratoconjunctivitis: Characterisitic lesion is a dendritic ulcer. May be visualized following staining with 1 % fluorescein.

P: Following primary viral infection the virus becomes dormant (classically in trigeminal or sacral root ganglia). Reactivation may occur in response to physical or emotional stresses or immunosuppression. The virus causes cytolysis of infected epithelial cells and vesicle formation.

I: Usually a clinical diagnosis and investigations are not warranted.

Vesicle fluid: Electron microscopy, PCR, direct immunofluorescence, growth of virus in tissue culture.

Diagnosis of HSV encephalitis (see Encephalitis)

M: Topical, oral or IV aciclovir (a nucleoside analogue phosphorylated by viral thymidine kinase to a monophosphate that, when converted to a triphosphate, causes chain termination of viral DNA synthesis). Valaciclovir is a prodrug of aciclovir with better bioavailability.

C: **Neonatal HSV:** Acquired during delivery. Skin vesicles, scarring eye disease, encephalitis. May be fatal. Treatment: caesarian section for mothers with active HSV infection. IV aciclovir to neonate.

HSV in immunocompromised: Severe local disease may disseminate involving the respiratory and GI tracts.

↑ Transmission of HIV in the presence of HSV2 genital lesions.

Erythema multiforme.

P: Infection is lifelong. Interindividual variation in frequency of reactivation. Tends to ↓ with ↑ age.

D: Infection with the HIV.

A: HIV is transmitted by:

1 *Sexual intercourse:* heterosexual is most common worldwide, but ↑ risk in homosexuals in the West.

2 *Blood (and other body fluids):* mother to child (intrauterine, childbirth or breastfeeding), needles (injecting drug users, health care workers), blood product transfusion, organ transplantation.

A/R: (see Aetiology).

E: Rising in Africa and Asia, >40 000 000 adults worldwide.

H & E: Three phases:

Seroconversion: (4–8 weeks postinfection), self-limiting: fever, night sweats, generalized lymphadenopathy, sore throat, oral ulcers, rash, myalgia, headache, encephalitis, diarrhoea.

Early/asymptomatic: (18 months to 15+ years), apparently well. Some patients may have persistent lymphadenopathy (>1 cm nodes, at 2+ extrainguinal sites for >3 months). Progressive minor symptoms, e.g. rash, oral thrush, weight loss, malaise.

AIDS: Syndrome of secondary diseases reflecting severe immunodeficiency or direct effect of HIV infection.

Direct effects of HIV infection:

Neurological: Polyneuropathy, myelopathy, dementia.

Lung: Lymphocytic interstitial pneumonitis.

Heart: Cardiomyopathy, myocarditis.

Haematological: Anaemia, thrombocytopenia.

GI: Anorexia, HIV enteropathy (malabsorption and diarrhoea), severe wasting.

Eyes: Cotton wool spots.

Some secondary infections arising from immunodeficiency:

Bacterial: Mycobacteria (lungs, GI, skin), e.g. *M. tuberculosis, M. avium intracellulare* (late), staphylococci (skin), *Salmonella*, capsulated organisms (*Streptococcus pneumoniae, Haemophilus influenzae*).

Viral: CMV (retinitis, oesophagitis, colitis, pneumonitis, adrenalitis, encephalitis), HSV (encephalitis), VZV (recurrent shingles), HPV (warts), papovavirus (progressive multifocal leucoencephalopathy with motor, intellectual and speech impairment), EBV (oral hairy leukoplakia on the side of the tongue).

Fungal: PCP, *Cryptococcus* (meningitis), *Candida* (oral, airway, genital, oesophageal), invasive aspergillosis.

Protozoal: Toxoplasmosis (cerebral abscess, chorioretinitis, encephalitis), cryptosporidia and microsporidia (diarrhoea).

Tumours: Kaposi's sarcoma (cutaneous or conjunctival vascular tumour caused by HHV8), squamous cell carcinoma (particularly cervical or anal), non-Hodgkin's B-cell lymphoma (brain, GI), Hodgkin's disease.

P: HIV enters the CD4 lymphocytes following binding of its envelope glycoprotein (gp120) to CD4 and a chemokine receptor. Reverse transcriptase (in viral core) reads RNA to manufacture DNA, which is incorporated into the host genome. Dissemination of virions lead to cell death and eventually to T-cell depletion.

I: **HIV testing** (after discussion and consent): HIV antibodies (usually positive by 12 weeks after exposure), PCR for viral RNA or incorporated proviral DNA. Monitor CD4 count and viral load.

Other investigations (as appropriate):
PCP: CXR bilateral perihilar/'ground glass' shadowing, bronchoalveolar lavage.
Cryptococcal meningitis: Brain CT or MRI, CSF microscopy (India ink staining), culture, ELISA for antigen.
CMV (colitis): Colonoscopy and biopsy (cytomegalic cells with inclusions).
Toxoplasmosis: Brain CT or MRI shows ring enhancing lesions.
Cryptosporidia/microsporidia: Stool microscopy.

M: **Highly active antiretroviral treatment (HAART):***
Two nucleoside reverse transcriptase inhibitors (e.g. zidovudine, lamivudine), plus either: one non-nucleoside reverse transcriptase inhibitor (e.g. nevirapine); or one protease inhibitor (e.g. ritonavir).
Aim for undetectable viral load and to increase CD4 counts. Test for resistance by genotyping.
Treatment of infections:
PCP: IV co-trimoxazole, steroids (severe cases).
Cryptococcus: IV amphotericin B or fluconazole and long-term oral fluconazole.
Aspergillus fumigatus: IV amphotericin B.
CMV: Ganciclovir.
Toxoplasmosis: Pyrimethamine and sulfadiazine, folinic acid.
Treatment of tumours:
Kaposi's sarcoma: Radiotherapy for localized and chemotherapy for systemic disease.
Social and psychological help.
Postexposure prophylaxis: 0.3 % risk without treatment. Triple therapy (4 weeks).
Prevention: Condoms and safe sex education, screening blood products, avoid sharing needles.

C: Complications of secondary infections, drug side-effects (e.g. myelosuppression with zidovudine, renal failure with amphotericin B, lipodystrophy with protease inhibitors), drug interactions (e.g. with TB treatments).

P: Viral load (plasma [HIV RNA]) and CD4 count are good predictors of disease progression, response to treatment and long-term prognosis.

*Indicated for CD4 count $< 350/mm^3$, rapidly falling CD4 count, rapidly rising viral load or serious symptomatic HIV-related illness. Treatment and pregnancy guidelines are available at the British HIV Association website, http://www.bhiva.org/guidelines.html

Huntington's disease

D: Autosomal dominant trinucleotide repeat disease characterized by progressive chorea and dementia, typically commencing in middle age.

A: The Huntington's disease (*HD*) gene is located on chromosome 4p and codes for the protein huntingtin. In the *HD* gene there is an extended trinucleotide repeat expansion (CAG) resulting in a toxic gain of function. The disease is inherited in an autosomal dominant pattern with full penetrance and exhibits anticipation (there is an earlier age of onset in each successive generation).

A/R: Family history. Parental consanguinity.

E: Worldwide prevalence 8 in 100 000. Average age onset 30–50 years.

H: Family history of Huntington's disease.
Insidious onset in middle age of progressive fidgeting and clumsiness, developing into involuntary, jerky, dyskinetic movements often accompanied by grunting and dysarthria.
Later in the course of the illness the patient may become rigid, akinetic and bed-bound.
Cognitive, emotional and behavioural changes followed by dementia.

E: Chorea and dysarthria.
Mental state examination reveals cognitive and emotional deficits.

P: **Anatomical:** Symmetrical atrophy of the striatum (particularly the caudate nuclei) and frontal cortex, with neuronal loss and an accompanying reactive gliosis.
Biochemical: General reduction in neurotransmitters in the basal ganglia (e.g. ↓ enzymes that synthesize ACh, GABA and GAD in the striatum. ↓ GABA, GAD, metenkephalin and ACE in the substantia nigra).

I: **Karyotype analysis:** Diagnostic if $\geq$ 38 CAG repeats in the *HD* gene.
Imaging: Brain MRI shows atrophy of the caudate nucleus and dilation of the lateral ventricles.
Electrophysiology: EEG shows slow wave α rhythms.

M: Genetic counselling of patient and relatives.
Psychological support.
Treatment of symptoms (e.g. antidepressants, antipsychotics), chorea may respond to phenothiazines.
Occupational therapy. Speech and language therapy.
Ultimately, the patient may require residential care.

C: 50 % of offspring will have Huntington's disease.

P: Death in 10–20 years after first onset of symptoms.

Hyperaldosteronism, primary

D: Characterized by autonomous aldosterone overproduction from the adrenal gland with subsequent suppression of plasma renin activity.

A: Excess aldosterone may be caused by adrenal adenomas (Conn's syndrome; 60 %) or bilateral adrenal hyperplasia (30 %).

A/R: Uncommon cause of hypertension.

E: Rare, ↑ prevalence in African-Americans. Adenomas are more common in females.

H: Usually asymptomatic and picked up on routine blood tests.
Symptoms of hypokalaemia: Muscle weakness, polyuria and polydipsia (nephrogenic diabetes insipidus secondary to hypokalaemia), paraesthesia, tetany.

E: Hypertension. Complications of hypertension (e.g. retinopathy).

P: **Pathophysiology:** Excess aldosterone results in:
1 ↑ Na and water retention causing hypertension;
2 ↑ renal K loss and hypokalaemia; and
3 suppression of renin because of NaCl retention.
Adrenal adenomas: Solitary, more common on the left, yellow cut surface.
Bilateral adrenal hyperplasia: Hyperplasia of zona glomerulosa-like cells interspersed with zona fasciculata nodules.

I: **Blood:** Plasma aldosterone (↑) and plasma renin activity (↓) (measured 2–5 weeks after stopping antihypertensives). *U&E:* ↑ Na^+, ↓ K^+.
CT or MRI (abdomen): Visualizes the adrenals.
Bilateral adrenal vein catheterization: Allows distinction between Conn's syndrome and bilateral adrenal hyperplasia by measuring adrenal vein aldosterone levels.
Adrenal scintigraphy: Allows distinction between Conn's syndrome and bilateral adrenal hyperplasia using ^{131}I or ^{75}Se-labelled aldosterone precursors. Unilateral uptake in Conn's and bilateral uptake in bilateral adrenal hyperplasia.
Diurnal and postural measurements of aldosterone and renin: Serum aldosterone, renin activity and cortisol are measured with patient recumbent at 8 a.m. The tests are repeated after 4 h of standing upright (at 12 noon). Allows distinction between Conn's syndrome and bilateral adrenal hyperplasia as adenomas are ACTH-sensitive and reduce aldosterone secretion from 8 a.m. until 12 noon, while hyperplastic adrenals respond to standing posture by increasing renin and aldosterone secretion.

M: **Conn's syndrome:** Surgery for removal of adenomas.
Bilateral adrenal hyperplasia: Aldosterone receptor antagonist (e.g. spironolactone) can be given but has notable side-effects such as impotence, gynaecomastia, menorrhagia. Alternatively, amiloride can be used.

C: Complications of hypertension (see Hypertension).

P: 70 % of patients with adrenal adenomas become normotensive 1 year after surgery.

Hyperlipidaemia

D: Elevation of one or more plasma lipid fractions.

A: **Primary:** Some have molecular genetic basis, but most are unknown.
Familial hypercholesterolaemia: ↓ Number of functional hepatic LDL receptors.
Familial hypertriglyceridaemia: Unknown. Autosomal dominant.
Hypertriglyceridaemia: Lipoprotein lipase or apo-CII deficiency.
Familial combined hyperlipidaemia: Unknown.
Remnant hyperlipidaemia: Apo-E2 genotype inheritance, accumulation of LDL remnants.
Secondary: Subdivided depending on the predominant abnormality.
↑ *Cholesterol:* Hypothyroidism, nephrotic syndrome, cholestatic liver disease, anorexia nervosa.
↑ *Triglycerides:* Diabetes mellitus, drugs (β-blockers, thiazides, oestrogens), alcohol, obesity, chronic renal disease, hepatocellular diseases.

A/R: Family history, diet (high fat and alcohol intake, low fibre), lack of exercise, conditions causing secondary hyperlipidaemia (see Aetiology).

E: 50 % of UK population have a cholesterol level high enough to be a risk for CHD .

H: Asymptomatic. Symptoms of CVS complications.
Enquire about other CVS risk factors: diabetes, family history, smoking, ↑ BP.

E: Usually normal. Examine for secondary causes.
Signs of lipid deposits: Around the eyes (xanthelasmas), cornea (arcus), tendons xanthomas (e.g. extensor tendons of the hands, Achilles tendon, patella tendon), tuberous xanthomas on knees and elbows, xanthomas in palmar creases (in remnant hyperlipidaemia), eruptive xanthomas and lipidaemia retinalis (pale retinal vessels) in severe hypertriglyceridaemia.
Signs of complications: e.g. ↓ peripheral pulses, carotid bruit, other cardiovascular risks: associated high BP.

P: LDL accumulates in intima of systemic arteries, taken up by LDL receptor on macrophages → formation of foam cell, part of atheromatous plaque. HDL acts as shuttle in periphery for transport of cholesterol esters back to the liver and is therefore cardioprotective.

I: **Blood:** Fasting lipid profile, exclude secondary causes: glucose, TFT, LFT, U&E.
Genotype analysis for possible primary aetiology.
Assess cardiovascular risk (other modifiable risk factors: smoking, BP, diabetes or insulin resistance, homocysteine levels). Various computer algorithms are available to calculate risk.
Check CK for patients on statins as they may very rarely cause rhabdomyolysis.

M: Treat secondary causes.
Advice: Exercise, lose weight, stop smoking, control BP, control diabetes, ↓ alcohol, dietary modification.
Lipid lowering drugs: Indicated for:

1 patients with multiple risk factors and no atherosclerosis (primary prevention) when risk for coronary heart disease > 20 % in 10 years (using Framingham scores *); and

*See back pages of *British National Formulary*.

2 those with any evidence of atherosclerosis, e.g. peripheral vascular disease, coronary heart disease, carotid artery disease and aortic aneurysms (secondary prevention).

(Guideline target: total cholesterol <5, LDL ≤ 3, triglycerides ≤ 2, HDL >1.)

↑ **LDL:** Statins (HMG-CoA reductase inhibitors) have been shown in a number of trials (e.g. '4S' trial) to lower mortality and CVS morbidity in hypercholesterolaemic high-risk coronary heart disease patients.

↑ **Triglycerides:** Fibrates (e.g. bezafibrate) stimulate lipoprotein lipase activity via specific transcription factors. Fish oil (Maxepa) is rich in omega-3 marine trigylcerides. (Note: it can aggravate hypercholesterolaemia.)

Other drugs: Anion-exchange resins (e.g. colestyramine, colestipol) bind bile acids and ↓ reabsorption, ↑ hepatic cholesterol conversion to bile acids and ↑ LDL receptor expression on hepatocytes.

Nicotinic acid: ↓ Hepatic VLDL release, ↓ triglycerides, ↓ cholesterol and ↑ HDL. Use is limited by side-effects (prostaglandin-mediated vasodilation, flushing, dizziness, palpitations). ↑ Glucose and urate.

C: Coronary artery disease, MI, peripheral vascular disease, strokes.
In hypertriglyceridaemia: pancreatitis and retinal vein thrombosis.

P: Depends on early diagnosis, treatment of hyperlipidaemia and control of other CVS risk factors. There is some evidence that lipid-lowering agents prevent cerebrovascular accidents.

D: **Primary:** ↑ Secretion of parathyroid hormone (PTH) unrelated to the plasma calcium concentration.
Secondary: ↑ Secretion of PTH secondary to hypocalcaemia.
Tertiary: Autonomous PTH secretion following chronic secondary hyperparathyroidism.

A: **Primary:** Parathyroid gland adenoma(s) or hyperplasia (80 % single adenoma, 18 % hyperplasia/multiple adenomas). Rarely, parathyroid carcinoma (2 %).
Secondary: Chronic renal failure, vitamin D deficiency.
Tertiary: Following chronic secondary hyperparathyroidism.

A/R: **Primary:** Multiple endocrine neoplasia (MEN),* neurofibromatosis, prior head and neck irradiation, postmenopausal women (five times increased risk).

E: **Primary:** Annual incidence is 5 in 100 000. Twice as common in females. Peak incidence 40–60 years.

H & E: **Hypercalcaemia:**
Bones: pain and fractures.
Stones: renal calculi, polyuria and polydipsia.
Groans: abdominal pain, nausea, constipation.
Moans: psychological depression, lethargy.
Primary: $\geq$50 % asymptomatic (exclude other causes of hypercalcaemia, e.g. sarcoidosis, malignancy, vitamin D excess).
Tertiary: Often only apparent when hypocalcaemia of secondary hyperparathyroidism treated (e.g. postrenal transplantation).
Hypocalcaemia (see Osteomalacia):
Muscle tetany.
Perioral paraesthesia.
Trousseau's sign.
Chvostek's sign.
Secondary: Ascertain cause, e.g. chronic renal failure, vitamin D deficiency.

P: **Primary:** Hypersecretion of PTH by parathyroid causes increases in bone resorption, renal tubular calcium reabsorption, 1α-hydroxylation of vitamin D and intestinal calcium absorption, leading to hypercalcaemia.
Secondary: Chronic hypocalcaemia (e.g. in chronic renal failure, secondary to ↓ vitamin D 1α-hydroxylation, ↓ tubular calcium reabsorption, bone PTH resistance) leading to compensatory hypersecretion of PTH.

I: **Blood:** *U&E:* Hyperchloraemic acidosis caused by PTH inihibition of renal tubular reabsorption of HCO_3^-. *Vitamin D:* May be ↓ in secondary disease. PTH, Ca^{2+}, albumin, PO_4^-, AlkPhos (see below).

	PTH	Ca^{2+} (corrected)	PO_4^-,	AlkPhos
Primary	↑	↑	↓	Normal
Secondary	↑↑	↓ or normal	↑	↑
Tertiary	↑	↑	↓	↑↑ (chronic osteomalacia)

*MEN type 1 (mutation in menin gene on chromosome 11): parathyroid adenoma or hyperplasia, pancreatic endocrine tumours, pituitary adenomas.
MEN type 2 (mutation in *RET* gene on chromosome 10): medullary thyroid carcinoma, phaeochromocytoma and either parathyroid hyperplasia (MEN-2A) or mucosal neuromas on the lips or tongue (MEN-2B).

In primary or tertiary hyperparathyroidism:
AXR: Renal calculi or nephrocalcinosis.
Hand X-ray radiograph: Subperiostial erosions of phalanges, brown tumours (osteolucent bone defects).
Skull X-ray radiograph: 'Pepper pot' skull (diffuse porotic mottling caused by demineralization).
Spine X-ray radiograph: Sclerosis of superior and inferior vertebral margins with central demineralization ('rugger jersey' spine).
Preoperative localization: ^{201}Th and ^{99m}Tc radioisotope subtraction scan of neck.

M: **Acute hypercalcaemia:**
Urgent IV fluid rehydration: Often 4–6 L/24 h.
Pamidronate infusion.
Corticosteroids: Not effective in hypercalcaemia caused by hyperparathyroidism but are sometimes helpful in sarcoidosis, myeloma and vitamin D excess.
Close monitoring: Temperature, pulse, respiratory rate, urine output, BP, sat O_2, ECG, U&E.
Treat the cause.
Primary or tertiary:
Surgical: Subtotal or total parathyroidectomy. Vitamin D to avoid post-operative hypocalcaemia. Indications for surgery include hypercalcaemia, previous episode of severe acute hypercalcaemia, hypercalciuria, marked symptoms (e.g. renal stones), impaired renal function.
Secondary:
Medical: Treat the underlying renal failure. Calcium and vitamin D supplements.

C: **Primary or tertiary:** Acute hypercalcaemia.
Secondary: Acute hypocalcaemia, acute pancreatitis (in 2 %).
Complications of surgery: Hypocalcaemia, recurrent laryngeal nerve palsy (< 1 %).

P: **Primary:** Surgery is curative for benign disease in most cases.
Secondary or tertiary: As for chronic renal failure.

D: Defined as systolic BP > 140 mmHg and/or diastolic BP > 85 mmHg measured on three separate occasions. Malignant hypertension is defined as BP ≥ 200/130 mmHg.

A: **Primary:** Essential or idiopathic hypertension (> 90 %).
Secondary:
Renal: Renal artery stenosis, chronic glomerulonephritis, chronic pyelonephritis, polycystic kidney disease, chronic renal failure.
Endocrine: Diabetes mellitus, hyperthyroidism, Cushing's syndrome, Conn's syndrome, hyperparathyroidism, phaeochromocytoma, congenital adrenal hyperplasia, acromegaly.
Cardiovascular: Aortic coarctation, ↑ intravascular volume.
Drugs: Sympathomimetics, corticosteroids, oral contraceptive pill.
Pregnancy: Pre-eclampsia.

A/R: Hypertension is one of the core cardiac and stroke risk factors. Essential hypertension may be associated with high alcohol intake, high sodium diet, insulin resistance, family history, obesity, poor exercise, low birth weight and stress.

E: Very common. 10–20 % of adults in the Western world.

H: Often asymptomatic.
Symptoms of complications (see Complications).
Symptoms of the cause.
Accelerated or malignant hypertension: Scotomas (visual field loss), blurred vision, headache, seizures, nausea, vomiting, acute heart failure.

E: Measure on 2–3 different occasions before diagnosing hypertension and record lowest reading.
There may be loud second heart sound, fourth heart sound.
Examine for end-organ damage, e.g. fundoscopy for retinopathy.
Keith–Wagner classification:
I 'Silver wiring'.
II As above, plus arteriovenous nipping.
III As above, plus flame haemorrhages and cotton wool exudates.
IV As above, plus papilloedema.
Examine for causes, e.g. radiofemoral delay (aortic coarctation), renal artery bruit (renal artery stenosis).

P: **Essential hypertension:** Fibrotic intimal thickening of the renal arteries, reduplication of elastic lamina, muscular hypertrophy and reduced kidney size. Arteriolar wall layers replaced by pink hyaline material with luminal narrowing (hyaline arteriosclerosis) leading to further hypertension.
Accelerated, malignant hypertension: Intimal cell proliferation and thickening in the renal arteries. Tunica medica and elastic lamina are largely unchanged. Fibrinoid necrosis of the arterioles causes renal damage, renin release and further hypertension.

I: **Blood:** U&E, glucose, lipids.
Urine dipstick: Blood and protein.
ECG: May show signs of left ventricular hypertrophy (deep S wave in V_{1-2}, tall R wave in V_{5-6}, inverted T waves in I, aVL, V_{5-6}, left axis deviation) or ischaemia.
Ambulatory BP monitoring (BP measured throughout the day): Excludes 'white coat' hypertension, allows monitoring of treatment response, assess preservation of nocturnal dip.

Others: Especially in patients <35 years or other suspected secondary cases (see relevant topics).

M: Assessment and modification of other cardiovascular risk factors.

Conservative: Stop smoking, lose weight, ↓ alcohol, reduce dietary Na^{+}.

Medical: *Treatment recommended for systolic BP ≥ 160 mmHg and/or diastolic BP ≥ 100 mmHg, or if evidence of end-organ damage. Other hypertension patients may still require treatment depending on other cardiac risk factors. Multiple drug therapies often necessary.

Thiazide diuretics (e.g. bendrofluazide): Recommended first line, especially in >60-year-olds.

β -Blockers: Recommended first line. Preferred in patients with previous MI or angina.

ACE inhibitors (e.g. ramipril): First line in diabetes, heart failure or left ventricular dysfunction.

Antigotensin II receptor antagonists: If ACE inhibitors not tolerated.

Ca^{2+} channel antagonists (e.g. nifedipine or amlodipine): Alternative to thiazide diuretics.

α-Blockers (e.g. doxazosin): First line in prostatism. May increase risk of heart failure.

Target BP:

$\leq$ 140/85 mmHg (non-diabetic).

$\leq$ 130/80 mmHg (diabetes without proteinuria).

$\leq$ 125/75 mmHg (diabetes with proteinuria).

Severe hypertension (diastolic BP $>$ 140 mmHg): Atenolol or nifedipine.

Acute malignant hypertension associated with encephalopathy, left ventricular failure or aortic dissection: IV sodium nitroprusside and/or β-blocker, or IV labetolol or IV hydralazine. Avoid very rapid lowering which can cause cerebral infarction.

C: Heart failure. Coronary artery disease and MI, CVA, peripheral vascular disease, emboli, retinopathy, renal failure, hypertensive encephalopathy, malignant hypertension.

P: Good, if blood pressure controlled. Uncontrolled hypertension linked with increased mortality (six times stroke risk and three times cardiac death risk). Treatment reduces incidence of renal damage, stroke and heart failure.

*See British Hypertension Society 1999 Guidelines and the National Service Framework for Coronary Heart Disease 2000 (available at http://www.prodigy.nhs.uk/ClinicalGuidance/ReleasedGuidance/).

Hyperthyroidism

D: Characterized by excess synthesis or release of thyroid hormones.

A: *Common:* Graves' disease (> 90 %).
Toxic multinodular goitre.
Toxic adenoma.
Thyroiditis (post-partum or de Quervain's thyroiditis, which is postviral).
Rare: Drugs (amiodarone, self-administration of T_4).
TSH-releasing tumours (↑ TSH).
Thyroid follicular carcinoma.
Choriocarcinoma (hCG is structurally similar to TSH).

A/R: Associated with autoimmune disorders and with *HLA-B8*, *DR3*, *DR4* and *DQ*.

E: Common. 1 % of population. ♀ : ♂ ~5 : 1. Peak incidence 20–40 years.

H: Heat intolerance, sweating, palpitations, anxiety and irritability.
Weight loss (despite good appetite), diarrhoea, pruritus.
Menstrual irregularities in females, ↓ libido, impotence in males.
Exertional dyspnoea (diaphragmatic weakness).
Graves' disease: Blurred vision, double vision, eye grittiness, eye protrusion, goitre.
de Quervain's thyroiditis: 'Flu-like illness, tender goitre.
Thyroid crisis: Hyperpyrexia, dehydration, tachycardia, restlessness, coma.

E: **General:** Slim, underweight, restless, irritable, sweating. There may be vitiligo.
Hands and arm: Warm, moist peripheries. Rapid or irregular pulse. Onycholysis, acropachy, palmar erythema, tremor, wide pulse pressure.
Ocular: Proptosis or exopthalmos (secondary to ↑ glycosaminoglycans from fibroblasts stimulated by cytokines).
Opthalmoplegia.
Optic nerve atrophy (caused by compression) or papilloedema.
Lid lag or retraction (caused by ↑ catecholamine sensitivity of levator palpebrae superioris).
Chemosis (conjunctival oedema) and ↑ tears.
Thyroid: Goitre or bruit.
Legs: Pretibial myxoedema (pink or purple plaques on the shins), proximal muscle weakness, hyper-reflexia.
Graves' disease: Thyroid acropachy (clubbing of digits with bony changes), periorbital oedema, proptosis.

P: **Graves' disease:** Plasma IgG to thyroid TSH receptor stimulates thyroid hyperplasia and thyroid hormone hypersecretion, causing exaggerated thyroid hormone action and autonomic overactivity.

I: **Blood:** *TFT:* Primary hyperthyroidism: ↑ T_4, ↑ T_3, ↓ TSH. Secondary hyperthyroidism: ↑ T_4, ↑ T_3, ↑ TSH.
Graves' disease: ↑ TSH receptor antibodies, ↑ microsomal and thyroglobulin antibodies.
Radioiodine (^{131}I) uptake scan: ↑ Uptake (diffuse in Graves'), absent uptake in de Quervain's.
MRI of orbit: Excludes orbital tumour in proptosis.

Note: in 'subclinical hyperthyroidism' TFT shows normal T_3, T_4 levels and ↓ TSH. There is long-term risk of atrial fibrillation and ↓ bone density.

M: **Acute thyroid crisis:** Prednisolone (inhibits peripheral conversion of $T_4 \rightarrow T_3$), propranolol, propylthiouracil or carbimazole. Oral iodine or iodide solution, rehydrate and control temperature. Treat the underlying cause.

Medical: Carbimazole or propylthiouracil (both inhibit thyroid peroxidase and hormone synthesis), β-blockers.

Radioactive iodine or surgery: For failure of drug treatment or if there are contraindications or complications.

Preoperative preparation: Patient must be euthyroid, stop propylthiouracil. Give oral potassium iodide and propranolol. Examination of vocal cords by ENT specialists. Patients may be hypothyroid postoperatively. Avoid pregnancy (4 months) and close contact with pregnant women and young children for 2 weeks after radioactive iodine therapy.

Dysthyroid eyes: Corneal protection (artificial tears or lateral tarsorrhaphy), surgery for realignment.

Advice: Carbimazole may cause agranulocytosis.

C: Thyrotoxic crisis, heart failure, osteoporosis, infertility, complications of surgery (recurrent laryngeal nerve palsy, hypothyroidism, hypoparathyroidism) or radioiodine (exacerbation of ophthalmopathy, hypothyroidism, recurrence).

P: 40 % single episode, others have a relapsing remitting course. Many eventually become hypothyroid.

D: Characterized by impairment of ovarian function.

A: **Primary hypogonadism (hypergonadotrophic):**
Gonadal dysgensis: Turner's syndrome (XO), XX and XY gonadal dysgensis (see Pathology).
Gonadal damage: Infection (e.g. mumps), autoimmune, surgery, radiation, drugs (e.g. cytotoxics).
Rare causes: Mutations in LH or FSH subunits, the receptors, enzymes involved in oestrogen synthesis (e.g. 17-hydroxylase deficiency), galactosaemia.
Secondary hypogonadism (hypogonadotrophic):
Pituitary or hypothalamic lesions: (see Hypopituitarism).
Genetic mutations: (see Hypogonadism, male).
Hyperprolactinaemia.
Systemic diseases: Cystic fibrosis, IBD, cirrhosis, chronic renal failure, malnutrition, thalassaemia (caused by regular blood transfusions).

A/R: (see Hypogonadism, male).

E: **Primary hypogonadism:** Responsible for 5 % of cases of anovulation and 10 % cases of amenorrhoea.
Secondary hypogonadism: Responsible for 40 % of cases of anovulation and > 50 % cases of amenorrhoea.
Risk of developing primary hypogonadism before 40 years ~0.6 %.

H: **Symptoms of oestrogen deficiency:** Night sweats, hot flush, vaginal dryness and dyspareunia.
↓ Libido, infertility.

E: **Prepubertal hypogonadism:**
Delayed puberty (primary amenorrhoea, absent breast development, no secondary sexual characteristics).
Eunuchoid proportions (e.g. long legs, ↑ arm span for height).
Postpubertal hypogonadism:
Regression of secondary sexual characteristics.
Loss of secondary sexual hair.
Breast atrophy.
Perioral and periorbital fine facial wrinkles.

P: In primary hypogonadism, karyotype analysis may show the following.
45 XO: One X chromosome (or occasionally part of it) is missing (Turner's syndrome).
46 XX: The cause of the defective ovarian development is not clear.
46 XY: Disruption of *SRY* gene on the Y chromosome, or its downstream pathway → genotypically male patients develop as undervirilized males or female patients, with abnormal gonads.
Mosaicism: XO/XY or XO/XX (variable phenotype).

I: **Blood:** Serum oestrogen/testosterone, SHBG, LH, FSH.
Investigations to determine the aetiology:
Primary: Karyotype, imaging of gonads (ultrasound, MRI), ovarian antibodies, ovarian biopsy.
Secondary: Pituitary function tests, 9 a.m. cortisol, TFT, MRI of brain, visual field testing, prolactin, smell tests for anosmia. Investigate for systemic diseases.

M: **Turner's syndrome:** (see Turner's syndrome).
Secondary hypogonadism in females: Treat the underlying cause.

To induce puberty: Low-dose ethinyloestradiol, gradually increasing dose over puberty. Simultaneously, give medroxyprogesterone acetate for first 2 weeks of each month.
In adults: Oestrogen/progesterone replacement (oral contraceptive pill).
To induce ovulation: Pulsatile GnRH or gonadotrophin replacement therapy (with pelvic ultrasound monitoring to avoid ovarian hyperstimulation).
Surgery: Surgical removal of gonads in patients with XY or XO/XY genotype caused by increased risk of neoplastic degeneration of the dysgenetic gonads.

C: Infertility. Unexpected pregnancy, complications of oestrogen deficiency: ischaemic heart disease, osteoporosis, thin skin, hair loss.

P: Good with early diagnosis and treatment. Prognosis varies with the underlying cause. Prognosis is poorer in those with anorexia nervosa.

D: Impaired testicular function and ↓ testosterone synthesis.

A: **Primary (hypergonadotrophic) hypogonadism:**
Gonadal dysgensis: Klinefelter's syndrome (XXY), undescended testes (cryptorchism).
Gonadal damage: Infection (e.g. mumps), torsion, trauma, autoimmune, surgery, radiation.
Rare causes: Mutations in LH or FSH subunits or their receptors, defects in enzymes involved in testosterone synthesis, myotonic dystrophy.
Secondary (hypogonadotrophic) hypogonadism:
Pituitary/hypothalamic lesions: (see Hypopituitarism).
*Genetic mutations.**
Hyperprolactinaemia.
Systemic/chronic diseases: Cystic fibrosis, malnutrition, malabsorption, chronic renal failure, Cushing's disease, thalassaemia (after regular blood transfusions).

A/R: Secondary hypogonadism may be seen in a number of rare syndromes.
Prader–Willi syndrome: Loss of a critical region on chromosome 15 causing obesity and short stature, small hands, almond-shaped eyes, learning difficulty/postnatal hypotonia.
Laurence–Moon–Biedl syndrome: Obesity, polydactyly, retinitis pigmentosa, learning difficulty.

E: Most common cause of primary hypogonadism is Klinefelter's syndrome (1 in 500–1000 live births).

H: ↓ Libido, impotence, infertility.

E: Measure testicular volume using Prader's orchidometer (ellipsoids of different sizes). Normal adult testicular volume is 15–25 mL.
Prepubertal hypogonadism:
Signs of delayed puberty (high-pitched voice, small or undescended testes, small phallus).
Eunuchoid proportions (continued growth of long bones secondary to delayed fusion of epiphyses).
Features of the underlying cause (e.g. cryptorchidism, anosmia in Kallmann's syndrome).
Postpubertal hypogonadism:
Regression of secondary sexual characteristics.
Scanty sexual (axillary/pubic) hair.
Gynaecomastia.
Soft and small testes, small phallus.
Fine perioral and perorbital facial wrinkles.

*Mutations that cause secondary hypogonadism:
KAL: Kallmann's syndrome (secondary GnRH deficiency and anosmia).
Isolated LH or FSH deficiency.
DAX 1: Secondary hypogonadism and CAH.
PROP 1: Absence of some pituitary hormones (GH, prolactin, TSH, LH, FSH).
PC1 (prohormone convertase 1): Secondary hypogonadism and defective prohormone processing.
HESX1: Associated with septo-optic dysplasia and pituitary hypoplasia.

P: **Primary:** Testosterone levels ↓ leading to a secondary rise in LH and FSH levels.

Secondary: Testosterone levels ↓ secondary to low LH and FSH levels.

I: **Blood:** Serum oestrogen or testosterone, LH and FSH.

Determine the site of defect:

Primary: Karyotyping, Imaging of gonads (ultrasound, MRI).

Secondary: Pituitary functional tests, SHBG, 9 a.m. cortisol), MRI of pituitary, visual field testing, prolactin, smell tests for anosmia.

M: **Primary hypogonadism:** To induce puberty and maintain secondary sexual characteristics: testosterone ester replacement therapy, gradually ↑ dose over puberty, monitor growth velocity and bone age.

Secondary hypogonadism: Treat the underlying cause. Induce puberty and maintain secondary sexual characteristics. Testosterone esters replacement therapy gradually ↑ dose over puberty. Monitor growth velocity and bone age. To induce testicular growth and spermatogenesis, use pulsatile GnRH therapy or gonadotrophin (hCG and FSH) replacement therapy.

C: Infertility (↓ sperm count), osteoporosis.

P: Normal life expectancy.

D: Deficiency of one or more of the hormones secreted by the anterior pituitary. Panhypopituitarism is deficiency of all pituitary hormones.

A: **Pituitary masses:** Most commonly adenomas. Other parapituitary tumours (e.g. craniopharyngioma, meningioma, glioma, metastases), cysts (arachnoid cyst, Rathke's cleft cyst).
Pituitary trauma: Radiation, surgery or skull base fracture.
Hypothalamus (functional): anorexia, starvation, severe exercise, weight loss.
Others: *Infiltration:* Tuberculosis, sarcoidosis, abscess, haemochromatosis, histiocytosis X.
Vascular: Pituitary apoplexy,* Sheehan's syndrome.†
Infection: Meningitis, encephalitis, syphilis (rare).
Genetic mutations: Pit-1 and *Prop-1* genes.

A/R: May be associated with 'empty sella syndrome' (enlarged sella turcica, not entirely filled by pituitary gland).

E: Annual incidence and prevalence of pituitary adenomas: ~1 in 100 000 and 9 in 100 000, respectively.

H & E: Symptoms and signs according to type of hormone deficiency.
GH: *Children:* Short stature (< third centile/not in keeping with parental height).
Adults: Low mood, fatigue, ↓ exercise capacity/muscle strength, ↑ abdominal fat mass.
LH or FSH: Delayed puberty.
Females: Loss of secondary sexual hair, breast atrophy, menstrual irregularities, dyspareunia, ↓ libido, infertility.
Males: Loss of secondary sexual hair, gynaecomastia, ↓ small or soft testes, ↓ libido, impotence.
ACTH: (see Adrenal insufficiency).
TSH: (see Hypothyroidism).
Prolactin: Absence of lactation (in Sheehan's syndrome).
Other symptoms or signs depending on aetiology (e.g. bitemporal hemianopia caused by a pituitary mass).
Pituitary apoplexy: Life-threatening hypopituitarism with headache, visual loss and cranial nerve palsies.

P: ↓ Synthesis, release, delivery of hypothalamic releasing or inhibiting factors to the pituitary or failure of secretion of pituitary hormone(s) despite adequate stimulation.

I: **Pituitary function tests:**
Basal tests: 9 a.m. cortisol, LH, FSH, testosterone, oestradiol, IGF-1, prolactin, free T_4 and TSH.
Dynamic tests (rarely performed): Insulin-induced hypoglycaemia (contraindicated in patients with epilepsy, IHD, hypoadrenalism). Give 0.15 U/kg IV insulin. In hypopituitarism, peak GH and cortisol response to insulin-induced hypoglycaemia are < 20 mU/L and < 550 nmol/L, respectively.
Short Synacthen test: (see Adrenal insufficiency).

*Pituitary apoplexy is the haemorrhage or infarction of a pituitary tumour.
†Sheehan's syndrome is pituitary infarction, haemorrhage and necrosis following post-partum haemorrhage.

MRI or CT of brain.
Visual field testing.

M: **Hormone replacement:**
Hydrocortisone: 20 mg in morning, 10 mg in evening (double oral dose for febrile illnesses, IM hydrocortisone at times of surgery). Should be provided with Medicalert bracelet and steroid card.
L-thyroxine: ~ 100 μg/day (always taken after hydrocortisone to avoid Addisonian crisis).
Sex hormones: Testosterone in males. Oestrogen ± progestogerone in females.
Growth hormone: SC 1.2 unit/day in adults. Children require specialist supervision.
In posterior pituitary deficiency: Desmopressin (vasopressin analogue) 10–20 μg/dayintranasally.
The patient must be monitored clinically.

C: Adrenal crisis, hypoglycaemia, myxoedema coma, infertility.
Osteoporosis; dwarfism (children).
Complications of the pituitary mass: Optic chiasm compression, hydrocephalus (third ventricular compression), temporal lobe epilepsy.

P: Lifelong hormone replacement.

D: The clinical syndrome resulting from thyroid hormone deficiency.*

A: **Primary** (↓ thyroid hormone production):
Acquired: Autoimmune (Hashimoto's thyroiditis).
Iatrogenic (post surgery, radioiodine, medication for hyperthyroidism).
Severe iodine deficiency or excess.
Drugs (e.g. lithium, amiodarone).
Congenital (cretinism):
Thyroid dysgenesis.
Iodine deficiency.
Dyshormogenesis (genetic deficiencies in thyroid hormone synthesis).
Secondary (< 5 % of cases):
Hypothalamic or pituitary disease: ↓ (TSH or TRH) and ↓ stimulation to thyroid hormone production.

A/R: Associated with other autoimmune diseases (e.g. Addison's disease, diabetes mellitus Type I, pernicious anaemia), vitiligo (depigmented skin patches caused by melanocyte destruction, seen in autoimmune diseases), POEMS syndrome.

E: Common. Prevalence is 10 in 1000. ♀ : ♂ ~6 : 1. Age of onset commonly > 40 years, but can occur at any age. Iodine deficiency is seen in mountainous areas (e.g. Alps, Himalayas).

H: Onset is usually insidious.
Cold intolerance, lethargy, weight gain, constipation, dry skin, hair loss, hoarse voice.
Mental slowness, depression, dementia, cramps, ataxia, paraesthesia.
Menstrual disturbances (irregular cycles, menorrhagia) in females.
History of surgery or radioiodine therapy for hyperthyroidism.
Myxoedema coma (severe hypothyroidism usually seen in the elderly): Hypothermia, hypoventilation, hypoglycaemia, hyponatraemia, heart failure, confusion and coma.

E: **Hands:** Bradycardia, cold hands.
Skin: Pale puffy face, periorbital oedema, loss of lateral eyebrows, hair loss, dry skin, vitiligo, large tongue.
Neck: Goitre.
Chest: Pericardial or pleural effusions.
Abdomen: Ascites.
Neurological: Slow relaxation of reflexes, carpal tunnel syndrome (see Carpal tunnel syndrome).

P: **Primary:** ↓ Secretion of thyroid hormone results in a compensatory increase in TSH.
Autoimmune: Cell- and antibody-mediated destruction of thyroid tissue, and can be either atrophic (thyroid gland is atrophic) or goitrous (with tissue regeneration following atrophy, resulting in a goitre).
Iodine deficiency: Iodine is essential for thyroid hormone synthesis.
Iodine excess (e.g. amiodarone): Causes reduced synthesis (Wolff–Chaikoff effect).
Secondary: (see Hypopituitarism).

*Subclinical hypothyroidism: normal serum free T_4 concentration and ↑ TSH. Risk of overt hypothyroidism is ~5 % risk per annum in those who are thyroid peroxidase antibody positive.

I: **Blood:** *TFT:* Primary: ↑ TSH and ↓ T_3/T_4. Secondary: ↓ TSH and ↓ T_3/T_4.
FBC: Normocytic anaemia.
U&E: May show ↓ Na^+.
Cholesterol: May be ↑.
Antithyroid antibodies: Against thyroglobulin and thyroid peroxidase. Not meaured routinely.
In suspected secondary cases: Pituitary function tests, pituitary MRI and TRH stimulation test.

M: **Myxoedema coma:** Oxygen, rewarming, IV T_3, IV hydrocortisone (in case hypothyroidism is secondary to hypopituitarism).
Chronic: L-thyroxine (25–200 µg/day). Rule out underlying adrenal insufficiency and treat before starting thyroid hormone replacement. Adjust dosage depending on TFT and clinical picture (monitor at 6 weeks). Thyroid function may take months to improve. In patients with ischaemic heart disease, start at low dose (25 µg/day) and gradually increase at 2–6 week intervals if ischaemic symptoms do not deteriorate.

C: Myxoedema coma, myxoedema madness (psychosis with delusions and hallucinations or dementia) in severe hypothyroidism (may be seen in the elderly after starting thyroxine treatment).

P: Lifelong thyroxine replacement therapy required. Myxoedema coma has 50 % mortality.

Immune thrombocytopenic purpura (ITP)

D: Syndrome characterized by immune destruction of platelets resulting in bruising or a bleeding tendency.

A: Often idiopathic. Acute ITP is usually seen after a viral infection in children, while the chronic form is more common in adults.

A/R: May be associated with infections (malaria, EBV, HIV), autoimmune diseases (e.g. SLE, thyroid disease), malignancies and drugs (e.g. quinine).

E: Acute ITP presents in children between 2 and 7 years. Chronic ITP is seen in adults, four times more common in ♀.

H: Easy bruising, mucosal bleeding, menorrhagia, epistaxis.

E: Visible petechiae, bruises (purpura or ecchymoses).
Typically, signs of other illness (e.g. infections, wasting, splenomegaly) would suggest other causes.

P: Autoantibodies that bind to platelet membrane proteins are produced, especially glycoprotein IIb/IIIa and Ib/IX in chronic ITP. This results in phagocytosis by macrophages of the reticuloendothelial system, especially as they pass through the spleen. Bone marrow megakaryocytes are not able to compensate for the extent of platelet loss and hence thrombocytopenia develops.

I: **Diagnosis of exclusion:** Exclude myelodysplasia, acute leukaemia, marrow infiltration.
Blood: FBC (↓ platelets), clotting screen (normal PT, APTT, fibrinogen), autoantibodies (antiplatelet antibody may be present but not used routinely for diagnosis, anticardiolipin antibody, antinuclear antibody).
Blood film: To rule out 'pseudothrombocytopaenia' caused by platelet clumping giving falsely low counts.
Bone marrow: To exclude other pathology. Normal or ↑ megakaryocytes.

M: **Medical:** Oral corticosteroids (IV in severe cases). Second-line therapy is IV infusion of immunoglobulin (IVIG). Platelet transfusions are usually contraindicated unless there is severe bleeding. In refractory cases, other immunosuppressants (e.g. azathioprine) may be used.
Surgery: Splenectomy has a 60 % cure rate in carefully selected patients.

C: Mucosal bleeding. Major haemorrhage is rare (< 1 %).

P: Usually self-limiting in children, with platelet counts recovering within 1–2 months.
ITP is less likely to resolve spontaneously in adults, but can be controlled medically in 60–90 % of cases.

Infectious mononucleosis

D: Infectious mononucleosis is the clinical syndrome caused by primary EBV infection. Also known as glandular fever or kissing disease.

A: EBV is a γ-herpes virus (dsDNA), present in pharyngeal secretions of infected individuals and is transmitted by close contact, e.g. kissing or sharing eating utensils.

A/R: (see Complications).

E: Common (UK annual incidence 1 in 1000).
2 age peaks: 1–6 years (usually asymptomatic) and 14–20 years.
$>$ 90 % adult population are EBV IgG positive.

H: Incubation period: 4–8 weeks.
May have abrupt onset: sore throat, fever, fatigue, headache, malaise, anorexia, sweating, abdominal pain.

E: Pyrexia.
Oedema and erythema of pharynx, fauces and soft palate, with white/creamy exudate on the tonsils which becomes confluent within 1–2 days, palatal petechiae.
Cervical/generalized lymphadenopathy, splenomegaly (50–60 %), hepatomegaly (10–20 %).
Jaundice (5–10 %), widespread maculopapular rash in patients who have received ampicillin.

P: **Pathogenesis:** EBV infection of the oropharyngeal epithelial cells leads to B cell infection with incorporation of the viral DNA into host DNA. Infected B cells disseminate and proliferate in lymphoid tissue throughout the body leading to lymphoid tissue enlargement. There is humoral (heteropile antibodies) and cellular (T cells or Downey cells) immune response resulting in atypical lymphocytosis and B cell lysis. EBV remains latent in lymphocytes. Reactivation may occur following physical or emotional stress or immunosuppression.

I: **Blood:** FBC (leukocytosis), LFT (↑ liver enzymes).
Blood film: Lymphocytosis ($>$ 20 % atypical lymphocytes).
Paul–Bunnell/Monospot test: Detects the presence of heterophile antibodies produced in response to EBV infection but are not actually against EBV antigens (10–15 % are heterophile Ab negative especially $<$ 14 years). ASO titres or bacterial throat swabs to exclude streptococcal tonsillitis.
Serology(rarely needed): IgM to EBV viral capsid antigen (VCA), IgG against VCA or EBNA (Epstein–Barr nuclear antigen).

M: **Medical:** Bed rest, aspirin gargle for sore throat, antipyretics. Corticosteroids may be indicated for severe cases (e.g. haemolytic anaemia, severe tonsilar swelling, obstructive pharyngitis).
Caution: Nearly 100 % of patients with infectious mononucleosis develop a widespread maculopapular rash when given amoxicillin or ampicillin.
Advice: Advise against contact sports for 2 weeks, as increased risk of splenic rupture (see Complications).

C: Lethargy for several months following the acute infection. Some postulate that chronic fatigue syndrome or myalgic encephalitis may be associated with EBV infection.
Respiratory: Airway obstruction by oedematous pharynx, secondary bacterial throat infections, pneumonitis.

Haematological: Haemolytic or aplastic anaemia, thrombocytopenia.
GI: Splenic rupture (caused by persistent splenomegaly), renal failure, fulminant hepatitis.
CNS: Guillain–Barré syndrome, encephalitis, viral meningitis, brachial plexitis.
EBV-associated malignancy: Burkitt's lymphoma (sub-Saharan Africa), nasopharyngeal carcinoma (China), post-transplant lymphoma, Hodgkin's lymphoma (usually mixed cellularity type).

P: Most make an uncomplicated recovery in 3–21 days. Immunodeficiency and death can occur very rarely.*

*Duncan's syndrome or X-linked lymphoproliferative (XLP) syndrome is the aberrant immune response to EBV leading to acute liver necrosis and permanent immunodeficiency. > 50 % of infected children die.

Infective arthritis

D: Joint inflammation resulting from articular infection.

A: **Bacteria:** *All ages: Staphylococcus aureus.*
< *4 years: Streptococcus pneumoniae* or *S. pyogenes, Neisseria meningitidis*, Gram-negative rods.
16–40 years: Mainly *Neisseria gonorrhoea*.
Mycobacterium tuberculosis can occur in any age group.
Viruses: Rubella, mumps, HBV, parvovirus B19.
Fungi: *Candida*.

A/R: Systemic infection allowing for haematogenous spread, orthopaedic procedures (particularly involving prosthetics), joint damage, osteomyelitis, diabetes, immunosuppression, alcoholism, IV drug abuse.

E: Most common in children and the elderly.

H: Excruciating joint pain, redness, swelling and loss of joint function. Usually affecting single large joint (polyarthritis in the immunosuppressed).
Fever.
TB arthritis is much more insidious and chronic.

E: Painful, hot, swollen and immobile joint with overlying erythema.
Severe pain prevents passive movement.
Pyrexia.
Look for signs of aetiology (e.g. small pustules near joint in *N. gonorrhoea*).

P: Joint can be infected directly (from bone in osteomyelitis) or indirectly (via haematogenous spread from another wound site). Multiplication in the synovium triggers an acute inflammatory response and attracts neutrophils. Neutrophil proteases destroy articular cartilage, while pus and inflammatory exudate leads to ↑ joint pressure and avascular necrosis of the cartilage.

I: **Joint aspiration** (very important): Aspirate is usually grossly purulent. Send synovial fluid for cytology, microscopy (for gout or pseudogout crystals), culture and sensitivity. PCR if suspected viral aetiology.
Blood: FBC (↑ WCC, ↑ neutrophils); ↑ CRP and ESR. Blood cultures for microscopy, culture and sensitivity. Viral serology may also be useful.
Plain radiographs: Affected joint may be normal early. Useful when assessing joint damage in later films.
Bone Scan: May highlight abscesses in bone.

M: Temporary joint immobilization with a splint. Analgesia. Immediate joint aspiration followed by antibiotic therapy (note that joint aspiration only provides symptomatic relief).
Medical: High-dose IV antibiotics for 7–14 days, then switch to oral for up to 4 weeks. A good starting empirical regimen would be flucloxacillin and fusidic acid. Change as appropriate once culture and sensitivity of aspirated synovial fluid is available. Viral arthritis is typically a self-limiting condition, no antiviral therapy required.
Physiotherapy: Best carried out as early as possible.

C: Septicaemia. Dislocation. Epiphyseal destruction in children. Ankylosis. Juxta-articular osteoporosis. Spinal cord compression in spinal tuberculosis (Pott's disease). Chronic osteomyelitis.

P: Complete recovery in 70 % of patients, especially with early appropriate antibiotic treatment. Full recovery may take several months. Risk of permanent joint damage in severe cases or if treatment is delayed.

D: Infection of intracardiac endocardial structures (mainly heart valves).

A: The endocardium can be colonized by virtually any organism, but the most common are as follow.

1. *Streptococci* (40 %): Mainly α-haemolytic *S. viridans* or *S. bovis*.
2. *Staphylococci* (35 %): *S. aureus* and occasionally *S. epidermis* (in IV drug users).
3. *Enterococci* (20 %): Usually *E. faecalis*.
4. *Other organisms:* HACEK (*Haemophilus, Actinobacillus, Cardiobacterium, Eikenella, Kingella*), *Coxiella burnetii, Histoplasma*.

A/R: Abnormal valves (e.g. congenital, post-rheumatic, calcification/degeneration), prosthetic heart valves, turbulent flow (e.g. patent ductus arteriosus or VSD), recent dental work, bacteraemia are known risk factors. *S. bovis* may be associated with GI malignancy.

E: Incidence 16–22 per million per year (UK).

H: Fever with sweats/chills/rigors (may be relapsing and remitting).
Inquire about recent dental surgery or IV drug abuse.
Malaise, arthralgia, myalgia, confusion (particularly in elderly).
Skin lesions.

E: Pyrexia, tachycardia, signs of anaemia.
Clubbing (if long-standing).
New murmur or muffled heart sounds (right-sided lesions may imply IV drug use). Splenomegaly.
Vasculitic lesions: Petechiae particularly on retinae (*Roth's spots*), pharyngeal and conjunctival mucosa; *Janeway lesions* (painless palmar macules, which blanch on pressure); *Osler's nodes* (tender nodules on finger/toe pads); *splinter haemorrhages* (nail-bed haemorrhages).

P: **Mechanism:** Vegetations form as a result of lodging of the organisms on the heart valves during a period of bacteraemia. These vegetations are made up of platelets, fibrin and infective organisms and are poorly penetrated by the cellular or humoral immune system as well as antibiotics. Vegetations proceed to destroy the valve leaflets, invade the myocardium or aortic wall leading to abscess cavities. Activation of the immune system also causes formation of immune complexes leading to cutaneous vasculitis, glomerulonephritis or arthritis.
Common sites: Mitral, aortic, tricuspid, pulmonary (in order of descending frequency).

I: **Blood:** FBC (↑ neutrophils, ↑ ESR and CRP, anaemia), U&E, rheumatoid factor positive.
Blood culture: At least three sets 1 h apart (ensure aseptic technique). Culture and sensitivity is vital, but empirical treatment should be started first.
Echocardiography: Transthoracic, transoesophageal sensitive for vegetations ≥ 1 cm.
Urinalysis: Microscopic haematuria, proteinuria.
Other investigations: ECG (abscesses can cause conduction changes), CXR (to exclude lung abscess).
Dukes' classification for diagnosis of endocarditis: (2 major, 1 major + 3 minor or all minor).
Major criteria:
Positive blood culture in two separate samples.

Positive echocardiogram (vegetation, abscess, prosthetic valve dehiscence, new valve regurgitation).
Minor criteria:
High grade pyrexia (temperature > 38°C).
Risk factors (abnormal valves, IV drug use, dental surgery).
Positive blood culture, but not major criteria.
Positive echocardiogram, but not major criteria.
Vascular signs.

M: **Medical:** Antibiotics (for 2 weeks if low-risk streptococcal infection, otherwise 4–6 weeks).*
On clinical suspicion: Benzylpenicillin + gentamicin (*Streptococci* and empirical treatment).
Streptococci: Continue above.
Staphylococci: Flucloxacillin/vancomycin + gentamicin.
Enterococci: Amoxicillin/ampicillin + gentamicin.
Future antibiotic prophylaxis, e.g. for dental procedures (individuals at risk).
Surgery: If poor response or deterioration, urgent valve replacement is indicated. In 'kissing' mitral valve vegetations, the mitral valve may be salvageable.

C: Valve incompetence, intracardiac fistulae or abscesses, aneurysm formation, heart failure, renal failure, glomerulonephritis, arterial emboli from the vegetations (brain, kidneys, lungs).

P: Fatal if untreated. 15–30 % mortality even when treated.

*See guidelines of the British Society of Antimicrobial Chemotherapy (1998) *Heart* **79**, 207–210.

Irritable bowel syndrome (IBS)

D: A functional bowel disorder defined as recurrent episodes (in the absence of detectable organic pathology) of abdominal pain/discomfort for >3 months of the previous year, associated with two of the following:
- relief with defecation;
- looser or more frequent stools; or
- harder or less frequent stools.

A: Unknown. Visceral sensory abnormalities, gut motility abnormalities, psychosocial factors (particularly stress), food intolerance (e.g. lactose) are all implicated.

A/R: Non-ulcer dyspepsia, chronic fatigue syndrome, psychological stress and affective disorders.

E: Common, prevalence 10–20 % of adults. More common in ♀ (2:1 ratio to ♂)

H: ≥3 month history abdominal pain (often colicky, in the lower abdomen and relieved by defecation or flatus).
Altered bowel frequency with ≥3 bowel motions daily or ≤3 motions weekly.
Abdominal bloating.
Change in stool consistency.
Passage with urgency or straining. Tenesmus.
Alarm symptoms (weight loss, anaemia or PR bleeding) are notably absent. Anyone >45 years with a change in bowel habit should be investigated to exclude colonic malignancy.

E: Normally nothing on examination. In some cases the abdomen may appear distended and be mildly tender to palpation in one or both iliac fossa.

P: Unknown. The most reproducible finding is a heightened visceral perception, demonstrated by balloon inflation in the ileum, colon and rectum causing discomfort or pain at lower pressures than in controls. This is postulated to result from a gut innervation anomaly or a CNS perceptual abnormality.

I: Diagnosis mainly by history.
Blood: FBC (for anaemia), LFT, ESR. Anti-endomysial antibodies (to exclude coeliac disease).
Stool examination: Microscopy and culture for parasites, cysts or other infective agents.
Endocscopy: Upper GI endoscopy, sigmoidoscopy or colonoscopy if other pathologies suspected.

M: **Advice:** Explanation and support with establishment of a positive doctor – patient relationship. Dietary modification (e.g. a higher fibre diet) may help with constipation, other approaches include exclusion diets and use of probiotics.
Medical: According to the predominant symptoms: antispasmodics (e.g. mebeverin), prokinetic agents (e.g. domperidone, metoclopramide), antidiarrhoeals (e.g. loperamide), laxatives (e.g. lactulose), low-dose tricyclic antidepressants (anticholinergic and may ↓ visceral awareness).
Psychological therapies: Often beneficial (e.g. cognitive – behavioural therapy, relaxation and psychotherapy).

C: Physical and psychological morbidity. ↑ Incidence of colonic diverticulosis.

P: A chronic relapsing and remitting course, often exacerbated by psychosocial stresses.

Ischaemic colitis

D: Inflammation of the colon caused by decreased colonic blood supply.

A: Occlusion of large vessels by thrombosis, embolism or iatrogenic ligation (particularly in abdominal aortic aneurysm surgery) or low flow states (hypovolaemia). In younger patients may be caused by small vessel vasculitis, vasospasm (e.g. cocaine) or hypercoagulable states.

A/R: Atherosclerosis, atrial fibrillation, history of cardiovascular or peripheral vascular disease, hypertension. Often associated with mesenteric vascular insufficiency (↓ blood flow to the small bowel).

E: Most commonly in the elderly (60–80 years) with equal gender distribution.

H: Symptoms may be acute or chronic in onset.
Crampy abdominal pain, may be post-prandial ('gut claudication') giving 'food fear'.
Fever, nausea, bloody diarrhoea (severe cases).

E: There may be a paucity of signs or symptoms.
Abdominal distension and tenderness, local peritonism (worse on left).
Fever and tachycardia, depending on severity of insult.
Proctoscopy typically shows normal rectal mucosa with blood from a higher source.

P: Ischaemia of the colonic mucosa and submucosa leads to early mucosal oedema, capillary dilation with inflammation, haemorrhage, necrosis and ulceration. The splenic flexure, the watershed between superior and inferior mesenteric artery territories, is the most common area affected.

I: **Blood:** FBC (↑ WCC), ↑ CRP, clotting screen (useful to exclude any coagulopathy).
AXR: Large bowel wall thickening or diffuse dilation, air in bowel wall or venous system.
CXR (erect): Air under diaphragm in cases of perforation.
Barium enema: 'Thumb printing' of colonic wall and ulceration (dangerous if there is a risk of perforation as barium is very irritant; gastrograffin contrast may be used as an alternative).
Endoscopy: To determine the source or site of bleeding. Upper GI endoscopy to rule out other causes of GI bleeding, colonoscopy will reveal mucosal erythema, friability and ulceration (potentially dangerous as colon can easily perforate).
CT: Thickening of colonic wall, irregular lumen, intramural air, portal or mesenteric venous air, occlusion in larger blood vessels.
Angiography: May be normal or show attenuated flow or site of occlusion.

M: **Medical:** *Conservative management:* IV fluids, nil orally, broad-spectrum antibiotics that cover enteric bacteria (e.g. cephalosporin and metronidazole). Specific treatment of the cause of the vascular insufficiency.
Surgical: Colonic resection may be required in cases of gangrenous or perforated bowel.
Long-term: Follow-up colonoscopy is used to assess recovery or stricture formation.

C: Acute ischaemia can lead to gangrene, perforation, sepsis and, occasionally, toxic megacolon or pyocolon. Chronic ischaemia can cause stricture formation with intestinal obstruction.

P: Outcome depends on severity, extent and timing of ischaemic insult. The majority of cases settle with conservative measures.

D: Group of systemic inflammatory disorders affecting children < 16 years old. Main types are as follow.
Pauci-articular onset: 4 or less joints involved (~ 50 %).
Polyarticular onset: > 4 joints involved (~ 30–40 %).
Systemic onset (Still's disease): Fever, rash and arthritis (~ 10–15 %).

A: Unknown. An autoimmune disease, possibly triggered by cross-immunity between an infectious agent in a genetically susceptible individual.

A/R: **Pauci-articular:** HLA types *B27*, *DR5*, *DR8*.
Polyarticular: *DR1*, *DR4*
Systemic: *DR4*.

E: Annual incidence is 16 in 100 000. Prevalence is 10–100 in 100 000. More common in females.

H: **Pauci-articular:** Young child with a limp or swollen joint (usually painless). Most commonly affecting the knee, then elbow, ankle and wrist.
Polyarticular: Older children (12–16 years) with painful symmetrical small joint swelling of insidious onset.
Systemic: Unwell, fever with rash, typically in evening returning to normal in morning for at least 2 weeks, painful joints.

E: **Pauci-articular:** Swollen joint. Systemically well. There may be uveitis and irregular pupil (posterior synechiae).
Polyarticular: Symmetrical small-joint swelling.
Systemic: Pyrexia (usually > 39.5°C), migratory salmon rash on trunk or thighs, Koebner phenomenon (rash developing following skin trauma), signs of arthritis, lymphadenopathy and organomegaly (up to 75 %).

P: Joint synovitis, villous hypertrophy and inflammatory infiltrate of lymphocytes (CD4 T-cells), plasma cells and macrophages. Features are fairly similar to adult rheumatoid arthritis.

I: Exclude infection, malignancy, rheumatic fever.
Blood: FBC (anaemia of chronic disease, ↑ WCC, ↑ platelets), ↑ ESR and CRP, ↑ ferritin in systemic onset, rheumatoid factor (10 % positive in polyarticular), antinuclear antibodies (40–70 % positive in pauci-articular).
Joint aspiration: Microscopy and culture.
Joint radiographs: Show soft-tissue swelling in early disease.

M: **Multidisciplinary approach** (involving paediatrician, rheumatologists, physiotherapists, occupational therapists, orthopaedic surgeons and opthalmologists): Treatment aims to relieve pain, preserve joint function, to prevent disability and complications and maintain normal growth and psychosocial development. Low doses of NSAIDs and paracetamol (for pain and stiffness). Corticosteroids, methotrexate, azathioprine, cyclophosphamide for systemic disease. Anti-TNFα treatment in polyarticular disease.

C: Poor developmental growth. Joint destruction requiring joint replacement.
Pauci-articular: Poor visual acuity, glaucoma, blindness.
Systemic: Serositis with pericardial involvement, pleurisy and pulmonary fibrosis.
Complications associated with treatment: (especially steroids).

P: Up to 50 % may have long-term disability. Death may occur as a result of pericarditis, amyloidosis or infection.
Pauci-articular: 80 % well after 15 years.
Polyarticular: If rheumatic factor positive, rheumatoid arthritis frequently develops as adults.
Systemic: Onset may last several years before remitting.

Klinefelter's syndrome

D: The constellation of symptoms and signs in a male with supernumerary X chromosome(s), most commonly 47 XXY.

A: Non-disjunction during the meiotic division of gametogenesis.

A/R: Increasing maternal age. In 60 % of cases, the error of disjunction is of maternal origin.

E: Common. 0.1–0.2 % of live male births.

H: **Childhood:** Mild learning difficulties, slow verbal development, clumsiness.
Failure of pubertal development and ↓ libido.

E: Tall stature (with relatively long legs, arm span > height).
Gynaecomastia.
Small, firm 'pea-like' testes, small penis.
Secondary sexual hair is sparse and in a female distribution (female escutcheon).
High-pitched voice.

P: The extra X chromosome(s) leads to seminiferous tubule dysgenesis and shortened lifespan of germ cells. By adulthood, Sertoli and germ cells are absent. There is an increased number of Leydig cells with ↓ function. The circulating testosterone levels are low and LH levels are raised (hypergonadotrophic hypogonadism).
Micro: Tubular atrophy, hyalinization, fibrosis and consequent azoospermia.

I: **Prenatal diagnosis:** Amniocentesis or chorionic villus sampling.
Postnatal: Buccal smear of squamous cells show Barr bodies.*
Karyotype analysis on peripheral blood lymphocytes.
Blood: Testosterone and dihydrotestosterone levels (↓), LH and FSH (↑), adrenal androgens (normal), oestradiol (↑).
Screen for complications (e.g. bone density scan).
Children: Psychosocial support for future development.

M: **Medical:** Testosterone ester replacement therapy (IM, oral or transdermal patch).
Advice: Counselling to address psychological issues.
Surgical: Correction of gynaecomastia, insertion of testicular prostheses into scrotum.

C: *Infertility.*
Malignancy: Increased risk of breast cancer (20 times > non-Klinefelter's men), germ cell tumours, bronchial cancer, acute lymphocytic leukaemia.
Autoimmune endocrinopathies (e.g. diabetes mellitus Type I and hypothyroidism).
Osteoporosis, obesity.
Mental retardation and subnormal IQ.

P: Life expectancy depends on the diagnosis and management of complications.

*Barr bodies are nuclear inclusion bodies representing inactivation of one of the two X chromosomes (normally seen only in females).

Leukaemia, acute lymphoblastic (ALL)

D: Malignancy of the bone marrow and blood characterized by the proliferation of lymphoblasts (primitive lymphoid cells).

A: Lymphoblasts (arrested at an early stage of development with varying cytogenetic abnormalities, gene mutations and chromosome translocations) undergo malignant transformation and proliferation, with subsequent replacement of normal marrow elements, leading to bone marrow failure and infiltration into other tissues.

A/R: **Environmental:** Radiation, viruses.
Genetic: Down's syndrome, Fanconi's anaemia, achondroplasia, ataxia telangiectasia, xeroderma pigmentosum, X-linked agammaglobulinaemia, ↑ risk in siblings.

E: Most common malignancy of childhood. Peak age of onset is 3–7 years, second peak in the elderly. Annual UK incidence is 1 in 70 000.

H: **Symptoms of bone marrow failure:** Anaemia (fatigue, dyspnoea), bleeding (spontaneous bruising, bleeding gums, menorrhagia), opportunistic infections (bacterial, viral, fungal, protozoal).
Symptoms of organ infiltration: Tender bones, enlarged lymph nodes, mediastinal compression (in T-cell ALL), meningeal involvement (headache, visual disturbances, nausea).

E: **Signs of bone marrow failure:** Pallor, bruising, bleeding, infection (e.g. fever, GI, skin, respiratory systems).
Signs of organ infiltration: Lymphadenopathy, hepatosplenomegaly, cranial nerve palsies, retinal haemorrhage or papilloedema on fundoscopy, leukaemic infiltration of the anterior chamber of the eye (mimics hypopyon), testicular swelling.

P: Subclassified using FAB (French–American–British) classification based on lymphoblast morphology:
L_1 Small lymphoblasts, scanty cytoplasm.
L_2 Larger, heterogenous lymphoblasts.
L_3 Large lymphoblasts with blue or vacuolated cytoplasm.

I: **Blood:** FBC (normochromic normocytic anaemia, ↓ platelets, variable WCC), ↑ uric acid, ↑ LDH, clotting screen.
Blood film: Lymphoblasts evident.
Bone marrow aspirate or trephine biopsy: Hypercellular with > 30 % lymphoblasts.
Immunophenotyping: Using antibodies for cell surface antigens to classify the cells into (e.g. CD20).
Cytogenetics: Karyotyping chromosomal abnormalities or translocations.
Cytochemistry: B- and T-lineage cells show up with PAS stain and acid phosphatase, respectively.
Lumbar puncture (and CSF analysis): For CNS involvement.
CXR: May show mediastinal lymphadenopathy, thymic enlargement, lytic bone lesions.
Bone radiographs: Mottled appearance with 'punched-out' lesions (e. g. skull caused by leukaemic infiltration).

M: **Medical:** Combination chemotherapy.
Remission induction: Prednisolone, vincristine, L-asparaginase (3–4 weeks).
Intensification or consolidation: Addition of cytosine arabinoside, daunorubicin.

Prophylaxis of CNS involvement: Intrathecal methotrexate, cranial irradiation now rarely used.
Maintenance (2–3 years): 6-mercaptopurine, methotrexate, vincristine or prednisolone.
Stem cell transplantation.
Supportive care: Antiemetics, central venous access (many chemotherapy agents need a central vein), blood product replacement, infection prophylaxis, counselling (especially in children, but also family).

C: **Secondary to treatment:** Tumour lysis syndrome (see AML).
Long-term sequelae of chemotherapy: Cardiotoxicity, fertility problems, malignancy (intracranial tumours, non-Hodgkin's lymphoma).

P: Childhood ALL has a 70 % cure rate, but adult ALL only has ~30 % cure rate.
Poor prognosis: Age (< 2 years, > 10 years), males, ↑ WCC, cytogenetics: translocation (4,11), translocation (9,22), CNS involvement at presentation.
Good prognosis: Translocation (12,21).

Leukaemia, acute myeloblastic (AML)

D: Malignancy of primitive myeloid lineage white blood cells (myeloblasts) with proliferation in the bone marrow and blood.

A: Myeloblasts, arrested at an early stage of development, with varying cytogenetic abnormalities (e.g. gene mutations and chromosome translocations), undergo malignant transformation and proliferation, with subsequent replacement of normal marrow elements, bone marrow failure.

A/R: AML can be primary or arise from myeloproliferative or myelodysplastic disease or previous chemotherapy.

E: Most common acute leukemia in adults. Incidence ↑ with age.

H: **Symptoms of bone marrow failure:** Anaemia (lethargy, dyspnoea), bleeding (thrombocytopenia or DIC), opportunistic or recurrent infections.

Symptoms of tissue infiltration: Gum swelling or bleeding, CNS involvement (headaches, nausea, diplopia), especially with M4 and M5 variants.

E: **Signs of bone marrow failure:** Pallor, cardiac flow murmur, ecchymoses, bleeding, opportunistic or recurrent infections (e.g. fever, mouth ulcers, skin infections, PCP).

Signs of tissue infiltration: Skin rashes, gum hypertrophy, deposit of leukaemic blasts may rarely be seen in the eye (chloroma), tongue and bone, in the latter may cause fractures.

P: Classified using the FAB (French–American–British) system into eight morphological variants M0–M7.

M0 Myeloblastic with no maturation.
M1 Myeloblastic with little maturation.
M2 Myeloblastic with maturation.
M3 Promyelocytic with coarse cytoplasmic granules. Characteristic Auer rods (crystallization of granules resembling bundle of sticks or 'faggots'). Associated with DIC.
M4 Granulocytic and monocytic differentiation (myelomonocytic).
M5 Monoblastic differentiation.
M6 Erythroblastic differentiation.
M7 Megakaryoblastic.

I: **Blood:** *FBC:* ↓ Hb, ↓ platelets, variable WCC.

↑ Uric acid, ↑ LDH, clotting studies, fibrinogen and D-dimers (when DIC is suspected in M3).

Blood film: AML blasts may show cytoplasmic granules or Auer rods (see Pathology).

Bone marrow aspirate or biopsy: Hypercellular with >30% blasts (immature cells).

Immunophenotyping: Antibodies against surface antigens to classify lineage of abnormal clones.

Cytogenetics: For diagnostic and prognostic information.

Cytochemistry: Myeloblasts granules are positive for Sudan black, chloroacetate esterase and myeloperoxidase, monoblasts are positive for non-specific and butyrate esterase.

M: **Emergency** (if DIC): FFP and platelet transfusions (see Disseminated intravascular coagulation).

Chemotherapy: Combination cytotoxic chemotherapy (e.g. cytosine arabinoside, daunorubicin, etoposide (topoisomerase inhibitor)). In the M_3 variant, all *trans*-retinoic acid is given as it induces differentiation of the cells involved.

Stem cell transplantation.

Supportive care: Central venous access, blood products, treatment and prophylaxis of infection.

C: Relapse, sequelae of chemotherapy: infertility, cardiotoxicity, malignancy. Tumour lysis syndrome (rapid cell death with initiation of chemotherapy may precipitate renal failure) is preventable with good hydration and allopurinol.

P: Prognosis depends on age. Overall cure rate is 40–50 % in < 60-year-olds on chemotherapy, but may be higher with bone marrow transplantation. 5–10 % long-term survival in > 60-year-olds.

Good prognosis: t(8,21) in M2, t(15,17) in M3, inversion 16 in M4 (70–90 % cure rate).

Poor prognosis: Monosomy 5, monosomy 7 and complex karyotypes (10–30 % cure rate).

Leukaemia, chronic lymphocytic (CLL)

D: Malignancy characterized by proliferation of small lymphocytes (relatively mature but poorly functioning) in the bone marrow and blood. There is an overlap between CLL and non-Hodgkin's lymphomas.

A: Aetiology is unknown but cell accumulation in blood, bone marrow, liver, spleen and lymph nodes is thought to be caused by impaired programmed cell death (apoptosis). Loss-of-function mutation in *P2X7* gene, encoding a pro-apoptotic protein, has recently been suggested to contribute to the pathogenesis of CLL.
Most common chromosomal changes include trisomy 12, 11q and 13q deletions.

A/R: No clearly defined risk factors.
Associated with autoimmune phenomena: haemolytic anaemia (10 %), thrombocytopenia or a combination of both (Evan's syndrome).

E: 90 % are > 50 years, ♂ > ♀. Rare in Asians.

H: **Asymptomatic:** Up to 40–50 % diagnosed on routine blood count.
Systemic symptoms: Lethargy, malaise, night sweats.
Symptoms of bone marrow failure: Recurrent infections (bacterial, viral, fungal), herpes zoster, easy bruising or bleeding (e.g. epistaxis).

E: Non-tender lymphadenopathy (often symmetrical), hepatomegaly, splenomegaly.
Later stages, signs of bone marrow failure: pallor, cardiac flow murmur, purpura/ecchymoses.

P: Immunophenotyping shows the malignant cell to be a relatively mature B cell with weak surface expression of monoclonal (κ or λ light chain only) IgM or IgD. Anaemia may be caused by bone marrow infiltration, hypersplenism or autoimmune haemolysis. T-cell variants of CLL are much rarer but more aggressive. Hairy cell leukaemia is a low-grade CLL variant with good prognosis showing monoclonal proliferation of 'hairy' B cells in blood, bone marrow and liver.

I: **Blood:** FBC (gross lymphocytosis, $5 - 300 \times 10^9$/L, anaemia, ↓ platelets), ↓ serum immunoglobulins.
Blood film: Shows small lymphocytes with thin rims of cytoplasm and smudge/smear cells.
Bone marrow aspirate or biopsy: Lymphocytic replacement (25–95 %) of normal marrow elements.
Special: Immunophenotyping (see Pathology), cytogenetics (provides some prognostic information).
CT scan: To stage disease.
Staging:
Rai:
0 Lymphocytosis.
I Above, plus lymphadenopathy.
II Above, plus organomegaly (hepatomegaly or splenomegaly).
III Above, plus anaemia (Hb < 10 g/dL).
IV Above, plus thrombocytopenia (platelets 100×10^9/L).
Binet:
A < 3 lymphoid areas (neck/axilla/groin lymph nodes, liver or spleen involvement).
B > 3 lymphoid areas.
C Anaemia and/or thrombocytopenia.

M: **Early stage:** Watch and wait, no survival benefit for treatment of early slowly progressive disease.
Symptomatic treatment in progressive disease: Traditionally, oral chlorambucil (alkylating agent), more recently IV purine analogue 2-chlorodeoxyadenosine or fludarabine (side-effect: ↓ CD4 cell count hence co-trimoxazole prophylaxis).
Other: Prednisolone for autoimmune phenomena. Immunoglobulin replacement. Antibiotic prophylaxis, blood products, splenectomy (in massive splenomegaly and hypersplenism). Monoclonal antibodies (anti-CD52, anti-CD20).
If transformation to Non-Hodgkin's lymphoma: Chemotherapy (see Lymphoma, non-Hodgkin's).
Stem cell transplantation: Allogeneic or autologous.

C: 10–15 % transform into a localized high-grade non-Hodgkin's lymphoma (Richter's transformation) or prolymphocytic leukaemia.*

P: Wide variation in prognosis, best for early stage disease. Not considered curable except in younger patients in whom a bone marrow transplant may be curative.

*Prolymphocytic leukaemia is characterized by larger malignant cells with prominent nucleoli, very high lymphocyte count, massive splenomegaly with little lymphadenopathy. Poor response to treatment.

D: Chronic myeloblastic leukaemia is a malignant clonal disease characterized by proliferation of granulocyte precursors in the bone marrow and blood, distinguished from AML by its slower progression.

A: Malignant proliferation of stem cells with characteristic (95 % of cases) chromosomal translocation t(9;22) resulting in the Philadelphia (Ph) chromosome. Variants include Ph-negative CML, chronic neutrophilic leukaemia and eosinophilic leukaemia.

A/R: Exposure to ionizing radiation is a risk factor.

E: Incidence increases with age, mean 40–60 years. Four times more common in males.

H: Asymptomatic in up to 40–50 % and is diagnosed on routine blood count.
Hypermetabolic symptoms: Weight loss, malaise, sweating.
Symptoms of bone marrow failure: lethargy, dyspnoea, easy bruising, epistaxis (infection is rare).
Abdominal discomfort and early satiety.
Occasionally presents with gout or hyperviscosity symptoms (visual disturbance, headaches, priapism).
May present during *blast crisis* with symptoms of AML or ALL.

E: *Splenomegaly:* Most common physical finding (90 %).
Signs of bone marrow failure: Pallor, cardiac flow murmur, bleeding or ecchymoses.

P: The Ph chromosome results in the fusion of the genes *BCR* and *ABL*. This results in transcription of a 210-kDa protein (BCR-ABL) with enhanced tyrosine kinase activity which drives cell replication.
Three phases: Relatively stable chronic phase of variable duration (average of 4–6 years) which transforms into an accelerated phase (3–9 months) and then an acute leukaemia phase (blast transformation).

I: **Blood:** FBC (grossly ↑ WCC, ↓ Hb, ↑ basophils/eosinophils/neutrophils, ↑ platelets but may be normal or ↓). Also ↑ uric acid, ↓ neutrophil alkaline phosphatase, ↑ vitamin B_{12} and B_{12}-binding protein (transcobalamin I).
Blood film: Shows immature granulocytes in peripheral blood.
Bone marrow aspirate or biopsy: Hypercellular with raised myeloid : erythroid ratio.
Special: Cytogenetics to demonstrate Philadelphia chromosome.

M: **Chronic phase:** Hydroxyurea or interferon-α, with allopurinol to prevent hyperuricaemia and gout.
New treatments: Tyrosine kinase inhibitors: STI 571 is a inhibitor of BCR-ABL.
Stem cell transplantation: Allogeneic or autogenous.
Acute phase: (see Leukaemia, acute myeloblastic and Leukaemia, acute lymphoblastic).

C: Transformation into acute leukemia (80 % AML, 20 % ALL).

P: Prognostic staging system of Sokal distinguishes between good and poor risk groups based on age, spleen size, percentage of blasts in blood and platelet count. Overall mean survival 5–6 years, with main cause of death transformation into acute leukaemia. 20 % survive > 10 years.

Liver abscesses and cysts

D: Liver Infection resulting in a walled off collection of pus or cyst fluid.

A: **Pyogenic:** *Escherichia coli*, *Klebsiella*, enterococcus, bacteroides, streptococci, staphylococci.
Amoebic: *Entamoeba histolytica*.
Hydatid cyst: Tapeworm *Echinococcus granulosis*.
Other: Tuberculosis.

A/R: **Pyogenic:** 60 % caused by biliary tract disease (gallstones, strictures, congenital cysts), cryptogenic (15 %).
Amoebic/hydatid: Foreign travel.

E: **Pyogenic:** Incidence 0.8 in 100 000, mean age 60 years, most common liver abscess in industrialized world.
Amoebic: Most common type worldwide (10 % of world's population have been infected).
Hydatid disease: common in sheep-rearing countries.

H: Fever, malaise, anorexia, night sweats, weight loss.
RUQ or epigastric pain, which may be referred to shoulder (diaphragmatic irritation). Jaundice, diarrhoea, pyrexia of unknown origin.

E: Fever (continuous or spiking), jaundice.
Tender hepatomegaly, right lobe affected more commonly than left.
Dullness to percussion and decreased breath sounds at right base of lung, caused by reactive pleural effusion.

P: **Pyogenic abscesses:** Typically polymicrobial, generated by an intense acute inflammatory response and are composed of neutrophils, macrophages, proteinaceous fluid and bacterial debris.
Amoebic abscesses: Contain 'anchovy sauce' fluid of necrotic hepatocytes and trophozoites.
Hydatid cysts: Grow slowly, can hold litres of fluid, produce tissue damage by mechanical means and contain millions of infective stages which are called hydatid sand (brood capsules and protoscolices).

I: **Blood:** FBC (mild anaemia, leukocytosis, ↑ eosinophils in hydatid disease), LFT (↑ AlkPhos, ↑ bilirubin), ↑ ESR, ↑ CRP, blood cultures, amoebic and hydatid serology.
Stool microscopy, cultures: For *E. histolytica* or tapeworm eggs.
Liver ultrasound or CT/MRI: Localizes structure of mass.
CXR: Right pleural effusion or atelectasis, raised hemidiaphragm.

M: **Pyogenic:** Percutaneous (under ultrasound or CT guidance) aspiration (if small sized) or catheter drainage (if moderate size) or surgical drainage (if large or multilocular abscesses). IV broad-spectrum antibiotics (e. g. ceftriaxone and metronidazole) then switch when sensitivities are known. Treatment of underlying cause.
Amoebic: Metronidazole and diloxanide furoate.
Hydatid: Surgical removal (pericystectomy) with mebendazole or albendazole to reduce risk recurrence.

C: Septic shock, rupture and dissemination (e.g. into biliary tract causing acute cholangitis, intrathoracic rupture or peritonitis), allergic sequelae or anaphylaxis on rupture hydatid cyst.

P: Untreated pyogenic liver abscesses often fatal, complications have high mortality, amoebic abscesses have a better prognosis and usually have a quick response to therapy, hydatid cysts may recur after surgery (10 %).

D: Severe liver dysfunction leading to jaundice, encephalopathy and bleeding diathesis.

Hyperacute liver failure: Jaundice with encephalopathy occurring in <7 days of onset.

Acute: Jaundice with encephalopathy occurring from 1 to 4 weeks of onset.

Subacute: Jaundice with encephalopathy occurring within 4–12 weeks of onset.

Acute-on-chronic: Acute deterioration (decompensation) in patients with chronic liver disease (see Cirrhosis).

A: **Viral:** Hepatitis A, B, D, E, 'non-A-E hepatitis'.

Drugs: Paracetamol overdose (see Paracetamol overdose), idiosyncratic drug reactions (e.g. anti-TB therapy).

Less commonly: Autoimmune hepatitis, Budd–Chiari syndrome, pregnancy-related, malignancy (e.g. lymphoma), haemochromatosis, mushroom poisoning (*Amanita phalloides*), Wilson's disease.

A/R: As above, paracetamol overdose is more dangerous in those who are malnourished or in those with experiencing liver enzyme induction caused by alcohol use or drugs such as phenytoin, barbiturates.

E: Can occur at any age, paracetamol overdose accounts for 50 % of acute liver failure in the UK.

H: The patient feels unwell, with fever, nausea and possibly jaundice.

Grading of encephalopathy:

Grade I Change of mood/behaviour.

Grade II Confusion, disorientation, drowsiness, slurred speech.

Grade III Incoherent speech, restlessness, stupor.

Grade IV Coma.

E: Jaundice, encephalopathy, liver flap (asterixis), fetor hepaticus ('pear drops' smell).

Ascites and splenomegaly (less common in acute or hyperacute).

Bruising or bleeding from puncture sites or GI tract.

Look for secondary causes (e.g. bronze skin colour, Kayser–Fleischer rings).

Pyrexia may reflect infection or liver necrosis.

Often no signs of chronic liver disease in acute liver failure.

P: **Pathogenesis of manifestations:**

Jaundice: ↓ Secretion of conjugated bilirubin.

Encephalopathy: ↑ Delivery of gut-derived products into the systemic circulation and the brain because of ↓ extraction of nitrogenous products of colonic bacteria by liver and portal systemic shunting. Ammonia and GABAergic transmission may play a part.

Bleeding diathesis: ↓ Synthesis of clotting factors, ↓ platelets (hypersplenism if chronic portal hypertension) or platelet functional abnormalities associated with jaundice or renal failure.

I: **Identify the cause:** Viral serology, paracetamol levels, autoantibodies (e.g. ASM, LKM antibody, immunoglobulins), ferritin, α_1-antitrypsin, caeruloplasmin and urinary copper (↓ and ↑, respectively in Wilson's disease).

Blood (in addition to above): *FBC:* ↓ Hb if GI bleed, ↑ WCC if infection. *U&E:* May show renal failure. Glucose, LFT (↑ bilirubin, transaminases, AlkPhos, γ-GT, ↓ albumin), ESR/CRP (inflammatory markers), coagulation screen (↑ PT, INR), ABG (to determine pH), group and save.

Ultrasound liver, CT scan: To image liver.

Ascitic fluid: Tap ascites and send for microscopy, culture, biochemistry (glucose, protein), cytology, > 250 neutrophil/mm^3 indicates spontaneous bacterial peritonitis.

Doppler scanning of hepatic or portal veins: To exclude Budd–Chiari syndrome.

Electroencephalogram: To monitor encephalopathy.

M: **Resuscitation** (according to airway, breathing, circulation): ITU care and specialist unit support essential.

Treat the cause if possible: *N*-acetylcysteine for paracetamol overdose, stop the suspected drug.

Monitor: Vital signs, PT, pH, creatinine, urine output and grade of encephalopathy.

Treatment/prevention of complications: Invasive ventilatory and cardiovascular support often required.

Encephalopathy: Lactulose and phosphate enemas.

Antibiotic and antifungal prophylaxis.

Hypoglycaemia treatment.

Coagulopathy treatment: IV vitamin K, FFP, platelet infusions if required.

Gastric mucosa protection: Proton pump inhibitors or sulcralfate.

Cerebral oedema: Nurse patient at 30°C, ↓ intracranial pressure by IV mannitol, hyperventilate.

Renal failure: Haemofiltration, nutritional support.

Avoid: Drugs metabolized by the liver or sedatives.

Surgical: King's College Hospital criteria for liver transplantation:

If due to paracetamol overdose:

- Arterial pH < 7.3, or
- PT > 100 s, creatinine > 300 µm and Grade III–IV encephalopathy.

For other causes (3 out of 5):

- Age < 10 or > 40 years.
- Bilirubin > 300 µm.
- Caused by non-A, non-E viral hepatitis or drugs.
- Interval from jaundice onset to encephalopathy > 7 days.
- PT > 100 s.

C: Infection, coagulopathy, hypoglycaemia, disturbances of electrolyte, acid–base and cardiovascular system, hepatorenal syndrome (concurrent hepatic and renal failure), cerebral oedema, ↑ intracranial pressure, respiratory failure.

P: Depends on the severity and aetiology of the liver failure, poor prognostic indicators are shown above under surgical management. The traditional prognostic score for surgical mortality is the Childs–Pugh score. See Cirrhosis.

D: Primary malignant neoplasm of the lung.
Three histological types: squamous cell carcinoma (35 %), adenocarcinoma (20 %) and large cell carcinoma (20 %).

A: Smoking is the leading cause of lung malignancies. Asbestos exposure. Adenocarcinomas are more common in non-smokers.

A/R: Occupational exposures (polycyclic hydrocarbons in petrochemical industry, nickel, chromium, cadmium, arsenic in metal refining and smelting, radon in miners), atmospheric pollution (urban > rural).

E: Most common fatal malignancy in the West. 35 000 deaths/year in the UK. ♂ : ♀ ~3:1 (mortality is increasing in women because of increasing numbers of female smokers).

H: May be asymptomatic and discovered on CXR (5 %).
Resulting from primary: Dyspnoea, new cough, a change in cough, haemoptysis, chest pain, recurrent pneumonia.
Systemic symptoms: Malaise, weight loss.
Resulting from local invasion: Brachial plexus (Pancoast's tumour) involvement causes shoulder and inner arm pain and can involve the sympathetic chain, left recurrent laryngeal nerve involvement (hoarseness and bovine cough), oesophagus (dysphagia).
Resulting from metastatic disease: Bone pain, pathological fractures, fits.
Paraneoplastic syndromes: (e.g. hypercalcaemia, neuromyopathies).

E: **Resulting from primary:** Fixed localized wheeze caused by partial obstruction of main airway, lymphadenopathy, signs of pleural effusion, lobar collapse or consolidation.
Resulting from local invasion: Superior vena cava compression (facial congestion, distension of neck veins, upper limb oedema). Brachial plexus (Pancoast's tumour) can cause wasting of the small muscles of the hand and Horner's syndrome (pupillary miosis, ptosis and facial anhydrosis).
Resulting from metastatic spread: Hepatomegaly, focal neurological signs, bone tenderness.
Resulting from paraneoplastic phenomena: Hypertrophic osteoarthropathy—clubbing, painful swollen wrists/ankles (periosteal new bone formation seen on X-ray).

P: **Macro:** Tumours usually arise in main or lobar bronchi. Adenocarcinomas tend to occur more peripherally.
Micro: Squamous cell carcinomas show keratin and intercellular bridges. Adenocarcinomas grow in tubular and papillary forms, produce mucin, and may arise in areas of old scarring. Bronchioloalveolar cell carcinoma spreads as cuboidal/columnar epithelium along the alveolar walls. Large cell tumours have abundant cytoplasm and large irregular nuclei.
Staging: Based on TNM system of tumour size, node involvement and presence of metastases.

I: **Sputum:** Cytology.
CXR: Coin lesions, lobar collapse, pleural effusion, features of lymphangitis carcinomatosis.*

*Lymphangitis carcinomatosis is the diffuse infiltration and obstruction of pulmonary parenchymal lymphatic channels by tumour. 80 % are caused by adenocarcinomas. CXR shows a reticulonodular opacification, but best seen with high-resolution CT. Very poor prognosis.

Bronchoscopy: Allows visualization of proximal tumours. Brushings or biopsy can be taken.
CT scan: Allows staging of tumour and planning for surgery. If peripheral, CT guided biopsy is possible.
Other: Lymph node biopsy, thoracoscopy, lung function tests.
Blood: FBC, U&E, Ca^{2+}, AlkPhos, LFT.

M: **Early:** Surgery may be curative (but < 20 % of patients eligible).
Non-operable: Combined modality therapy with radiotherapy and chemotherapy improves survival.
Palliative care: Laser therapy to bronchial tumours and endobronchial stents can prolong patency of bronchi. Management of complications and pain control.

C: Pneumonia, metastases to brain, bone, liver, adrenals, skin. Paraneoplastic syndromes.

P: Prognosis depends on stage, but generally poor.
Overall 5-year survival < 5 %. After resection for early stage disease ~25 %.

D: Malignant neoplasm of neuroendocrine Kulchitsky cells of the lung with early dissemination. Also known as oat cell carcinoma.

A: **Major:** Smoking.
Others: Occupational and environmental exposures (see Lung cancer, non-small cell)

A/R: **Associated with paraneoplastic syndromes:** Syndrome of inappropriate ADH secretion (SIADH in 7–10 % of patients), Cushing's syndrome (ACTH secretion, 1 %), Eaton–Lambert myaesthenic syndrome (< 1 %).

E: Accounts for 20 % of lung cancers.

H: May be asymptomatic with radiographical abnormality found.
Caused by primary tumour: Cough, haemoptysis, breathlessness, chest pain.
Caused by metastatic disease: Weight loss, fatigue, bone pain.
Caused by paraneoplastic syndromes: Weakness, lethargy, seizures, muscle fatiguability.

E: May be no signs or a fixed wheeze on auscultation of the chest.
Signs of lobar collapse or pleural effusion.
Signs of metastases, e.g. supraclavicular lymphadenopathy or hepatomegaly.
Signs of paraneoplastic syndrome.

P: **Staging:** Divided into limited (confined to one hemithorax and regional lymph nodes) and extensive disease (60 % at presentation).
Macro: Typically found around major bronchi, greyish tumours with areas of haemorrhage and necrosis, extend along lymphatics and spread into the lung parenchyma.
Micro: Sheets of uniform ovoid hyperchromatic cells with scanty cytoplasm that stain with neuroendocrine markers such as chromogranin, neurone-specific enolase, synaptopysin and have neurosecretory granules and neurofilaments on electron microscopy.

I: **Diagnosis:** Sputum cytology, bronchoscopy with brushings and biopsy or percutaneous biopsy, thoracoscopy.
Staging: CT of chest, abdomen and head. Isotope bone scan.
Other: Lung function tests, FBC, U&E, Ca^{2+}, Alkphos, LFT.

M: **Limited disease:** Combination chemotherapy and radiotherapy. Cisplatin and etoposide is a common regimen and chest irradiation results in a 5 % improvement in 3-year survival. Prophylactic cranial irradiation also improves survival in those who achieve a complete remission or have limited stage disease.
Extensive disease: Chemotherapy, e.g. cisplatin and etoposide.
Palliation: Radiotherapy to metastasis.

C: Pneumonia, superior vena caval compression.
Metastases: Most commonly to brain, liver, adrenals, skin.
Endocrine: Ectopic ACTH (gynaecomastia, Cushing's syndrome), ectopic ADH production (SIADH), hypercalcaemia (bony metastases or PTH-related peptide secretion).
Skin (more common in non-small cell tumours): Acanthosis nigricans (pigmented thickened skin in axilla or neck), herpes zoster, dermatomyositis, thrombophlebitis migrans. *See also* Lung cancer, non-small cell.

P: Poor. Even with limited disease, 5-year survival rate is only 15–20 %.

Lyme disease

D: Tick-borne spirochaete infection with clinical manifestations involving several organ systems including skin, joints, CNS and heart. Also known as Bannwarth's syndrome (particularly in European cases).

A: Spiral-shaped *Borrelia* bacteria. (USA: *B. burgdorferi*; Europe: *B. garinii*. or *B. afzelii*). Transmitted to humans by the bite of infected ticks (*Ixodes* species) whose normal hosts are small rodents, deer and pheasants.

A/R: Forestry/agricultural workers, outdoor activities in wooded or grassy areas in endemic areas.

E: Endemic in North America, Europe and Russia.

H: Skin rash (erythema migrans) present in 60–80 %, expanding out from site of tick bite (although most unaware of bite), with fever, malaise, headache, muscle or joint aches.
After days–weeks, disseminated disease causes secondary skin lesions, neurological manifestations: headache, neck stiffness, facial paralysis, numbness, migratory joint and muscle pain.
Late disseminated disease: joint swelling, personality change, sleep disorder, palpitations, syncope, fatigue.

E: Erythema migrans (annular flat erythematous lesion with demarcated border and central clearing).
Meningism (positive Kernig's sign).
Mononeuritis multiplex (VII nerve palsy, motor or sensory nerve palsies).
Cardiac arrhythmias (especially heart block).

P: *B. burgdorferi* resides in the gut of infected ticks and is transmitted when an infected tick feeds on a susceptible individual. The bacteria disseminate to certain target organs, with the resulting immune-mediated inflammatory response causing tissue damage and clinical manifestations. Autoimmune mechanisms may be responsible for late complications.

I: **Serology:** For diagnosis by ELISA or indirect fluorescent antibody testing on acute and convalescent serum samples. May be negative in early disease. PCR available in some laboratories.
Lumber puncture: Lymphocytosis.

M: **Prevention:** Protective clothing/footwear, prompt removal of ticks (if attached for < 24 h low likelihood of transmission), recombinant spirochaete's outer surface protein A vaccine is available for those at high risk but is unstable and only works in North American cases.
Medical: Antibiotic treatment based on clinical suspicion and rash, even if serology is negative. Oral amoxicillin or doxycyline in early disease for 2–3 weeks, later disease high-dose IV ceftriaxone for 4 weeks.

C: Atrioventricular conduction defects, myocarditis, encephalitis, post-Lyme disease syndrome (paraesthesias, fatigue, cognitive deficits), chronic arthritis, chronic skin disease (acrodermatitis chronicum atrophicans).

P: 20 % achieve remission after early disease, most develop other disease manifestations which generally resolve. Rarely fatal, one episode does not protect against reinfection.

Lymphoma, Hodgkin's

D: Lymphomas are neoplasms of lymphoid cells, originating in lymph nodes or other lymphoid tissues (see Lymphoma, non-Hodgkin's). Hodgkin's lymphoma (~15% of lymphomas) is diagnosed histopathologically by the presence of Reed–Sternberg cells (a cell of B lymphoid lineage).

A: Unknown. Likely to be a result of an environmental trigger in a genetically susceptible individual. EBV genome has been detected in ~50% of Hodgkin's lymphomas, but role in pathogenesis unclear.

A/R: Higher socioeconomic groups, occasionally familial aggregation, past history of infectious mononucleosis.

E: Bimodal age distribution, with peaks 20–30 years and >50 years. More common in males. Annual European incidence is 2–5 in 100 000.

H: Painless enlarging mass (most often in neck, occasionally in axilla or groin).
May become painful after alcohol ingestion.
'B' symptoms: Fevers >38°C (if cyclical referred to as Pel–Ebstein fever).
Night sweats.
Weight loss >10% body weight in last 6 months.
Other: Pruritus, cough or dyspnoea with intrathoracic disease.

E: Non-tender firm rubbery lymphadenopathy: cervical, axillary or inguinal.
Splenomegaly, occasionally hepatomegaly.
Skin excoriations.
Signs of intrathoracic disease (e.g. pleural effusion, superior vena cava obstruction).

P: **Histological subtypes:**
1 Nodular sclerosing (70%);
2 Mixed cellularity (20%);
3 Lymphocyte predominant (5%);
4 Lymphocyte depleted (5%).
The **Reed–Sternberg** cell is pathognomonic. It is a large cell with abundant pale cytoplasm and two or more oval lobulated nuclei containing prominent 'owl-eye' eosinophilic nucleoli (can appear as lacunar or 'popcorn' cells).

I: **Blood:** *FBC:* Anaemia of chronic disease, leucocytosis, ↑ neutrophils, ↑ eosinophils. Lymphopenia with advanced disease. ↑ ESR and CRP, LFT (↑ LDH, ↑ transaminases if liver involved).
Lymph node biopsy.
Bone marrow aspirate and trephine biopsy: Involvement seen only in very advanced disease.
Imaging: CXR, CT of thorax, abdomen and pelvis, gallium scan, PET scans.
Staging (Ann Arbor):
I Single lymph node region.
II Two or more lymph node regions on one side of the diaphragm.
III Lymph node regions involved on both sides of diaphragm.
IV Extranodal involvement (liver or bone marrow).
A Absence.
B Presence of B symptoms.
E Localized extranodal extension.
S Involvement of spleen.

M: **Stage I and IIA:** Radiotherapy (e.g. 'mantle' field above the diaphragm, 'inverted Y' below the diaphragm) with or without adjuvant chemotherapy.

Stage III and IV: Cyclical chemotherapy (e.g. ABVD regimen of Adriamycin, bleomycin, vinblastine and dacarbazine) with or without adjuvant radiotherapy.

Stem cell transplantation for relapsed disease.

C: *Secondary malignancy after treatment:* Acute myeloid leukaemia (1 % at 10 years), non-Hodgkin's lymphoma or solid tumours.

Inverted Y irradiation: Infertility, premature menopause, skin cancers.

Mantle irradiation: Adverse effects on thyroid, cardiac (accelerated coronary artery disease), pulmonary function (fibrosis), skin cancer.

P: **Stage I and II:** 80–90 % cure rate.

Stage III and IV: 50–70 % cure rate.

Prognosis less good with B symptoms, older age or lymphocyte-depleted type.

D: Lymphomas are malignancies of lymphoid cells originating in lymph nodes or other lymphoid tissues (see Lymphoma, Hodgkin's). Non-Hodgkin's lymphomas are a diverse group consisting of 85 % B cell, 15 % T cell and NK cell forms, ranging from indolent to aggressive disease and referred to as low, intermediate and high grades.

A: Probable environmental trigger in a genetically susceptible individual results in DNA mutations or translocations leading to uncontrolled proliferation of lymphoid cells.

A/R: Associated with inherited and acquired immunodeficiency syndromes (e.g. HIV), EBV, autoimmune disease. Known associations: HTLV-1 and adult T cell leukaemia or lymphoma, EBV and Burkitt's lymphoma, *H. pylori* and stomach MALT lymphomas, previous treatment with chemotherapy or radiotherapy.

E: Incidence increases with age. More common in the West. More common in males.

H: Painless enlarging mass (often in neck, axilla or groin).
Systemic symptoms (less frequent than in Hodgkin's): Fever $>38°C$, drenching night sweats, weight loss $>10\%$ body weight, symptoms of hypercalcaemia.
Symptoms related to organ involvement (extranodal disease is more common in non-Hodgkin's lymphoma than in Hodgkin's disease): Skin rashes, abdominal discomfort, sore throat, headache, testicular swelling.

E: *Painless firm rubbery lymphadenopathy:* Cervical, axillary or inguinal. Often only clinical sign.
Oropharyngeal (Waldeyer's ring of lymph nodes) involvement.
May present with abdominal mass.
Skin rashes: Mycosis fungoides (well-defined thickened indurated scaly plaque-like lesions with raised ulcerated nodules caused by cutaneous T-cell lymphoma) and Sezary's syndrome.
Hepatosplenomegaly.
Signs of bone marrow involvement (e.g. anaemia, infections or purpura).

P: Non-Hodkgin's lymphomas are classified according to the Revised American and European Lymphoma (REAL) classification based on clinical, biological and histological criteria.

I: **Blood:** FBC (anaemia, neutropenia and thrombocytopenia if bone marrow involved), ↑ ESR and CRP, LFT (↑ LDH, ↑ transaminases with liver involvement), Ca^{2+} (may be raised).
Blood film: Lymphoma cells may be visible in some patients.
Bone marrow aspirate and biopsy.
Other: Lymph node biopsy, immunophenotyping, cytogenetics.
Imaging: CXR, CT thorax, abdomen, pelvis.
Staging: As for Hodgkin's (less related to prognosis than histological type).

M: Depends on lymphoma subtype:
Aggressive:
Localized (stage I and II): Radiotherapy and adjuvant chemotherapy. Many regimens, e.g. CHOP (cyclophosphamide, hydroxy daunorubicin, oncovincristine and prednisolone).
Advanced: Chemotherapy followed by radiotherapy to sites of bulky disease.

Indolent: Conservative approach ('just watch and wait'). Single agent chemotherapy, radiotherapy or combined modality treatment.
Relapse: Autologous or allogeneic stem cell transplantation.

C: **Resulting from treatment:** Bone marrow suppression, nausea and vomiting, mucositis, infertility, tumour lysis syndrome, secondary malignancies.

P: Dependent on histological type. Other factors include age, stage, extranodal sites and LDH level.

D: Infection with protozoan *Plasmodium* (*P. falciparum, P. vivax, P. ovale* and *P. malariae*). The most serious is *P. falciparum*, which is potentially fatal.

A: The *Plasmodium* species are transmitted by the bite of the female *Anopheles* mosquito.
The protozoa infect RBCs and grow intracellularly. Haemolysis and release of pigment and inflammatory cytokines, e.g. TNF, produces the symptoms.

A/R: Certain groups have some innate immunity, such as sickle cell trait, thalassaemias, G6PD deficiency, pyruvate kinase deficiency and lack of Duffy RBC antigen.

E: Endemic in tropics. Affects 250 million people worldwide yearly.
There are about 2000 reported cases and 10 deaths caused by malaria (mainly *P. falciparum*) annually in the UK.

H: High degree of clinical suspicion in any feverish traveller (incubation up to 1 year, but usually 1–2 weeks).
Cyclical symptoms of high fever, 'flu-like symtoms, severe sweating and shivering cold/rigors.
Peak temperature may coincide with rupture of the intra-erythrocytic schizonts:

- every 48 h for *P. falciprum* (malignant tertian);
- every 72 h for *P. malariae* (benign quartan); and
- every 48 h for *P. vivax* and *P. ovale* (benign tertian).

Note that these terms are now rarely used.
Cerebral malaria: Headache, disorientation, coma.

E: Pyrexia/rigors, anaemia, hepatosplenomegaly.

P: *Plasmodium* life cycle:

1. Injection of sporozoites into the bloodstream by the bite of the female *Anopheles* mosquito.
2. Invasion and replication in hepatocytes (exoerythrocytic schizogeny). *P. vivax* and *ovale* may develop into dormant hypnozoites and cause relapse within months or even years.
3. The parasites may reinvade the blood (at this point they are called merozoites). Inside RBCs, parasites develop from ring forms (trophozoites) to multinucleated schizonts (erythrocytic schizogeny).
4. The RBCs rupture and release merozoites, which may reinfect new RBCs. Some differentiate into male and female gametocytes. These are taken up by the *Anopheles* mosquitoes, develop into sporozoites in their gut and migrate to the salivary gland of the mosquito to be transmitted in their bite.

I: **Thick/thin blood film** (using Field's or Giemsa's stain): Detection and quantitative count of level of intracellular ring forms. Should be taken daily. Has to be negative for 3 days to exclude malaria. $>2\%$ in *P. falciparum* malaria is severe.
Blood: FBC (Hb, platelets), U&E, LFT, ABG (pH).
Urinalysis: Test for blood or protein.
Quantitative buffy coat (QBC) test: Acridine orange stains blood parasite nucleus.
Immunochromatographic (ICT) test: Detects histidine-rich protein 2 found only in *P. falciparum*, allowing distinction from *P. vivax*.

M: *P. malariae:* Chloroquine.
P. vivax and P. ovale: Chloroquine + primaquine (to destroy the parasites in the liver and prevent relapse; beware of G6PD deficiency).
P. falciparum:
1 Quinine + doxycycline or Fansidar (pyrimethamine + sulfadoxine); or
2 Mefloquine or Malarone (proguanil + atovaquone).
Other drugs are available if resistance is a problem, e.g. artmethinin.
Prophylaxis: Depends on the resistance of the *Plasmodium* species in the area of travel. Examples include:
- Malarone: (– 1 day to + 7 day);
- (Chloroquine + proguanil) or mefloquine: (– 3 days to + 28 days).

Public health: Personal awareness and protection (netting, long sleeves, time of day, insect repellants). Malaria is a notifiable disease.

C: *P. falciparum* can cause cerebral malaria, Blackwater fever (intravascular haemolysis → haemoglobinuria → renal failure), DIC and shock, metabolic acidosis, hypoglycaemia, splenic rupture.
Pregnancy: abortion, stillbirth and low birth weight.

P: *P. falciparum* malaria is life threatening. The others are more benign.

D: Autosomal dominant inherited disorder of connective tissue, characterized by abnormalities in musculoskeletal, cardiovascular and ocular systems.

A: Mutation in fibrillin-1 (*FBN1*) gene located on chromosome 15q. 25 % are spontaneous new mutations and occur anywhere on the gene.

A/R: Mutations in *FBN1* causes other rare Marfan-like disorders (e.g. Shprintzen–Goldberg syndrome).

E: Annual incidence is 1 in 10 000.

H: Musculoskeletal problems (e.g. frequent joint dislocations).
Visual difficulties (e.g. sudden visual deterioration as a result of lens dislocation).
Cardiovascular complications (e.g. heart failure).
May be asymptomatic and present as a result of family history.

E: Tall stature, long thin extremities. Arm span > height. Long spidery fingers (arachnodactyly).
Kyphoscoliosis, chest deformities (pectus excavatum or carinatum).
Joint hypermobility common, skin striae.
High arched palate, crowding of teeth.
Lens dislocation.
Signs of mitral valve prolapse or aortic regurgitation (see Mitral regurgitation and Aortic regurgitation).

P: Fibrillin-1 is a main component of extracellular microfibrils which are abundant in elastic tissue especially of skin, blood vessels, perichondrium and ciliary zonules of the eye. Mutations are predicted to disrupt the structural organization of the microfibrils.

I: Skeletal examination and family history is often sufficient to diagnose the condition.
Slit lamp examination: To examine for signs of lens dislocation.
Echocardiography: Screens for valve disease.
Genetic analysis: Useful for research purposes and to confirm diagnosis.

M: Best managed by a specialist centre.
Lifestyle adaptations: Avoidance of strenuous exercise and contact sports, supports when exercising.
Eyes: Annual slit lamp examination and orthopaedic assessments.
Cardiac: Regular ECG, echocardiograms to monitor changes in valves and aortic diameter, antibiotic prophylaxis for dental work. β-Blockers may slow rate of aortic root dilation by reducing blood pressure.
Surgery: Mitral valve repair, aortic root surgery when diameter > 50–60 mm.
Genetic counselling and careful monitoring during pregnancy.

C: Heart failure as a result of mitral regurgitation or aortic root dilation and aortic regurgitation, aortic dissection, dysrhythmias, bacterial endocarditis, spontaneous pneumothorax, upward dislocation of the lens, myopia and, less commonly, retinal detachment.

P: Lifespan is shortened because of cardiovascular complications. Mean survival is in the fourth decade, but may be extended with good care and heart surgery.

Melanoma, malignant

D: Malignancy arising from neoplastic transformation of melanocytes, the pigment-forming cells of the skin. The leading cause of death from skin disease.

A: DNA damage in melanocytes caused by ultraviolet radiation results in neoplastic transformation. Inherited mutations have been identified in *CDKN2A* and *CDK4* (tumour suppressor genes) in the rare familial melanoma syndrome (autosomal dominant).

A/R: Ultraviolet light exposure (sun exposure, especially history of blistering burning, use of tanning lamps, PUVA).
Fair skin, freckles, red/blond hair.
Family history (10 %), giant congenital naevi.
Dysplastic naevus syndrome (multiple pigmented naevi, many >5 mm, mainly on the trunk).
Congenital (e.g. xeroderma pigmentosum*).

E: Steadily increasing incidence, 6000/year diagnosed in UK, lifetime risk 1 in 80 in USA. White races have 20 times increased risk to non-white races.

H: Change in size, shape or colour of a pigmented skin lesion, redness, bleeding, crusting, ulceration.

E: **ABCD criteria for examining moles:**
A Asymmetry.
B Border irregularity/bleeding.
C Colour variation.
D Diameter >6 mm.
E Elevation.

P: 50 % arise in pre-existing naevi, 50 % in previously normal skin. Four histopathological types:
1 *Superficial spreading (70 %):* Typically arises in a pre-existing naevus, expands in radial fashion before vertical growth phase.
2 *Nodular (15 %):* Arises *de novo*, aggressive, no radial growth phase.
3 *Lentigo maligna (10 %):* More common in elderly with sun damage, large flat lesions, follow a more indolent growth course. Usually on the face.
4 *Acral lentiginous (5 %):* Arise on palms, soles and subungual areas. Most common type in non-white populations.

I: **Excisional biopsy:** For histological diagnosis and determination of Clark's levels or Breslow thickness.
Lymphoscintigraphy: Radioactive compound is injected around lesion and dynamic images are taken over the course of 30 min to trace the lymph drainage and the sentinel node(s).
Sentinel lymph node biopsy (if primary and <1 mm depth): Sentinal lymph nodes are dissected and histologically examined for metastatic involvement.
Staging: Imaging by ultrasound, CT or MRI, CXR.
Blood: LFT (liver is a common site of metastases).

M: **Primary prevention:** Limit sun overexposure, avoid sunburn.
Wide local excision, margin dependent on depth of invasion (<1 mm: 1 cm, 1–4 mm: 2 cm margin). Skin grafting may be required.
Staging: (see Investigations).

*Defect in DNA repair after UV light damage.

Metastatic disease: Chemotherapy with dacarbazine (~20 % respond). Immunotherapy (interferon α-2b, IL-2).
Regular follow-up is essential to detect recurrence or spread of disease.

C: Lymphoedema may result after block dissection of lymph nodes.

P: 5-year survival 90–95 % for lesions < 1.4 mm, 40 % with node-positive disease and mean survival of 9 months with metastatic disease.
Poorer prognostic indicators: ulceration, ↑ mitotic rate, trunk lesions compared to limb. Males poorer prognosis than females.

Ménière's disease

D: Inner ear disorder characterized by recurrent episodes of tinnitus, paroxysmal vertigo* and unilateral fluctuating hearing loss.

A: Underlying cause unknown, thought to arise as a result of disturbed homoeostasis of endolymph, the fluid within the inner ear (idiopathic endolymphatic hydrops).

A/R: None.

E: Annual incidence of 15–20 in 100 000. Peak incidence in 40–50-year-olds.

H: Episodes of:
Tinnitus: Roaring, buzzing or ringing sound in ear, may worsen before an episode of vertigo.
Vertigo: Sudden loss of balance, room appears to rotate at speed. Nausea and vomiting.
Hearing loss: Typically fluctuates from day to day, episodes last from minutes to hours, with abrupt onset, often preceded by a sense of pressure or fullness in affected ear, asymptomatic between attacks. May feel weak and off balance for 1–2 days afterwards. All features may not appear in early attacks.

E: During an attack, nystagmus (fast phase towards the affected ear).
Careful ear examination should be carried out to rule out infection.

P: **Pathogenesis:** Oversecretion or malabsorption of endolymph causes ballooning or rupture of Reissner's membrane, resulting in mixing of endolymph and perilymph with loss of endocochlear potentials and hair cell injury in the cochlea and semicircular canals.

I: No specific test will confirm the diagnosis.
Audiogram: Low-frequency sensorineural hearing loss. May fluctuate on repeat testing.
Special: Electronystagmography, brainstem-evoked response audiometry, electrocochleography, MRI to rule out other causes if history is not typical.

M: **Medical:** Anticholinergics, antihistamines, benzodiazepines may be needed for acute attacks.
To reduce frequency of attacks: salt restriction and diuretics are first-line treatment, betahistine is sometimes used (appears to act by improving microcirculation in inner ear).
Surgical: Labyrinthectomy may be warranted for failed medical management or if hearing loss complete (can be performed surgically or by intratympanic injection of gentamicin). Vestibular neurectomy can be attempted to spare any hearing. Endolymphatic shunts and sac decompression are controversial.

C: Hearing loss may become progressive and permanent, becomes bilateral in 10–25 %.

P: Medical management controls symptoms in 80 % of individuals. 15 % develop symptoms in contralateral ear.

*Vertigo is defined as a sensation of movement when no movement is occurring.

Meningitis

D: Inflammation of the leptomeningeal (pia mater and arachnoid) coverings of the brain, most commonly caused by infection.

A: **Bacterial:**
Neonates: Group B *Streptococci, Escherichia coli, Listeria monocytogenes.*
Children: Haemophilus influenzae, Neisseria meningitidis, Streptococcus pneumoniae.
Adults: Neisseria meningitidis (meningococcus), *Streptococcus pneumoniae*, tuberculosis.
Elderly: Streptococcus pneumoniae, risk groups are alcoholics and post-splenectomy.
Specific types: Lyme disease, syphilis.
Viral: Enteroviruses, mumps, HSV, VZV, HIV.
Fungal: *Cryptococcus* (associated with HIV infection).
Others: Malignancy, drugs (e.g. trimethoprim).

A/R: Close communities (e.g. dormitories), basal skull fractures, mastoiditis, sinusitis, inner ear infections, immunodeficiency, alcoholism, splenectomy, sickle cell anaemia, CSF shunts, intracranial surgery.

E: Variation according to geography, age, social conditions. UK Public Health Laboratory Service receives ~2500 notifications/year. More common in recent visitors to the Haj (meningococcal serogroup W135), epidemics occur in the meningitis belt of Africa (meningococcal serogroup A).

H: Severe headache, photophobia, neck or backache, irritability, drowsiness, vomiting, high-pitched crying or fits (common in children), clouding of consciousness, fever.

E: Signs of meningism: photophobia, neck stiffness (Kernig's sign: with hips flexed, pain/resistance on passive knee extension; Brudzinski's sign: flexion of hips on neck flexion).
Signs of infection: fever, tachycardia and hypotension, skin rash (petechiae with meningococcal septicaemia), altered mental state.

P: In bacterial meningitis:
Macro: Congested meningeal vessels with purulent exudate within the subarachnoid space with foci of haemorrhage.
Micro: Vasodilation and infiltration of neutrophils (early) and macrophages (later).

I: **Blood:** Blood cultures (do not delay antibiotic).
Imaging: CT to exclude mass lesion before lumbar puncture.
Lumbar puncture (if no evidence ↑ ICP: ↓ consciousness, papilloedema, focal neurological signs): For CSF microscopy with Gram staining, cytology, biochemistry, culture and sensitivity.
Bacterial: Cloudy CSF, ↑ neutrophils, ↑ protein, ↓ glucose.
Viral: ↑ Lymphocytes, ↑ protein, normal glucose.
TB: Fibrinous CSF, ↑ lymphocytes, ↑ protein, ↓ glucose.
Staining of petechiae scrapings may detect meningococcus ~70 %.

M: **Acute:** Immediate antibiotics if meningitis suspected (before lumbar puncture or CT, especially if rash or shock is evident).
Neonates: Ampicillin with gentamicin/cefotaxime.
Adolescents and adults: Cefotaxime/ceftriaxone to adults (IM benzylpenicillin if urgent).
Elderly: Cefotaxime/ceftriaxone for older patients.

Resuscitation: Patient is best managed in ITU.
Corticosteroids: Dexamethasone if Gram-negative coccobacilli on CSF examination in children > 2 years. Steroids may ↓ complications: hearing loss (*H. influenza*) and death (*S. pneumoniae*).
Prevention (only applicable to meningococcal meningitis): Household and other close contacts should be given antibiotic prophylaxis after discussion with Public Health (rifampicin for 2 days). Vaccination against meningococcal serogroups A and C. (Note that there is no vaccine for serogroup B, the most common serological group isolated in UK.)

C: Septicaemia, shock, DIC, renal failure, fits, peripheral gangrene, cerebral oedema, cranial nerve lesions, cerebral venous thrombosis, hydrocephalus, Waterhouse–Friderichsen syndrome (bilateral adrenal haemorrhage).

P: Mortality rate from bacterial meningitis is high (10–40 % with meningococcal sepsis). In developing countries mortality rate often higher. Viral meningitis self-limiting.

D: Severe episodic headache that may have a prodrome of focal neurological symptoms (aura) and is associated systemic disturbance. Classified as migraine with aura (classical) or without (common migraine) and migraine variants (familial hemiplegic, opthalmoplegic, basilar, migraine equivalents and childhood periodic syndromes).

A: Unknown. Mutations in the P/Q-type calcium channel implicated in rare familial hemiplegic migraine.

A/R: Family history. Triggers include stress, exercise, lack of sleep, oral contraceptive pill, certain foods (e.g. alcohol, cheese, chocolate).

E: Prevalence is 6 % in males and 15–20 % in females. ♀ : ♂ = 3 : 1. Onset in adolescence or early adulthood.

H: **Headache:** Pulsating. Bilateral (in 30–40 %). Duration 4–72 h.
Associated with nausea, vomiting, photophobia, phonophobia or lightheadedness.
May be **preceded by aura** that may include visual disturbance, flashing lights, spots, blurring, zigzag lines (fortification spectra) or blindspots (scotomas) or other sensory symptoms such as tingling or numbness in limbs. Patients prefer to be in a quiet darkened room during an attack.

E: Usually no specific physical findings.
Examination of mental state, neurological examination, fundi, sinuses, cervical spine, general examination to look for other causes of symptoms (e.g. meningoencephalitis, subarachnoid haemorrhage, space-occupying lesion, temporal arteritis).

P: Precise pathophysiological mechanism poorly understood.
Neurovascular hypothesis: Early aura of cortical spreading depression associated with intracranial vasoconstriction resulting in localized ischaemia. This is followed by meningeal and extracranial vasodilation mediated by 5-HT, bradykinin and the trigeminovascular system.

I: Diagnosis based on history. Investigations may be needed to exclude other diagnoses.
Blood: FBC, ESR.
CT/MRI: If suspicion of space-occupying lesion.
Lumbar puncture: If suspicion of meningitis. Do not perform until space-occupying lesion excluded.

M: **Advice:** Stop oral contraceptive pill, encourage regular meals and sleep, caffeine restriction, measures to reduce stress, avoid triggers, symptom diary. Rest in quiet dark room during episode.
Medical: Beware of NSAID-induced headaches as many patients use OTC preparations.
Acute: NSAIDs, paracetamol, codeine, antiemetics (e.g. metoclopramide), 5-HT_1 agonists (sumatriptan, zolmitriptan) and ergotamine.
Prophylaxis (if $>$ 2/month, 50 % patients benefit): Pizotifen (5-HT_2 antagonist), β-blockers, amitriptyline, antihistamines (cyproheptadine), calcium-channel blocker (flunarizine) and sodium valproate.

C: Disruption of daily activities. Frequent attacks can substantially reduce quality of life.

P: Usually chronic, but majority of cases can be managed well by preventative/early treatment measures.

Mitral regurgitation

D: Retrograde flow of blood from left ventricle to left atrium during systole.

A: Caused by mitral valve damage or dysfunction:
- Rheumatic heart disease (most common).
- Infective endocarditis.
- Mitral valve prolapse. Prolapse of mitral valve leaflets into the left atrium during systole.
- Papillary muscle rupture or dysfunction. Secondary to ischaemic heart disease and cardiomyopathy.
- Chordal rupture and floppy mitral valve associated with connective tissue diseases (see Associations).
- Functional mitral regurgitation may be secondary to left ventricular dilation.

A/R: Connective tissue diseases (e.g. pseudoxanthoma elasticum,* osteogenesis imperfecta,† Ehlers–Danlos syndrome,‡ Marfan's syndromes, SLE).
Mitral valve prolapse is associated with ischaemic heart disease, rheumatic heart disease, Marfan's syndrome, thyrotoxicosis, polycystic kidney disease.

E: Affects ~5% of adults. Mitral valve prolapse is more common in young females.

H: Chronic mitral regurgitation: may be asymptomatic or present with exertional dyspnoea, palpitations (if in atrial fibrillation) and fatigue (↓ cardiac output).
Acute (decompensated) mitral regurgitation presents with symptoms of left ventricular failure.
Mitral valve prolapse: Asymptomatic or atypical chest pain or palpitations.

E: Pulse may be normal or irregularly irregular (atrial fibrillation).
Apex beat may be laterally displaced and thrusting (left ventricular dilation).
Pansystolic murmur, loudest at apex, radiating to axilla (palpable as a thrill).
S_1 is soft, S_3 is heard in left ventricular failure (caused by rapid ventricular filling in early diastole).
Acute mitral regurgitation: Signs of left ventricular failure.
Mitral valve prolapse: Mid systolic click and late systolic murmur. The click moves towards the first heart sound on standing and moves away on lying down.

P: **Acute mitral regurgitation** (e.g. following MI, endocarditis): ↑ Left atrial and pulmonary venous pressure from loss of atrial input to ventricular filling resulting in pulmonary oedema.
Chronic mitral regurgitation: Enlargement of left atrium and left ventricle.

*Collagen/elastic tissue disorder characterized by yellow papules on the skin in the flexures, ischaemic heart disease, GI bleeding and angioid streaks on fundoscopy (caused by degeneration of Bruch's membrane).
†Group of autosomally dominant inherited disorders caused by mutations in collagen type I gene causing brittle, deformed bones, blue sclerae, hypermobile joints and heart valve disorders.
‡A group of ~10 genetic disorders characterized clinically by joint hypermobility and skin hyperlasticity. May result from mutations in several genes including type II collagen, fibronectin and elastin.

I: **ECG:** Normal, may show broad bifid p wave (known as p mitrale) or atrial fibrillation.

CXR: Acute mitral regurgitation produces signs of left ventricular failure. Chronic mitral regurgitation shows left atrial enlargement, cardiomegaly (caused by left ventricular dilation) or mitral valve calcification in rheumatic cases.

Echocardiography, Doppler ultrasonography: To assess severity.

Cardiac catheterization: Rarely required.

M: **Medical:** ACE-inhibitors (especially with ventricular dysfunction), β-blockers (for chest pain and palpitations in valve prolapse), furosemide (frusemide) to relieve pulmonary congestion, digoxin for control of ventricular rate, anticoagulation for atrial fibrillation, antibiotic cover for dental or other invasive procedures. Vasodilator therapy may slow progression of heart failure.

Advice: Lose weight, stop smoking.

Surgical: Mitral valve repair or replacement if severe (↓ ejection fraction or ventricular dilation).

C: Atrial fibrillation (and resultant systemic embolism), pulmonary oedema, pulmonary hypertension, right heart failure, infective endocarditis.

P: Prognosis depends on aetiology, severity and state of left ventricular function.

Acute mitral regurgitation resulting from rupture of a cusp or papillary muscle has a poor prognosis.

Rheumatic mitral regurgitation may slowly deteriorate over 10–20 years.

Mitral stenosis

D: Mitral valve narrowing causing obstruction to blood flow from the left atrium to the ventricle.

A: Most common cause is rheumatic heart disease (90 %).
Less common are congenital mitral stenosis, SLE, rheumatoid arthritis, endocarditis and atrial myxoma (rare cardiac tumour).

A/R: Lutembacher's syndrome: Mitral stenosis and atrial septal defect.

E: Incidence is declining in industialized countries because of declining incidence of rheumatic fever.

H: May be asymptomatic.
Presents with fatigue, shortness of breath on exertion or lying down (orthopnoea). Palpitations (related to atrial fibrillation).
Rare: Cough, haemoptysis (late finding, caused by rupture of dilated bronchial veins), hoarseness caused by compression of the left laryngeal nerve by an enlarged left atrium.

E: May have peripheral or facial cyanosis (malar flush).
Pulse normal or small volume in severe stenosis or irregularly irregular (atrial fibrillation).
Apex beat undisplaced and tapping.
Parasternal heave secondary to right ventricular hypertrophy and pulmonary hypertension.
Loud first heart sound with opening snap.
Mid diastolic murmur (presystolic accentuation if in sinus rhythm).
Evidence of pulmonary oedema on lung auscultation (if decompensated).

P: The normal area of the mitral valve orifice is 4–6 cm^2. Critical mitral stenosis occurs when the opening is reduced to 1 cm^2, most commonly because of inflammation and subsequent healing in rheumatic heart disease. Left atrial pressure rises to maintain a normal cardiac output. This increase raises pulmonary venous and capillary pressures, resulting in exertional dyspnoea, chronically leading to pulmonary hypertension and eventual right heart failure.

I: **ECG:** May be normal, broad bifid p wave (p mitrale) caused by left atrial hypertrophy, atrial fibrillation or evidence of right ventricular hypertrophy in cases of severe pulmonary hypertension.
CXR: Left atrial enlargement, cardiac enlargement, pulmonary congestion, mitral valve may be calcified in rheumatic cases.
Echocardiography and Doppler ultrasonography: To assess functional and structural impairments. Transoesophageal gives better valve visualization.
Cardiac catheterization: Measures severity of heart failure.

M: **Lifestyle:** Advise to stop smoking and lose weight.
Medical: Anticoagulation and digoxin for atrial fibrillation. Diuretics. Treat heart failure. Antibiotic cover for dental/invasive procedures.
Surgical: Mitral valvuloplasty, valvotomy or replacement if severe.

C: Atrial fibrillation and systemic embolism, pulmonary oedema, pulmonary hypertension and right heart failure, infective endocarditis.

P: Prognosis fair, worse if pulmonary hypertension or right heart failure.

D: A progressive neurodegenerative disorder of cortical, brainstem and spinal motor neurones (lower and upper motor neurone). Also known as amyotrophic lateral sclerosis (ALS) or Lou Gehrig's disease.

A: Unknown. Free radical damage and glutamate excitotoxicity have been implicated. Mutations in superoxide dismutase (*SOD1* gene, chromosome 21) affect ~20 % with familial motor neurone disease.

A/R: 5–10 % have family history with autosomal dominant inheritance.

E: Rare, annual incidence is about 2 in 100 000. Mean age of onset is 55 years.

H: Weakness of limbs (focal or asymmetrical).
Speech disturbance (slurring or reduction in volume).
Swallowing disturbance (e.g. choking on food, nasal regurgitation).

E: Combination of upper motor neurone (UMN) and lower motor neurone (LMN) signs often affecting several regions asymmetrically.
LMN: Muscle wasting, fasciculations, flaccid weakness (↓ tone and power), depressed or absent reflexes.
UMN: Spastic weakness (↑ tone and ↓ power), brisk reflexes and extensor plantar responses.
Sensation: Unimpaired.
A number of variants:

1. *Progressive muscular atrophy variant* (10 %): Only LMN signs.
2. *Progressive bulbar palsy variant:** Dysarthria and dysphagia with wasted fasciculating tongue (LMN) and brisk jaw jerks (UMN).
3. *Primary lateral sclerosis variant:* UMN pattern of weakness, brisk reflexes, extensor plantar responses, without LMN signs.

P: Progressive injury and death of motor neurones. Neurones may exhibit mitochondrial damage, proximal accumulation of neurofilaments or inclusion bodies but no changes are pathognomonic.

I: **Blood:** CK (mild ↑), anti-GM1 ganglioside antibodies should be negative.
EMG: Widespread denervation and reinervation.
Nerve conduction studies: To exclude motor neuropathy.
MRI: To exclude cord or root compression, brainstem lesion in progressive bulbar palsy variant. May show high signal in motor tracts on T2 imaging.

M: Because of grave prognosis, must exclude other potentially treatable conditions (e.g. myasthenia gravis).
Medical: Riluzole (glutamate release inhibitor) has a modest effect on prolonging survival. Symptomatic treatment of spasticity (e.g. baclofen), salivation (anticholinergics), cramps (quinine).

*Bulbar palsy: any lesion affecting cranial nerves (IX–XII) at nuclear, nerve or muscle level, presenting with nasal speech, nasal regurgitation of food, especially fluids (palatal weakness), ↓ gag reflex, absent jaw jerk, wasted fasciculating tongue. Pseudobulbar palsy: any UMN (corticobulbar) lesion to the lower brainstem, presenting with monotonous or explosive speech, dysphagia, ↑ gag reflex, brisk jaw reflex, shrunken immobile tongue, emotional lability, UMN limb spasticity and weakness.

Multidisciplinary management: Psychological support, physiotherapy, walking aids, home adaptations, speech and language therapy, communication aids, swallowing assessment, dietitian input. Percutaneous endoscopic gastrostomy (PEG) in marked bulbar palsy. Hospice care in terminal stages.

C: Depression, emotional lability, frontal type dementia.
Weight loss and malnutrition (resulting from dysphagia).
Immobility-related problems: DVT, aspiration pneumonia.
Respiratory failure because of weakness of ventilatory muscles (usual cause of death).

P: Relentless progression. Mean survival is about 3 years. Bulbar onset and young onset have worse prognosis.
Those with only LMN signs have a better prognosis.

Multiple myeloma

D: Haematological malignancy characterized by proliferation of plasma cells resulting in bone lesions and production of a monoclonal immunoglobulin (paraprotein, usually IgG or IgA).

A: Unknown. Postulated viral trigger. Chromosomal aberrations are frequent, certain cytokines (e.g. IL-6) act as potent growth factors for plasma cell proliferation.

A/R: Ionizing radiation, agricultural work or occupational exposures (benzene).

E: Incidence is 4 in 100 000/year, peak age in 70-year-olds. Afro-Caribbeans > white people > Asians.

H: May be diagnosed incidentally on routine blood tests.
Bone pain: Often in back, ribs. Sudden and severe if caused by pathological fracture or vertebral collapse.
Infections: Often recurrent.
General: Tiredness, thirst, polyuria, nausea, constipation, mental change (resulting from hypercalcaemia).
Bleeding, headaches, visual disturbance (because of blood hyperviscosity).

E: Pallor, tachycardia, flow murmur, signs of heart failure, dehydration.
Purpura, hepatosplenomegaly, macroglossia, carpal tunnel syndrome and peripheral neuropathies.

P: Lytic lesions caused by tumour expansion and osteoclast activation because of excess production of a protein known as osteoprotegerin ligand. Recurrent infections as a result of impaired humoral immunity and opsonization (encapsulated bacteria are the most prevalent pathogens). Bleeding tendency caused by impaired platelet and coagulation factor function, thrombocytopenia in late stages.
Durie/Salmon staging: Based on serum Hb, immunoglobulin, Ca^{2+}, creatinine levels and number of radiographical bone lesions on the skeletal survey.

I: **Blood:** FBC (↓ Hb, normochromic normocytic), ↑ ESR, ↑ CRP (CRP may be normal with elevated ESR), U&E (↑ creatinine, ↑ Ca^{2+} in 45 %), typically normal AlkPhos.
Blood film: Rouleaux formation with bluish background (↑ protein).
Bone marrow aspirate and trephine: ↑ Plasma cells (identified as large cells with a perinuclear halo, eccentric nuclei, blue cytoplasm): usually > 20 %.
Serum or urine electrophoresis: Serum paraprotein (two-thirds IgG, one-third IgA), Bence-Jones protein (free light chains, κ or λ in 70 % cases).
Chest, pelvic or vertebral X-ray: Osteolytic lesions without surrounding sclerosis. Pathological fractures.
MRI: To identify any cord compression.

M: **Emergency:** Rehydration. Consider dialysis and/or plasmapheresis. Radiotherapy if there is bone pain or cord compression. Treat pathological fractures normally.
Medical: Chemotherapy is the core strategy. Melphalan and prednisolone (50–60 % respond) or VAD regimen (vincristine, Adriamycin, dexamethasone). Interferon-α prolongs remissions or plateau phase achieved by chemotherapy. High-dose therapy with bone marrow or stem cell transplantation is an option in selected patients.

Supportive: Hydration, allopurinol (protects against hyperuricaemia and gout), antibiotics, blood components, bisphosphonates, erythropoietin.

C: Pathological fractures, renal failure (in up to one-third of patients), spinal cord compression, carpal tunnel syndrome and polyneuropathies (amyloidosis).

P: Median survival is 4–6 years from diagnosis. Important prognostic parameters are β_2-microglobulin, plasma cell labelling index, CRP, creatinine and age. Monosomy of chromosome 13 associated with poor prognosis.

D: Chronic inflammatory demyelinating disease of the central nervous system.

A: Unknown. Autoimmune basis with postulated environmental trigger in a genetically susceptible individual.

A/R: Associated with *HLA-A3, A7, DR2, DQ1*. Concordance: monozygotic twins 25 %, dizygotic twins 3 %.
Devic's disease (neuromyelitis optica) is a variant of MS with optic neuritis and transverse myelitis.

E: Prevalence in UK is 1 in 1000. ♀ : ♂ 2 : 1. Presents at 20–40 years. Geographical variation (temperate > tropical).

H: Varies depending on site of inflammation.
Visual: Blurred vision, pain on eye movement.
Sensory: Pins and needles, numbness, burning.
Motor: Limb weakness, spasms, stiffness, heaviness.
Autonomic: Urinary urgency, hesitancy, incontinence, impotence.
Psychological: Depression, psychosis.
Uhthoff's phenomenon: Temporary ↑ or recurrence of symptoms precipitated by rise in body temperature.

E: **Visual (most common):** ↓ Acuity, loss of coloured vision.
Visual field testing: Central scotoma (optic nerve) or field defects (optic radiations).
Relative afferent pupillary defect: Tested with a swinging torch test. Both pupils contract when light is shone on the unaffected side, both pupils dilate when light is 'swung' to the diseased (eye).
Fundoscopy: Pink swollen (papillitis) or pale disc (optic atrophy).
Eye movements: Loss of smooth pursuit.
Internuclear opthalmoplegia: Successful abduction on attempted lateral gaze but failure of adduction of the other eye. Nystagmus greater in the abducting eye. This indicates that the contralateral medial longitudinal fasciculus is affected.
Sensory: Paraesthesia (vibration and joint position sense loss more common than pain and temperature).
Motor: UMN signs (e.g. spastic weakness, brisk reflexes, extensor plantars).
Cerebellar: *Finger – nose – finger test:* intention tremor, dysmetria (inability to judge distance) and past-pointing, dysdiadochokinesis, cerebellar rebound (stretched arm overshoots and oscillates when tapped), ataxic wide-based gait, scanning speech, uncoordinated heel – knee – shin test.
Lhermitte's phenomenon: Shock-like sensation in arms and legs precipitated by neck flexion pressure sores.
Dementia, mood disorders (euphoria, depression).

P: Episodes of perivascular inflammation, loss of myelin and later gliosis. Immune-mediated damage to myelin sheaths in white matter of CNS results in impaired conduction along nerve fibres.

I: Diagnosis based on two or more CNS lesions with corresponding symptoms, separated in time and space.
Lumbar puncture: CSF electrophoresis shows oligoclonal bands.
MRI: Plaque detection is highlighted as high-signal lesions.
Electrophysiological studies: Visual, auditory or somatosensory evoked potentials (delayed central conduction and ↑ latency).

M: **Multidisciplinary management:** Need to involve neurologists, specialist nurses, physiotherapists, occupational therapists and pain team for treatment of symptoms.
Relapses: Corticosteroids hastens recovery but not degree of recovery. Interferon β reduces frequency and severity of relapses.
Bladder disturbances: Anticholinergics (e.g. oxybutynin), intermittent self-catheterization.
Spasticity: Baclofen, dantrolene, tizanidine or diazepam.
Seizures: Antiepileptics (e.g. carbamazepine, phenytoin).
Cerebellar tremor: Clonazepam, gabapentin.
Depression: Psychological support, antidepressants.
Erectile dysfunction: Intracorporeal papaverine, prostaglandins.
Care of pressure areas.
Speech and language therapy.

C: Disability, impaired mobility, psychological problems.

P: Life expectancy slightly ↓. Disability is a major issue. 80 % relapsing – remitting disease: after initial resolution, subsequent episodes leave residual disability, eventually entering secondary progressive phase, 10 % benign course, 10 % primary progressive disease.

Muscular dystrophy

D: Genetically determined, degenerative class of muscle disorders, characterized by progressive muscle weakness and wasting of variable distribution and severity.

A: Caused by insufficiency of or defects in muscle proteins. Classified according to distribution of predominant muscle weakness and mode of inheritance as shown below.

X-linked: e.g. Duchenne (severe), Becker (benign), Emery–Dreifuss (benign with early contractures).

Autosomal recessive: e.g. Limb girdle, childhood type (resembling Duchenne).

Autosomal dominant: e.g. Facioscapulohumeral, scapuloperoneal.

Duchenne muscular dystrophy (DMD) is the most common form.

A/R: Not applicable.

The remainder of the information below relates to DMD.

E: Duchenne occurs in 1 in 3500 live male births. One-third of cases are caused by new mutations.

H: The child appears healthy at birth, but motor milestones are delayed.

Waddling gait, difficulty with running, climbing stairs or getting up from a seated or lying position.

In some cases (< 20 %), there is an associated learning difficulty.

E: Muscle weakness that is symmetrical and more prominent in the pelvic and shoulder girdles.

Calf muscles shows pseudohypertrophy (resulting from excessive adipose replacement of muscle fibres).

Gower's sign: The use of hands to climb up thighs, pushing down on them, in order to overcome proximal muscle and pelvic girdle weakness on standing up from seated position.

Later the patient may develop muscle contractures, exaggerated lumbar lordosis and thoracolumbar scoliosis.

P: **Pathomechanism:** DMD is caused by mutations in a gene on Xp21, which results in absence of dystrophin (a protein that forms part of a membrane-spanning protein complex of the muscle sarcolemma which connects the cytoskeleton to the basal lamina). Muscle fibre necrosis is thought to result from uncontrolled entry of calcium into the cells. Becker muscular dystrophy is a less severe form of disease caused by an insufficiency rather than lack of dystrophin.

Micro: Variation in muscle fibre size, segmental necrosis of fibre groups. Initially, fibre regeneration occurs which later fails, leading to loss of muscle and replacement by adipose cells and connective tissue.

I: **Blood:** High levels of creatinine kinase are present in serum from birth.

EMG: Establishes the myopathic nature and excludes neurogenic causes of weakness.

Muscle biopsy and immunostaining for dystrophin.

Genetic testing: Identification of the specific mutation or defect can be carried out in specialized centres.

M: **General:** Supportive care including physiotherapy with moderate physical exercise, mobility aids, night splints, spinal supports, care of pressure areas. Attention to educational, social and psychological needs is paramount. Respiratory care and assisted respiration in the form of non-invasive intermittent positive pressure ventilation in later stages. Genetic counselling of female family members.

Medical: Steroids have shown to have a beneficial effect in controlled studies, helping to maintain mobility for a further 2–3 years. Early detection of a cardiomyopathy enables treatment.
Surgical: Surgery can be used at later stages for the correction of contractures and also correction of scoliosis to help preserve lung function.

C: Loss of mobility, limb contractures, scoliosis, respiratory insufficiency and infection, cardiomyopathy.

P: Progressive muscle weakness and heart failure. A child with DMD loses the ability of independent ambulation by ~12 years. Respiratory insufficiency occurs in the second decade, few live beyond the late twenties. In Becker muscular dystrophy, disease develops later and less rapidly.

D: An autoimmune disease affecting the neuromuscular junction producing weakness of voluntary muscles.

A: Autoantibodies against the nicotinic acetylcholine receptor is the central feature. It has been proposed that a possible infectious trigger causes breakdown in immune tolerance (molecular mimicry). Lambert–Eaton myasthenic syndrome* is a particular rare paraneoplastic subtype.

A/R: Associated with other autoimmune conditions (e.g. pernicious anaemia) and thymoma development.

E: Prevalence is 8–9 in 100 000. In younger ages, ♀ > ♂, with increased age, ♀ = ♂.

H: Muscle weakness that worsens with repetitive use or towards end of day. Facial weakness ('myasthenic snarl'), drooping eyelids, diplopia.
Disturbed hypernasal speech, difficulty in smiling, chewing or swallowing (nasal regurgitation of fluids).

E: **Ptosis:** Usually bilateral and asymmetrical.
Tests for muscle fatigue: Ask patient to sustain upward gaze for 1 min and watch for progressive ptosis. Reading aloud may provoke dysarthria or nasal speech after 3 min.
May be **generalized** (affecting many muscle groups) or **ocular** (affecting only the eyes).

P: Breakdown in immune tolerance thought to arise in thymus (75 % have either thymic hyperplasia or thymoma). Autoantibodies directed against the nicotinic acetylcholine receptor cause postsynaptic receptor loss leading to reduced efficiency of neuromuscular transmission.

I: **Blood:** Serum acetylcholine receptor antibody (positive in 80 %), TFT (associated hyperthyroidism), antistriated muscle antibody (may be positive in those with thymoma).
Tensilon test: Short-acting anticholinesterase (e.g. edrophonium) increases acetylcholine levels by blocking its metabolism and causes rapid and transient improvement in clinical features (atropine and cardiac resuscitation equipment must be kept at hand, in case of bradycardia and hypotension).
EMG: Repetitive stimulation demonstrating decrements of the muscle action potential. Differentiates between myasthenic gravis and Lambert–Eaton myasthenic syndrome.
CT or MRI scan or lateral CXR: To visualize thymoma in the mediastinum or malignancies in the lung.

M: **Medical:** *Symptomatic treatment:* Cholinesterase inhibitors (e.g. pyridostigmine, neostigmine).
Immunosuppresssion: Prednisolone (for restricted ocular myasthenia gravis and severe cases), azathioprine, ciclosporin. IV immunoglobulin and plasma exchange is used in sudden worsening of symptoms or on a chronic intermittent basis in patients refractory to other treatment.
Surgical: Thymectomy is beneficial in those with a thymoma or early-onset generalized myasthenic gravis. 50 % improvement after 2 years.

*Lambert–Eaton myasthenic syndrome presents similarly to myasthenia gravis and is caused by autoantibodies against presynaptic calcium ion channels. This reduces acetylcholine release and produces the same sort of weakness. It is associated with malignancies (particularly small cell bronchocarcinoma).

C: **Myaesthenic crisis** (respiratory failure requiring intubation and mechanical ventilation) may be caused by infections, aspiration, physical and emotional stress, and changes in medication.

Cholinergic crisis caused by excessive cholinesterase inhibitor use presents as agitation, sweating, fever, flush, hypersalivation, pupillary miosis, muscle fasciculations and muscle weakness.

Fetal or neonatal myasthenia (caused by transplacental antibodies transfer from mother with myasthenia gravis).

P: Maximum extent of involvement in an individual patient usually manifests itself within the first 5–7 years, although the disease may wax and wane in severity.

D: Group of acquired clonal disorders of bone marrow stem cells.

Five subgroups	Blasts in bone marrow (%)
Refractory anaemia (RA)	< 5
RA with ring sideroblasts (RARS)	< 5 (> 15 % RS)
RA with excess blasts (RAEB)	5–20
RAEB in transformation (RAEB-t)	20–30
Chronic myelomonocytic leukaemia (CMML)	Any of above + promonocytes

A: May be primary, or arise in patients who have received chemotherapy or radiotherapy for previous malignancies.

A/R: Chromosomal abnormalities (partial or total loss of chromosomes 5, 7, 8 or Y). *Ras* oncogene mutations, Down's syndrome.

E: Mean age diagnosis is 65–75 years, more common in males. Twice as common as acute myeloid leukemia.

H: **Asymptomatic**: Diagnosed after routine blood count (50 %).
Symptoms of bone marrow failure: Malaise, dizziness, recurrent infections, easy bruising, epistaxis.

E: **Signs of bone marrow failure:** Pallor, cardiac flow murmur, infections, purpura or ecchymoses.
Spleen not enlarged, except in CMML, also may have gum hypertrophy and lymphadenopathy.

P: Ineffective erythropoiesis results in low levels of all blood cellular components, accompanied by a hypercellular marrow with morphological changes in all three lineages.

I: **Blood:** FBC (pancytopenia).
Blood film: Red cells macrocytic, dimorphic, normoblasts, ↓ granulocytes with lack of granulation or exhibiting the Pelger abnormality (a single or bilobed nucleus), monocytes (CMML), myeloblasts.
Bone marrow aspirate or biopsy: Hypercellularity, ring sideroblasts with dyserythropoietic features, abnormal granulocyte prescursors and megakaryocytes. 10 % show marrow fibrosis.

M: **Low risk** (< 5 % blasts): Largely supportive. Red cell and platelet transfusions, antibiotics, growth factors, ciclosporin, antilymphocyte globulin.
High risk (> 5 % blasts): Supportive (see Low risk), single agent chemotherapy or intensive combination chemotherapy (e.g. FLAG; fludarabine, cytosine arabinoside and growth factor G-CSF).
Stem cell transplantation.

C: Pancytopenia causes complications such as opportunistic infections and haemorrhage.
~20 % progress to acute leukaemia (see Leukaemia, acute myeloblastic).
Iron overload can result from repeated transfusion with iron chelation therapy required.

P: Depends on type. Blast cells predict risk of developing acute leukemia.

Myelofibrosis

D: Disorder of haematopoietic stem cells characterized by progressive marrow fibrosis in association with extramedullary haematopoiesis and splenomegaly.

A: Primary stem cell defect is not known, but results in increased numbers of abnormal megakaryocytes (platelet precursor cells) with stromal proliferation as a secondary reactive phenomenon to growth factors from the megakaryocytes.

A/R: ~30 % of patients have previous history of polycythaemia rubra vera or essential thrombocythaemia.

E: Rare. Annual incidence ~0.4 in 100 000. Peak onset 50–70 years.

H: Asymptomatic: diagnosed after abnormal blood count.
Systemic symptoms: *Common:* Weight loss, anorexia, fever and night sweats, pruritus.
Uncommon: Left upper quadrant abdominal pain, indigestion (caused by massive splenomegaly).
Bleeding, bone pain and gout are less common complaints.

E: Splenomegaly (massive in 10 %) is the main physical finding, hepatomegaly present in 50–60 %.

P: Abnormal megakaryocytes release cytokines (e.g. PDGF, PF4 and TGF-β) which stimulate fibroblast proliferation and collagen deposition in bone marrow, with resulting extramedullary haematopoiesis in liver and spleen.

I: **Blood:** FBC (variable Hb, WCC and platelets initially, but later anaemia, leucopenia and thrombocytopenia). LFT (abnormal).
Blood film: Leucoerythroblastic changes (circulating red and white cell precursors) with characteristic 'tear drop' poikilocyte red cells.
Bone marrow aspirate or biopsy: Aspiration usually unsuccessful ('dry tap'). Trephine biopsy shows fibrotic hypercellular marrow, with dense reticulin fibres on silver staining.

M: No therapy has been shown to reverse/halt disease process.
Supportive therapy: Red cell transfusion, folic acid, allopurinol.
Chemotherapy: Hydroxyurea for splenomegaly and hypermetabolic symptoms.
Radiotherapy: Short-term palliation of splenomegaly.
Surgery: Splenectomy for severe cases. Stem cell transplantation can be curative for selected patients.

C: Heart failure, infections. Iron overload resulting from blood transfusions. Transformation to AML occurs in 10–20 %.

P: Median survival is 3–5 years, with wide variation. The degree of anaemia (Hb < 10 g/dL) is the most important prognostic factor.

Myocardial infarction

D: Cardiac muscle necrosis resulting from ischaemia caused by sudden occlusion of a coronary artery (see Angina pectoris).

A: Rupture of atheromatous plaque (see Pathology) in coronary artery results in thrombus formation that occludes the artery.

A/R: Hypertension, hyperlipidaemia, diabetes, family history, smoking, age, male gender, ethnicity.

E: Common. Annual incidence in UK is 5 in 1000. More common in males.

H: Central crushing chest pain radiating to left arm or jaw.
May be associated with breathlessness, sweating, nausea and vomiting.
May be silent in elderly or in diabetics.

E: May have no clinical signs. Pale, sweating, restless, low-grade pyrexia.
Arrhythmias, disturbances of blood pressure.
New heart murmurs (e.g. pansystolic murmur of mitral regurgitation from papillary muscle rupture or VSD).
Signs of acute heart failure, cardiogenic shock (hypotension, cold peripheries, oliguria).

P:

Time from onset	Macro	Micro
< 24 h	Minimal change	Minimal change
24–36 h	Pale	Acute inflammation with neutrophils
Days	Pale and hyperaemic border	Organization (granulation tissue)
Weeks–months	White scar	Fibrosis (collagenous scar tissue)

Degree of injury depends on the extent and duration of ischaemia and ranges from subendocardial infarction (with ↑ cardiac enzymes but no ST segment elevation or Q waves) to transmural infarction (with ST segment elevation and Q waves).
Atherosclerosis: Endothelial injury is followed by migration of monocytes into subendothelial space and differentiation into macrophages. Macrophages accumulate LDL lipids insudated in the subendothelium and become foam cells. Macrophages also release growth factors which stimulate smooth muscle proliferation, production of collagen and proteoglycans. This leads to the formation of an atheromatous plaque.

I: **Blood:** FBC, U&E, cholesterol, cardiac enzymes: CK-MB and troponin-T (increased after 12 h) (AST and LDH increase after 24 and 48 h, respectively; used only to make retrospective diagnosis).
ECG: *Q-wave MI:* Hyperacute T waves, ST elevation (> 1 mm in limb leads, > 2 mm in chest leads), new onset LBBB. Later: T inversion (hours) and Q waves (days).
Non-Q wave MI: T wave inversion and ST depression.

Location of infarct	Changes in leads
Inferior infarct	II, III, aVF
Anterior infarct	V_2-V_6
Lateral infarct	I, II, aVL
Posterior infarct	Tall R wave, ST depression in V_1–V_3

CXR: To look for signs of heart failure. Useful to look for differentials (e.g. aortic dissection).

Follow-up investigations: Exercise ECG, angiography, echocardiography, myocardial perfusion scan.

M: **Resuscitate** (according to Airway, Breathing and Circulation): Best managed in a specialist Coronary Care Unit.

Initial:

Aspirin: 300 mg.

Oxygen, diamorphine and metoclopramide (antiemetic).

β -Blockers: If not contraindicated.

Nitrates: Only symptomatic benefit.

Thrombolysis: Streptokinase or recombinant tissue plasminogen activator if within 12 h of chest pain with ECG changes (ST elevation, new onset LBBB or posterior infarction).

Contraindications: Recent surgery, trauma, haemorrhage, bleeding diathesis, history of recent CVA with residual disability, suspected aortic dissection, severe hypertension, previous allergic reactions, active peptic ulcer, active pulmonary disease with cavitation, acute pancreatitis, pregnancy, coma.

Heparin: IV infusion as an adjunct to tissue plasminogen activator, SC LMW heparin if not receiving thrombolysis.

Insulin: Insulin – glucose sliding scale if glucose $> 11.0\,\mu m$.

Angioplasty: Consider if thrombolysis contraindicated or continued pain or ST elevation after thrombolysis.

Monitor: Pulse, BP, sat O_2, BP, K^+, serial ECG and cardiac enzymes.

Secondary prevention: Antiplatelet agents (aspirin, clopidogrel if aspirin contraindicated), ACE-inhibitors, β-blockers and statins. Control other risk factors (smoking, diabetes, hypertension).

Advice: Not to drive for 1 month. Lifestyle changes (e.g. exercise, stop smoking, changing diet).

Surgical: Coronary artery bypass graft for patients with left main stem or three-vessel disease.

C: **Early (24–72 h):** Cardiogenic shock, death, heart failure, ventricular arrhythmias, heart block, pericarditis, myocardial rupture, thromboembolism.

Late: Ventricular wall (or septum) rupture, valvular regurgitation, ventricular aneurysms, tamponade, Dressler's syndrome (pericarditis), thromboembolism.

P: High mortality, but this is now decreasing as a result of therapeutic advances. Many patients die before reaching hospital. Inpatient mortality ~10 %. Worse prognosis with multivessel coronary disease, left ventricular dysfunction, comorbidity or ↑ age.

Note: clinical trials suggesting benefits for the drugs used in MI: ISIS-2, aspirin and streptokinase; ISIS-4, ACE-inihibitors; ISIS-1, β-blockers; GUSTO-1, IV heparin with tissue plasminogen activator; DIGAMI, insulin–glucose infusions.

D: Acute inflammation and necrosis of cardiac muscle (myocardium).

A: Usually unknown (idiopathic).
Infection: *Viruses:* e.g. Coxsackie B virus, echovirus, EBV, CMV, adenovirus, influenza, HIV.
Bacterial: e.g. *Chlamydia*, diphtheria, Lyme disease, *Meningococcus*, poststreptococcal.
Fungal: e.g. Candidiasis.
Protozoal: e.g. Trypanosomiasis.
Helminths: e.g. Trichinosis.
Non-infective: Systemic disorders (SLE, sarcoidosis, polymyositis), hypersensitivity myocarditis (e.g. sulphonamides).
Others: Cocaine abuse, heavy metals, radiation.

A/R: May be associated with pericarditis (myopericarditis).

E: True incidence is unknown, as many cases are not detected at the time of acute illness. Coxsackie B virus is a common cause in Europe and USA. Chagas' disease is a common cause in South America.

H: Prodromal 'flu-like illness, fever, malaise, fatigue, lethargy.
Breathlessness (pericardial effusion/myocardial dysfunction).
Palpitations.
Sharp chest pain (suggesting associated pericarditis).
Symptoms of complications.

E: Signs of pericarditis or complications: heart failure, arrhythmia.

P: **Macro:** May be normal or may show dilation of all chambers, with patchy diffuse haemorrhagic mottling.
Micro: Myocyte necrosis and inflammatory infiltration.
Hypersensitivity myocarditis: interstitial infiltrate with prominent eosinophils and little myocyte necrosis.
Idiopathic giant cell myocarditis: focal myocyte necrosis and granulomas.

I: **Blood:** FBC (↑ WCC in infective causes), U&E, ↑ ESR or CRP, cardiac enzymes (may be ↑). To identify the cause: viral or bacterial serology, anti-streptolysin O titre, ANA, serum ACE, TFT.
ECG: Non-specific T wave and ST changes, widespread saddle-shaped ST elevation in pericarditis.
CXR: May be normal or show cardiomegaly with or without pulmonary oedema.
Pericardial fluid drainage: Measure glucose, protein, cytology, culture and sensitivity.
Echocardiography: Assesses systolic/diastolic function, wall motion abnormalities, pericardial effusion.
Myocardial biopsy: Rarely required, as the result does not influence management.

M: **Supportive:** Bed rest, treatment of complications (heart failure, arrhythmias), pericardial drainage for compromising pericardial effusion.
Steroids and immunosuppressants have been used in severe cases but are of unproven benefit.
Surgical: Cardiac transplantation for severe cases.

C: Severe cases can lead to chronic inflammation, cardiac failure. Resolution of inflammation with different degrees of residual dilated cardiomyopathy, arrhythmias and death.

P: Usually mild and self-limiting. Recovery is variable in patients with severe acute myocarditis.

Myotonic dystrophy

D: Autosomal dominant condition characterized by muscle wasting, weakness and myotonia (abnormal sustained contraction of muscle).

A: Caused by expansion of CTG nucleotide triplet repeats at the 3′ untranslated region (UTR) of the myotonic dystrophy gene (myotonin-protein kinase: chromosome 19). The disease has earlier onset or increased severity in the offspring than in the parents as a result of further triplet repeat expansion in succeeding generations. This phenomenon is called anticipation.

A/R: Associated with cataracts, frontal baldness, diabetes mellitus, hypogonadism, cardiomyopathy, cardiac conduction defects, cholecystitis.

E: Most common form of adult-onset muscular dystrophy. Annual incidence 1 in 8000. Usual onset age 20–50 years.

H: Progressive weakness (hands, legs, sternomastoids) and myotonia.
Inability to release the grip.
Mental impairment.
Symptoms of associated conditions, e.g. cataracts, hypogonadism.

E: Facial muscle wasting and weakness gives 'myopathic facies' with lack of facial expression.
Wasting of frontalis and temporalis.
Frontal balding (in men), bilateral ptosis, weakness of sternomastoids.
Unable to release the grip.
Percussion myotonia: Striking the thenar eminence provokes slow flexion of the thumb.
Signs of associated conditions, e.g. cataracts, testicular atrophy.

P: The pathological changes are variable and may show features of dystrophy. Atrophy of type I fibres and hypertrophy of type II fibres, internally situated nuclei and ring fibres with circumferential concentration of heavily stained cytoplasm (containing myofibrils). Muscle spindles with fibre splitting, necrosis and regeneration.

I: **EMG:** Characteristic abnormal spontaneous electrical discharge during insertion of the electrode into the muscle. The spontaneous discharge ↓ with time.
DNA mutation analysis: Expansion of the CTG triplet repeat in the 3′ UTR of the gene.
Blood: Creatine kinase (may be raised).

M: Myotonia is treated with quinine, phenytoin or procainamide.
Genetic counselling.

C: Neurological, endocrine and cardiac complications as above.

P: Most patients do not live past 50 years.

D: Characterized by proteinuria (> 3 g/24 h), hypoalbuminaemia (< 30 g/L), oedema and hypercholesterolaemia.

A: All causes of glomerulonephritis can cause nephrotic syndrome (see Associations/Risk factors for other associations).

A/R: Diabetes mellitus, sickle cell disease, amyloidosis, malignancies (lung and GI adenocarcinomas), drugs (NSAIDs), Alport's syndrome (haematuric nephritis and sensorineural deafness, caused by an inherited mutation in the gene coding for collagen type IV), HIV infection.

E: Most common cause of nephrotic syndrome in children (90 %): minimal change glomerulonephritis (usually seen in boys < 5 years, rare in black populations).
Most common causes of nephrotic syndrome in adults: diabetes mellitus, membranous glomerulonephritis.

H: Family history of atopy in those with minimal change glomerulonephritis, family history of renal disease.
Swelling: facial, abdominal, limb, genital.
Symptoms of the underlying cause (e.g. SLE).
Symptoms of complications (e.g. renal vein thrombosis: loin pain, haematuria).

E: Oedema: periorbital, peripheral, genital.
Ascites: fluid thrill, shifting dullness.

P: Proteinuria may be caused by structural damage to the glomerular basement membrane as well as reduction of its negatively charged components, which repel negatively charged proteins. Hypoalbuminaemia is mediated by proteinuria and ↑ breakdown of filtered albumin in the kidney. Pathogenesis of oedema is not clear, but may be related to defective intrarenal Na^+ retention/excretion.

I: **Blood:** FBC, U&E, LFT (↓ albumin), ESR/CRP, glucose, lipid profile (secondary hyperlipidaemia), immunoglobulins, complement (C3, C4).
Tests to identify the underlying cause of glomerulonephritis:
SLE: ANA, anti-dsDNA.
Infections: Group A β-haemolytic streptococcal infection (ASOT), HBV infection (serology), *Plasmodium malariae* (thick/thin blood film).
Goodpasture's syndrome: Antiglomerular basement membrane antibodies.
Vasculitides: e.g. Wegener's and microscopic polyarteritis (ANCA).
Urine: Urinalysis (protein, blood), microscopy, culture, sensitivity, 24-h collection (to calculate creatinine clearance and 24-h protein excretion).
Renal ultrasound: Excludes other renal diseases that may cause proteinuria, e.g. reflux nephropathy.
Renal biopsy: In all adults and in children who have unusual features or do not respond to steroids.
Other imaging: Doppler ultrasound, renal angiogram, CT or MRI are options if renal vein thrombosis is suspected.

M: **Treat oedema:** Bed rest, fluid restriction (~ 1 L/day), Na^+ restriction (~50 mmol/day), diuretics (e.g. oral furosemide (frusemide) ± metolazone or spironolactone). Occasionally, IV diuretics and salt-poor albumin may be required for initiation of diuresis.
Monitor: BP, U&E, weight, fluid balance.

Treat the cause:
Minimal change glomerulonephritis: High-dose steroids (60 mg for 2 months) and gradually ↓ the dose, treat relapses (~40 % within 3 years) with steroids, immunosuppressants: cyclophosphamide or ciclosporin for steroid non-responders or those with frequent relapses. In membranous glomerulonephritis the benefit of steroids and immunosuppressants is uncertain.
SLE: steroids, cyclophosphamide.
Prevention of complications: avoid prolonged bed rest, prophylactic SC heparin.

C: Renal failure (caused by hypovolaemia especially following diuretics, renal vein thrombosis, progression of underlying renal disease), ↑ susceptibility to infection (e.g. peritonitis, pneumococcal because of loss of immunoglobulins and lipid content in the urine), thrombosis (e.g. renal vein and DVT caused by hypovolaemia and hypercoagulable state caused by loss of antithrombin in the urine and ↑ synthesis of fibrinogen in the liver), hyperlipidaemia (possibly caused by ↑ synthesis of trigylcerides and cholesterol along with albumin in the liver).

P: Varies according to the underlying condition and presence of complications.

D: Autosomal dominant genetic disorder affecting cells of neural crest origin resulting in the development of multiple neurocutaneous tumours (tumours may affect brain, spinal cord and peripheral nerves).
Type 1 (von Recklinghausen's disease): Characterized by peripheral neurofibromas, multiple *café au lait* spots, freckling (axillary/inguinal), Lisch nodules (on iris), skeletal deformities and optic nerve glioma.
Type 2: Characterized by schwannomas, e.g. bilateral vestibular schwannomas (acoustic neuromas), meningiomas, gliomas.

A: Associated with mutations in tumour suppressor genes, **NF1** neurofibromin; **NF2** merlin or schwannomin.

A/R: Associated with ↑ risk of epilepsy, phaeochromocytomas and renal or carotid artery dysplasia (NF1).

E: Incidence is 1 in 4000 births (NF1), 1 in 40 000 (NF2). No gender or racial predilection.

H: Positive family history (but 50 % are caused by new mutations).
NF1: Skin lesions, learning difficulties (in 40 %), headaches, disturbed vision (optic gliomas, in ~15 %).
NF2: Hearing loss developing in teenage years, tinnitus, balance problems, headache, facial pain or numbness.

E: **NF1:** >5 *café au lait* macules of >5 mm (children) or >15 mm (adults), neurofibromas appear as cutaneous nodules or complex plexiform neuromas, freckling in armpit or groin. Lisch nodules (tan nodules on iris, hamartomas), spinal scoliosis.
NF2: Few or no skin lesions, sensorineural deafness with facial nerve palsy or cerebellar signs if schwannoma large (see Acoustic neuroma).

P: Neurofibromin is a GTPase-activating protein (GAP) and is present in all tissues, with increased concentrations in neural tissues. The mutated form has been shown to interact with the oncogene *Ras*, resulting in excessive activity. Less is known about merlin, but it appears to act as a negative growth regulator or as a tumour suppressor. Multiple mutations have been described in both genes.

I: Opthalmological assessment. Audiometry.
MRI brain and spinal cord: For vestibular schwannomas, meningiomas and nerve root neurofibromas.
SXR: Sphenoid dysplasia in NF1.
Genetic testing: Possible but difficult as the NF1 gene is very long.

M: Education and genetic counselling. Surveillance for complications.
NF1: Monitoring physical development, skin lesions, blood pressure, vision, hearing, signs of learning disability and scoliosis.
NF2: Regular hearing assessment and MRI follow-up of CNS lesions.
Surgery: Removal of vestibular schwannomas, removal of painful or disfiguring tumours, treatment of scoliosis or bone deformities.

C: **NF1:** Sarcomatous change (neurofibrosarcoma) occurs in 2–5 %, indicated by pain and weakness in muscle innervated by involved nerve. Tumours can compress spinal nerve roots (dumbbell tumours) or stenose aqueduct of Sylvius (obstructive hydrocephalus).
NF2: Schwannomas of other cranial or peripheral nerves, cataracts.

P: If no complications develop lifespan may be normal. Prognosis may be worse in those with manifestations before the age of 10 years and those with plexiform neurofibromas of the head and neck. If neurofibrosarcoma develops, prognosis is poor (5-year survival ~15 %).

Non-ulcer dyspepsia

D: Recurrent or persistent pain or discomfort in the upper abdomen for > 3 months in the year, in the absence of biochemical, endoscopic or ultrasonographical evidence of organic disease. Also known as functional dyspepsia.

A: Unknown. Abnormal gastric motility (e.g. delayed gastric emptying or gastroparesis), heightened sensitivity to gastric acid, ↑ visceral awareness and mild gastro-oesophageal reflux have all been suggested.

A/R: Psychosocial stress, IBS, affective or anxiety disorders, somatoform disorders. There is no clear association with *Helicobacter pylori* infection.

E: Common. Affecting mainly < 40-year-olds. ♀ : ♂ ~ 2:1.

H: Long-standing epigastric or diffuse abdominal pain.
Heartburn typically unresponsive to antacids.
Nausea, bloating, early satiety.
Alarm symptoms of unexplained weight loss, dysphagia, repeated vomiting and anaemia should be absent.

E: Usually normal.
There may be some epigastric abdominal tenderness or distention.
There should be no evidence of anaemia, abdominal mass or lymphadenopathy.

P: No structural or biochemical abnormality has been demonstrated. Visceral hypersensitivity, altered motility and impaired gut–brain axis may be involved.

I: In < 45-year-olds without alarm symptoms: either endoscopy or a non-invasive test for *H. pylori* may be carried out.
In > 45-year-olds with new onset dyspepsia, or in those with alarm symptoms: upper GI endoscopy.
Upper GI endoscopy: Should be normal by definition.
Others: *Blood:* FBC (to check for anaemia), U&E and LFT normal.
Ultrasound: To exclude gallstones.
More specialized tests include gastric emptying studies (with ^{99m}Tc-labelled mashed potato) or electrogastrogram to monitor gastric motility.

M: **Advice:** Explanation and advice. Dietary advice, e.g. avoidance of fatty foods which may slow stomach emptying, eating small frequent meals and avoidance of foods that aggravate an individual's symptoms.
Medical: *H. pylori* eradication has been controversial in this area, but may be beneficial. Antacid treatments and prokinetic agents (e.g. domperidone, metoclopramide) may help. Low-dose tricyclic antidepressants (e.g. amitriptyline) may also be beneficial. Some patients may require psychological or psychiatric treatment.

C: Interference with quality of life. High physical and psychological morbidity.

P: Usually a chronic relapsing and remitting course, often exacerbated by psychosocial stresses.

D: Characterized by recurrent collapse of the pharangeal airway and apnoea (defined as cessation of airflow for > 10 s) during sleep, followed by arousal from sleep. Also known as Pickwickian syndrome.

A: Obstructive apnoeas occur when the upper airway narrows because of collapse of the soft tissues of the pharynx when tone in pharangeal dilators decreases during sleep. Associated with:

- excessive weight gain, smoking, alcohol or sedative use;
- enlarged tonsils or adenoids in children; and
- macroglossia, Marfan's syndrome, craniofacial abnormalities.

A/R: (see Aetiology).

E: Common. Affects 5–20 % of men, 2–5 % of women > 35 years. Prevalence increases with age.

H: Excessive daytime sleepiness (at work, driving).
Unrefreshing or restless sleep.
Morning headaches or dry mouth, difficulty concentrating, irritability or mood changes.
Partner reporting snoring, nocturnal apnoeic episodes or nocturnal choking.

E: Large tongue, enlarged tonsils, long or thick uvula, retrognathia (pulled back jaws).
Neck circumference (> 42 cm males, > 40 cm females) strongly correlated.
Obesity and hypertension is common.

P: Important factors are upper airway anatomy (defines upper airway caliber), neuromuscular factors (especially tone of genioglossus, the chief pharangeal dilator) and state of arousal.

I: Video or audiotaping of episodes.
Sleep study: Managed by sleep study centre for polysomnography or diagnostic sleep studies with monitoring of airflow, respiratory effort, pulse oximetry and heart rate.
Blood: Thyroid function tests, ABG.

M: **Mild:** Advice on sleep positions (sleep on side rather than on back), weight loss, smoking cessation, avoidance of alcohol, sedatives and late night meals.
Moderate: Mandibular advancement splints.
Severe: Nasal CPAP: pneumatically dilates upper airways and prevents their closure.
Surgery: Used in severe cases with variable success (e.g. uvulopalatopharyngoplasty). Removal of nasal polyps, deviated nasal septum, tonsillar hypertrophy may be less invasive.

C: Risk of accidents when driving or working. Worsening of congestive heart failure. Linked to ↑ risk of coronary artery disease and stroke.

P: Short-term prognosis good with symptom improvement with CPAP. Compliance with advice or CPAP may be poor in long term.

Oesophageal carcinoma

D: Malignant tumour arising in the oesophagus. Two major types: squamous cell commonly arising in the upper two-thirds and adenocarcinoma in the lower third.

A: Proposed environmental insults in a genetically susceptible individual results in accumulated genetic mutations and tumour development. It is presumed that a sequence of oesophagitis, local metaplasia, dysplasia and carcinoma occurs.

A/R: **Squamous:** Alcohol, tobacco, iron-deficiency anaemia and oesophageal webs,*achalasia, scleroderma, coeliac disease, certain nutritional deficiencies and dietary toxins also implicated.
Adenocarcinoma: Gastro-oesophageal reflux disease and Barrett's oesophagus.†

E: Eighth most common cause of cancer deaths. ♂ : ♀ ~3:2. Annual incidence is 7000 in UK.
Squamous: High incidence in northern Iran, southern Russia, China, Japan, South Africa.
Adenocarcinoma of the distal oesophagus is increasing in the West (*H. pylori* eradication suggested as a possible contributing factor).

H: Progressive dysphagia, initially worse for solids then progressing to liquids.
Regurgitation, cough or choking after food, hoarseness, pain, weight loss.

E: No physical signs may be evident.
Metastases: Supraclavicular lymphadenopathy, hepatomegaly, hoarse voice caused by recurrent laryngeal nerve involvement, signs of bronchopulmonary involvement.

P: **Macro:** Ulcerative, polypoid, fungating or infiltrative tumours.
Micro: *Squamous:* Oval or polygonal sheets of cells with keratinization and intercellular prickles.
Adenocarcinoma: Glandular patterns, reduced cytoplasmic : nuclear ratio and ↑ mitoses.

I: **Imaging:** Barium swallow, CXR, CT chest, abdomen.
Endoscopy: Brushings or biopsy, endoscopic ultrasound to help in tumour staging.
Other: Bronchoscopy (in case of tumour invasion), lung function tests and ABGs (if surgery is planned).

M: Only 30–40 % patients are deemed suitable for attempted curative resection, the remainder are treated with combined modality chemotherapy and radiotherapy.
Palliative: Oesophageal dilation or stent insertions by endoscopy. PEG, laser thermal ablation or photodynamic therapy provide relief of dysphagia.
Surgery: Vital to have good preoperative nutritional support and physiotherapy. Operative approach depends on tumour location. Neoadjuvent chemotherapy or radiotherapy may be helpful.

*Paterson–Kelly–Brown (also known as Plummer–Vinson syndrome) is characterized by a postcricoid web, iron-deficiency anaemia, glossitis and angular stomatitis.
†See Gastro-oesophageal reflux disease (footnote).

C: Malnutrition, aspiration pneumonia, oesophageobronchial fistula. **Postoperative:** Pneumonia, anastamotic leakage, chylothorax, recurrent laryngeal nerve damage.

P: Very poor (5-year survival < 10 %). Attempted curative resection only raises survival rate to 20–25 %.

Osteoarthritis

D: Age-related synovial joint disease when cartilage destruction exceeds repair, causing pain and disability.

A: Osteoarthritis can also be classified according to distribution of joint sites involved.

Primary: Aetiology unknown. Likely to be multifactorial; 'wear and tear' concept proposed in the past.

Secondary: Other diseases can cause altered joint architecture and stability. Commonly associated diseases include the following.

1 Developmental abnormalities (e.g. hip dysplasia, Perthes' disease, slipped femoral epiphysis).
2 Trauma (e.g. previous fractures).
3 Inflammatory (e.g. rheumatoid arthritis, gout, septic arthritis).
4 Metabolic (e.g. alkaptonuria, haemochromatosis, acromegaly).

A/R: Age, family history (especially in general nodal osteoarthritis), joint injury, obesity (especially affecting the knees), strenuous physical occupation.

E: Common, with 25 % of those > 60 years symptomatic (70 % have radiographical changes). More common in females, white people and Asians.

H: Joint pain or discomfort, usually use-related, stiffness or gelling after inactivity.

Difficulty with certain movements or feelings of instability.

Restriction walking, climbing stairs, manual tasks.

Systemic features are typically absent.

E: Local joint tenderness.

Bony swellings along joint margins, e.g. Heberden's nodes (at distal interphalangeal joints).

Bouchard's nodes (at proximal interphalangeal joints).

Crepitus and pain during joint movement, joint effusion.

Restriction of range of joint movement.

P: Synovial joint cartilage fissuring and fibrillation. Eventually, there is loss of joint volume as a result of altered chondrocyte activity, subchondral sclerosis, bone cysts, osteophyte formation, patchy chronic synovial inflammation and fibrotic thickening of the joint capsules.

I: **Joint X-ray:** Radiographs of involved joints typically show four classic features.

1 Joint space narrowing (resulting from cartilage loss).
2 Subchondral cysts.
3 Subchondral sclerosis.
4 Osteophytes.

Note that the severity of radiological changes is not a good indicator of symptom severity.

Synovial fluid analysis: Clear synovial fluid, viscous with low cell count and possibly cartilage fragments.

M: Treatment goals include symptom relief, optimizing joint function, minimizing disease progression and limiting disability.

Medical: Analgesia with paracetamol, codeine, NSAIDs, COX-2 inhibitors, quinine and glucosamine. Topical NSAIDs or capsaicin provide benefit in some. Intra-articular injection of steroids and hyaluronic acid provides good symptomatic relief. Tidal irrigation (intra-articular instillation of normal saline) is not very effective.

Supportive: Patient education. Encourage lifestyle changes (e.g. weight loss, exercise). Physiotherapy, occupational therapy and psychosocial support.

Surgical: Various techniques can provide benefit, such as arthroscopic irrigation, osteophyte removal, joint replacement (arthroplasty) and joint fusion (arthrodesis).

C: Pain and disability, nerve entrapment syndromes, falls and fractures caused by reduced mobility.

P: Although symptoms may improve or worsen in phases, disease evolution is usually slow, with the natural history depending on the joint site involved.

Osteomalacia and rickets

D: Characterized by defective mineralization of skeletal osteoid. When this occurs before epiphyseal closure in children it is termed rickets.

A: **Vitamin D deficiency:***

- Lack of sunlight exposure.
- Dietary deficiency or malabsorption.
- Liver disease (↓ production of 25-hydroxylated vitamin D and malabsorption of vitamin D).
- Drugs (e.g. phenytoin, carbamazepine, rifampicin).
- Renal disease (e.g. inactivating mutation in L-hydroxylase gene: 'type I vitamin D-resistant rickets').
- Vitamin D resistance (mutations in the vitamin D receptor gene, 'type II vitamin D-resistant rickets').

Hypophosphataemia: Caused by ↑ urinary phosphate excretion.

- Fanconi's syndrome (phosphaturia, glycosuria, amino aciduria).
- Renal tubular acidosis.
- Hereditary hypophosphataemic rickets (X-linked or autosomal dominant).
- Tumour-induced osteomalacia.†

A/R: House-bound elderly, Asian, coeliac disease, Crohn's disease, primary biliary cirrhosis, chronic renal failure.

E: Now uncommon in industrialized countries, more common in females.

H: **Osteomalacia:** Vague bone pain (especially axial skeleton), weakness, malaise.

Rickets: Ill child with bone pain, weakness, difficulty in walking, lethargy, bony deformities, poor growth.

E: **Osteomalacia:**

Bone tenderness, proximal muscle weakness, waddling gait.

Signs of hypocalcaemia may be present:

Trousseau's sign: Inflation of the sphygmomanometer cuff to above the systolic pressure for > 3 min causes tetanic spasm of wrist and fingers.

Chvostek's sign: Tapping over the facial nerve causes twitching of the facial muscles.

Rickets:

Bossing of frontal and parietal bones.

Swelling of costochondral junctions (rickety rosary).

Harrison's sulcus of rib cage (caused by inward pull by diaphragm).

Bow legs in early, 'knock knees' in later childhood.

Short stature.

P: Excess osteoid covering trabecular bone surfaces, often with evidence of increased resorption as a result of secondary hyperparathyroidism.

*Vitamin D is a prohormone obtained from normal dietary intake or synthesized in the skin from 7-dehydrocholesterol. Vitamin D is activated by hydroxylation into 1,25-$(OH)_2$ vitamin D in the liver and kidney.

†Caused by ↑ fibroblast growth factor-23 (FGF-23) which causes ↑ renal phosphate loss ('phosphate diabetes').

I: **Blood:** ↓ Ca^{2+} (but normal in > 50 %), ↓ Po_4^{3-}, ↑ AlkPhos, ↑ PTH, ↓ 25-(OH) vitamin D. Also FBC, U&E (renal function), ABG (acid–base balance, severe hypercholaemic acidosis suggests renal tubular disease).
Urinalysis: ↓ Ca^{2+} and ↑ Po_4^{3-} excretion.
Iliac crest biopsy: After two courses of oral tetracycline separated by 10–21 days.
X-ray radiographs:
Rickets: Show ragged and concave growth plate with cupped epiphyseal cartilage (saucer deformity).
Osteomalacia: May appear normal or show osteopenia. Later Looser's zones or pseudofractures (radiolucent bands) in ribs, scapula, pubic rami or upper femur. May have evidence of hyperparathyroidism with subperiosteal erosions of phalanges.

M: Vitamin D and calcium replacement, monitoring Ca^{2+} to avoid hypercalcaemia.
Treat the underlying cause (e.g. advice on diet and sunlight exposure).
X-linked hypophosphataemia: Oral phosphate and 1,25 $(OH)_2$ vitamin D.

C: Bone deformities, epileptic seizures, cardiac arrhythmias, hypocalcaemic tetany, depression.

P: Improvement of symptoms and radiological appearances occur within weeks of treatment. Bone deformities in children tend to be permanent.

D: Reduced bone density (defined as < 2.5 standard deviations below peak bone mass achieved by healthy adults) resulting in bone fragility and increased fracture risk.

A: **Primary:** Idiopathic (< 50 years), postmenopausal.
Secondary:
Malignancy: Myeloma, metastatic carcinoma.
Endocrine: Cushing's disease, thyrotoxicosis, primary hyperparathyroidism, hypogonadism.
Drugs: Corticosteroids, heparin.
Rheumatological: Rheumatoid arthritis, ankylosing spondylitis.
Gastrointestinal: Malabsorption syndromes (e.g. coeliac disease, partial gastrectomy), liver disease (primary biliary cirrhosis), anorexia.

A/R: Risk factors include age, family history, low BMI, low calcium intake, smoking, lack of physical exercise, low exposure to sunlight, alcohol abuse, late menarche, early menopause, hypogonadism.

E: Common. In > 50-year-olds, one-third of women, one-twelfth of men. Causes > 200 000 fractures annually in UK (especially hip fractures). More common in caucasians than in afro-carribeans.

H: Often asymptomatic until characteristic fractures occur.
Femoral neck fractures (commonly after minimal trauma).
Vertebral factures (loss of height or stooped posture or acute back pain after lifting).
Colles' fracture of the distal radius after fall onto outstretched hand.

E: Often no signs until complications develop:
- tenderness on percussion (over vertebral fractures);
- thoracic kyphosis (if multiple vertebral fractures); and
- severe pain with leg shortened and externally rotated (in a femoral neck fracture).

P: Reduction of both organic matrix and mineral content affecting mainly trabecular bone.

I: **Blood:** Ca^{2+}, Po_4^{3-} and AlkPhos are normal (unless a result of secondary causes).
X-ray radiography: Usually to diagnose fractures when symptomatic. Often normal (> 30 % loss in density before showing radiolucency, abnormal trabeculae or cortical thinning evident), biconcave vertebrae, crush fractures. Isotope bone scans can highlight stress or microfractures.
Bone densitometry (dual-energy X-ray absorptiometry): Measure T and Z scores.
T-score: The number of standard deviations the bone mineral density measurement is above or below the young normal mean bone mineral density. T-score is used to define osteoporosis.
Z-score: The number of standard deviations the measurement is above or below the age-matched mean bone mineral density. Z-score may be helpful in identifying patients who may need a work-up for secondary causes of osteoporosis.

M: **Primary prevention:** Regular weight-bearing exercise, calcium-rich diet, avoidance of smoking and excess alcohol, hormone replacement therapy (if not contraindicated).
Medical:
Hormone replacement therapy: In postmenopausal women.

Bisphosphonates (e.g. alendronate): Pyrophosphate analogues that adsorb onto bone surfaces and exert an inhibitory effect on osteoclasts and decrease bone turnover.
Calcium supplements (> 1 g/day), *nasal calcitonin* (side-effects: nausea/flushing).
Vitamin D supplements.
Testosterone replacement: For hypogonadal men.
Consider selective oestrogen receptor modulators (e.g. raloxifene) in women who have a strong family history of breast cancer or who are unwilling or otherwise unable to take oestrogen.
Currently, all available treatments are antiresorptive. New treatments being developed stimulate bone formation, e.g. PTH (not licensed in the UK at present).

C: Pain, disability, loss of independence with fractures; 20 % of those sustaining hip fractures will need long-term residential care.

P: Further loss of bone density can be stopped or slowed with treatment.

Paget's disease of bone

D: Characterized by excessive bone remodelling at one (monostotic) or more (polyostotic) sites resulting in bone that is structurally disorganized.

A: Uncertain, postulated to be caused by a slow viral infection.

A/R: Family history, various candidate gene loci associated (e.g. chromosome 18 q).

E: Common in older age, 3 % of all > 50-year-olds, 10 % of all > 80-year-olds. ♂ : ♀ ratio is 2 : 1.

H: May be asymptomatic. May present with insidious onset pain, dull constant ache, aggravated by weight bearing and movement (may be caused by Pagetic process, associated degenerative joint disease or stress fractures), headaches, deafness, increasing skull size.

E: Bitemporal skull enlargement with frontal bossing. Spinal kyphosis.
Anterolateral bowing of femur, tibia or forearm (bowed 'sabre' tibia).
Skin over involved bone is warm (as a result of ↑ vascularity).
Sensorineural deafness (compression of vestibulocochlear nerve).

P: Affected bone contains increased numbers of osteoclasts which are abnormally large with more nuclei, involved in accelerated bone resorption with compensatory osteoblastic bone formation that is disorganized and hypervascular. The presence of intranuclear inclusions in Pagetic osteoclasts has led to the hypothesis that a slow virus is the cause.

I: **Bloods:** ↑ Alk Phos, but Ca^{2+} and PO_4^{3-} normal (except if immobilized).
Bone radiographs: enlarged, deformed bones with mixed lytic/sclerotic appearance, osteoporosis circumscripta in skull, cortical thickening, bowing, microfractures, enlargement of the skull (frontal and occipital areas) associated with a 'cotton wool' appearance.
Bone scan (^{99m}Tc MDP): to assess distribution of disease.
Resorption markers (for monitoring of disease activity): urinary hydroxyproline, pyridinoline crosslinks.

M: **Medical:** Bisphosphonates (e.g. etidronate, pamidronate) reduce bone turnover, calcitonin (SC or intranasal) can be used to reduce blood flow preoperatively. Stress fractures are treated by bed rest, analgesia, low-dose bisphosphonates and physiotherapy.
Surgical: Decompression indicated for neurological complications if medical treatment fails. Fracture fixation, joint replacement for associated degenerative joint disease.

C: Stress fractures, accelerated osteoarthritis.
Skull enlargement, which can cause sensorineural deafness, platybasia (upward bulging of the floor of the posterior cranial fossa in the region of foramen magnum) and hydrocephalus.
Neurological deficits from impingement of spinal cord and foramina.
High-output cardiac failure.
Osteosarcoma (or other sarcoma) develops in ~1 % of patients (suggested by increasingly severe bone pain).

P: Bisphosphonate treatment can result in prolonged remission. Sarcoma development is associated with very poor prognosis.

D: Malignant neoplasm of pancreas, mostly arising from exocrine ductal epithelium (adenocarcinoma).

A: Unknown. Aberrations of growth factor signalling, transcription factors and cell cycle control are implicated.

A/R: Age, smoking, dietary fat, hereditary pancreatitis, family history (4–16 %).

E: Fourth leading cause of cancer death in West. Annual UK incidence is 10 in 100 000. ♂ : ♀ ~2 : 1. Mean age 60–70 years.

H: Anorexia, early satiety, weight loss, fatigue.
Epigastric pain radiating into back pain (worse on lying flat).
New-onset diabetes mellitus.
Painless jaundice with dark urine, pale stools and pruritus.

E: Epigastric tenderness or mass, jaundice.
Gallbladder may be palpable (according to Courvoisier's law, a palpable gallbladder in the presence of painless jaundice is unlikely to be caused by gallstones).
Signs of extrapancreatic spread: Hepatomegaly, left supraclavicular lymphadenopathy, ascites.

P: **Macro:** 70 % arise in the pancreatic head, an important differential is periampullary carcinoma which has a better prognosis, 20 % in body and 10 % in tail (present at a later stage).
Micro: Majority are ductal cell adenocarcinomas (90 %), other types include adenosquamous, mucinous or cystadenocarcinoma tumours.
Staging: TNM system.

I: **Blood:** FBC, U&E, LFT (abnormalities may be caused by obstructive cholestasis or tumour metastases), glucose, clotting, Ca^{2+}, tumour markers (CA19-9 and CEA to monitor progression and response to treatment).
Ultrasound: To assess obstruction of biliary tree.
CT or MRI scan: Stages tumour and assesses size.
MRCP or ERCP: To assess obstruction of biliary tree.

M: Those with limited disease should be offered surgery if fit.
Surgery: Pancreaticoduodenectomy (Whipple's procedure) can be curative for localized disease (< 3 cm, no nodal metastases; however, < 15 % of patients eligible), should be performed in specialized centres. Chemotherapy trials can be attempted on patients who are not eligible.
Palliation: Alleviation of pain and improving quality of life. Biliary decompression by endoscopic stenting or surgical bypass, gastric outlet obstruction by gastrojejunostomy, pain control by medication and coeliac plexus block, nutritional supplementation, radiotherapy to symptomatic metastases.

C: Obstructive jaundice (caused by compression of common bile duct or metastases to nodes at the porta hepatis), diabetes, pancreatitis, GI bleeding, splenic vein thrombosis, malignant ascites.

P: Very poor, 5-year survival rate of 1 %. Mean survival from diagnosis is 3 months. With chemotherapy or chemoradiotherapy ~6–12 months. With resection in Stage I disease, 5-year survival is about 20 %.

Pancreatitis, acute

D: Acute inflammation of the pancreas.

A: **Most common:** Gallstones, alcohol.
Others: Drugs (e.g. steroids, azathioprine, thiazides, valproate), trauma, ERCP or abdominal surgery, infective (e.g. mumps, EBV, CMV, coxsackie B, *Mycoplasma*), hyperlipidaemia, hyperparathyroidism, anatomical (e.g. pancreas divisum, annular pancreas), idiopathic.

A/R: See above.

E: Common. Annual UK incidence ~10 in 10 000.

H: Severe epigastric or abdominal pain (radiating to back, relieved by sitting forward, aggravated by movement).
Associated with anorexia, nausea and vomiting.
There may be a history of gallstones.

E: Epigastric tenderness, fever.
Shock, tachycardia, tachypnoea.
Jaundice.
↓ Bowel sounds (resulting from ileus).
If severely haemorrhagic, Grey Turner's sign (flank bruising) or Cullen's sign (periumbilical bruising).

P: Varies in severity from mild glandular and interstitial oedema to frank parenchymal necrosis and haemorrhage with release of inflammatory mediators into the systemic circulation. Saponification may be seen as a result of the action of lipases and proteases on pancreatic tissue.

I: **Blood:** ↑ Amylase (usually > 3 times normal), ↑ serum lipase, FBC (↑ WCC, ↑ haemactocrit), U&E, ↑ glucose, ↑ CRP, ↓ Ca^{2+}, LFT (deranged if caused by gallstone pancreatitis or alcohol), ABG (for hypoxia or metabolic acidosis). See modified Glasgow criteria below.
Ultrasound: For gallstones or biliary dilation.
Erect CXR: Mainly to exclude other causes of an acute abdomen. There may be a pleural effusion.
AXR: Mainly to exclude other causes of an acute abdomen. There may be loss of psoas shadow.
Assessment of severity: Modified Glasgow* (Imrie) or Ranson's criteria† (for alcohol-induced pancreatitis), CRP. Note: amylase level does not correlate with disease severity.

*Modified Glasgow criteria:
WCC > 15 × 10^9/L, Glucose > 10 mmol/L, Urea > 16 mmol/L, AST > 200 unit/L, PO_2 < 8 kPa, Albumin < 32 g/L, Ca^{2+} < 2 mmol/L, LDH > 600.
†Ranson's criteria:
On admission: WCC > 16 × 10^9/L, age > 55 years, AST > 250, LDH > 350, glucose > 11 mmol/L.
During first 48 h: PO_2 < 8 kPa, Ca^{2+} < 2mmol/L, urea > 16 mmol/L, base deficit < 4.

M: **Intensive supportive care:** Fluid and electrolyte resuscitation and close monitoring. Urinary catheter and nasogastric tube. Analgesia. All patients should be nil-by-mouth. Nutritional support may be necessary. Prophylactic antibiotics have not been shown to reduce mortality. If gall-stone pancreatitis, stone removal by ERCP can be attempted.
Early detection and treatment of complications: Monitor respiratory function, renal function and clotting. Management in ITU may be necessary for severe cases.
Surgery: For necrotizing pancreatitis, drainage and débridement of all necrotic tissue.

C: **Local:** Pancreatic necrosis, pseudocyst, abscess, pancreatic ascites. In the long term, chronic pancreatitis (with diabetes and malabsorption).
Systemic: Multiorgan dysfunction, sepsis, renal failure, ARDS.

P: 20 % follow severe fulminating course with high mortality (pancreatic necrosis associated with 70 % mortality), 80 % run milder course (but still 5 % mortality).

Pancreatitis, chronic

D: Chronic inflammation of the pancreas with permanent structural changes leading to impaired endocrine and exocrine function and recurrent abdominal pain.

A: **Major:** Alcohol.
Others: Idiopathic in 20 %. Malnourishment, a variety of exogenous food toxins, cystic fibrosis, haemachromatosis, α_1-antitrypsin deficiency, pancreatic duct obstruction (acute pancreatitis, pancreas divisum, pancreatic duct anomalies), hyperparathyroidism.

A/R: See above.

E: Annual UK incidence is about 1 in 100 000; prevalence is about 3 in 100 000. Mean age 40–50 years in alcohol-associated disease.

H: Recurrent severe epigastric pain, often radiating to back, relieved by sitting forward. Exacerbated by eating or after an episode of binge drinking. Associated with nausea and vomiting.
May also be associated with bloating, pale offensive stools difficult to flush away (steatorrhoea).
Diarrhoea, weight loss, thirst and polyuria.

E: Epigastric tenderness.
There may be epigastric fullness (caused by pseudocyst).
Signs of weight loss, malnutrition and alcohol abuse.

P: Disruption of normal glandular architecture as a result of chronic inflammation and fibrosis, calcification, ductal dilation, cyst and stone formation.

I: **Blood:** Glucose (↑ may indicate endocrine dysfunction), amylase and lipase (usually normal), LFT (↑ if there is obstruction of the common bile duct).
Ultrasound: Percutaneous or endoscopic. Visualizes biliary duct dilation.
ERCP or MRCP: Early changes include main duct dilation. Late manifestations are duct strictures with alternating dilation ('chain of lakes' appearance).
AXR: Pancreatic calcification may be visible.
CT scan: Pancreatic cysts, calcification.
Tests of pancreatic endocrine function: Rarely performed, e.g. Lundh meal, faecal fat content.

M: **General:** Dietary advice and alcohol abstinence. Liaison with alcohol treatment and other support services.
Acute: Management of exacerbations of pain with analgesia.
Chronic: Pain management may need specialist pain clinic, treatment of diabetes (e.g. insulin). Pancreatic enzyme replacements (e.g. Creon, Pancrease). Endoscopic stenting of strictures may be possible.
Pain control: As the majority of sensory nerves to the pancreas transverse the coeliac ganglia and splanchnic nerves, both coeliac plexus block and transthoracic splanchnicectomy offer variable degrees of pain relief.
Surgery: Indicated if medical management has failed. Options include proximal resection (pancreatico-duodenectomy) or lateral pancreaticojejunal drainage (Puestow procedure).

C: **Local:** Pseudocysts, biliary duct stricture, duodenal obstruction, pancreatic ascites, pancreatic carcinoma.
Systemic: Diabetes mellitus, steatorrhoea, hypoglycaemic coma, narcotic dependency.

P: Surgery improves in 60–70 % but results are often not sustained. Life expectancy reduced by 10–20 years.

D: Excessive ingestion of paracetamol causing toxicity.

A: Maximum recommended dose: two 500 mg tablets four times in 24 h. Intake of > 12 g or > 150 mg/kg can cause hepatic necrosis.

A/R: Chronic alcohol abusers or those on enzyme-inducing drugs (which ↑ cytochrome P450 activity, e.g. anticonvulsants or anti-TB drugs), malnourished, anorexia nervosa, HIV are more susceptible to toxic effects of paracetamol. Overdose of paracetamol is commonly associated with ingestion of other substances, e.g. alcohol.

E: Most common intentional drug overdose in UK, 70 000/year, ♀ > ♂, causing ~100 deaths/year, this has been reduced by legislation in 1998 restricting pack sizes.

H: Very important to ascertain timing and quantity of overdose.
0–24 h: Asymptomatic or mild nausea, vomiting, lethargy, malaise.
24–72 h: RUQ abdominal pain, vomiting.
> 72 h: Increasing confusion (encephalopathy), jaundice.

E: **0–24 h:** No signs are evident.
24–72 h: Liver enlargement and tenderness.
> 72 h: Jaundice, coagulopathy, hypoglycaemia and renal angle pain.

P: **Pathogenesis:** At therapeutic levels, paracetamol is metabolized in the liver by conjugation with glucuronate or sulphate and excreted by the kidneys. A proportion (< 7 %) is metabolized by cytochrome P450 mixed function oxidases to a toxic highly reactive intermediate *N*-acetyl-*p*-benzoquinoneimine (NAPQI) which can be inactivated by conjugation with glutathione. At toxic levels the conjugation pathway and glutathione stores are overwhelmed, leading to NAPQI-induced oxidative damage and acute liver necrosis.
Micro: Acute liver necrosis in a centrilobular pattern is visible in moderate overdoses and entire lobules are affected in severe overdoses.

I: **Blood:** Paracetamol levels, 4 h post ingestion (absorbed rapidly, hence peak plasma levels are usually within 4 h). Assess need to treat based on normogram (see UK National Poisons Information Service guidelines). FBC, U&E, glucose, LFT (severe if peak ALT > 1000 IU/L) clotting studies (may be deranged by necrosis), ABG (for degree of acidosis).

M: **See UK National Poisons Information Service guidelines.**
Patient presenting within 8 h of overdose: If level within toxic range, antidote should be given: IV *N*-acetylcysteine (NAC). Caution: NAC can cause anaphylactoid reactions (treated with antihistamines). A less effective alternative is oral methionine.
Patient presenting > 8 h after overdose: If dose > 150 mg/kg then start NAC immediately before waiting for levels (efficacy of NAC is more limited after 15 h). Continue NAC until PT is normalized.
Patient with hepatotoxicity: Good supportive care with management of complications. Liver transplantation indications are PT > 100 s, creatinine > 300 μm, arterial pH < 7.3 (36 h post overdose), Grade III encephalopathy.

C: Acute hepatic failure, hypoglycaemia, cerebral oedema, GI bleeding, coagulation defects, metabolic acidosis, pancreatitis, acute tubular necrosis and renal failure (25 % if severe damage).

P: Depends on dose ingested and time of presentation. Early treatment with NAC may be lifesaving.

Parkinson's disease

D: Neurodegenerative disease of the dopaminergic neurones of the substantia nigra, characterized by a triad of bradykinesia, rigidity and tremor.

A: **Sporadic and idiopathic** (most common): Unknown. Environmental toxins and oxidative stress have been proposed (e.g. pesticides, wood pulp). Susceptibility gene, α-synuclein, has been identified on chromosome 4.
Secondary: Neuroleptic therapy (e.g. in schizophrenia), MPTP toxin from illicit drug contamination, post encephalitis (e.g. influenza) and repeated head injury (e.g. boxing) produce a very similar clinical picture.
Familial forms: Juvenile autosomal recessive associated with parkin gene (chromosome 6).

A/R: Other idiopathic akinetic –rigid syndromes have parkinsonian features.*

E: Very common: 1–2 % of > 60-year-olds. Annual incidence is 20 in 100 000. Mean age of onset is ~ 57 years.

H: Insidious onset.
Tremor at rest, usually noticed in hands.
Stiffness and slowness of movements.
Difficulty getting out of a chair or rolling over in bed, clumsiness, frequent falls.
Smaller hand writing (micrographia).
Insomnia, mental slowness (bradyphenia).

E: **Tremor:** Classically 'pill rolling' rest tremor in the hands of about 4–6 Hz frequency. Decreased on action or flexed posture. Usually asymmetrical.
Rigidity: ↑ Tone (lead pipe rigidity), with superimposed tremor (cogwheel rigidity). Rigidity can be enhanced by asking the patient to keep raising and lowering the other arm (sinkinesis). Normal power and reflexes.
Gait: Stooped, 'simian', shuffling, small-stepped gait with reduced arm swing. Freezing (difficulty in initiation of walking). Falls easily with little pressure from the back (propulsion) or the front (retropulsion).
Cranial nerve impairments: Mild impairment of upgaze. Glabellar tap sign (repeated taps on the forehead causes reflex blinking without fatigue). Tremulous eyelids (blepharoclonus).
Psychiatric: Depression is very common. Cognitive problems and dementia may occur in late disease.
Others: Mask-like face (hypomimia) with ↓ spontaneous blinking, soft monotonous voice (hypophonia) and tendency to drool (sialorrhoea). Greasy skin and seborrhoeic dermatitis is common.

P: **Macro:** Reduced melanin pigmentation in the substantia nigra (as dopamine is a precursor to melanin).
Micro: Degeneration of midbrain dopaminergic neurones projecting from the substantia nigra (pars compacta) to the basal ganglia (specifically, caudate nucleus and putamen). Symptoms appear only after > 70 % neuronal loss. Surviving neurones often contain eosinophilic cytoplasmic inclusions (Lewy bodies).

*Diffuse Lewy body disease: parkinsonism, cerebral cortical dysfunction, fluctuations and visual hallucinations.
Multiple system atrophy (Shy–Drager syndrome): autonomic failure, cerebellar and pyramidal features.
Progressive supranuclear palsy: failure of voluntary gaze (downgaze first, then upgaze), dementia.

I: Diagnosis is clinical. Dopamine treatment trial (e.g. timed walking after apomorphine) may be informative.
Blood: Serum ceruloplasmin (excludes Wilson's disease in young onset).
CT or MRI brain: Excludes other areas of neurodegeneration. Usually unnecessary.
PET: Shows uptake abnormalities in basal ganglia. Usually unnecessary.

M: Neurodegenerative process is still not treatable.
Medical: Symptomatic therapy by dopamine replacement. L-DOPA with peripheral DOPA decarboxylase inhibitor (carbidopa, benserazide) or dopamine receptor agonists (e.g. pergolide, ropinirole, pramipexole) are the main treatment options in the early stages of the disease but long-term therapy has serious complications. Anticholinergics (e.g. benzatropine) have a mild effect and mainly on tremor. MAO-B inhibitor (e.g. selegiline) and COMT inhibitor (e.g. entacapone) may reduce end-of-dose deterioration.
Surgery: Stereotactic thalamotomy, pallidotomy, deep brain stimulation and fetal cell transplantation have produced results in small studies.
Other: Physiotherapy, occupational and speech therapy is vital in maintaining a reasonable quality of life.

C: Depression, dementia, autonomic dysfunction (postural hypotension, constipation, urinary retention or overflow incontinence, erectile dysfunction), death (usually from pneumonia or pulmonary embolism).
Treatment complications (develops gradually over years on L-DOPA therapy): 'On–off' motor fluctuations and tardive dyskinesias (involuntary twisting or turning), painful sustained contractions (e.g. the foot). These can be minimized by frequent small doses, controlled release preparations or using dopamine agonists.

P: Progressive but variable in rate. Optimal treatment can delay impact of disability by 5–10 years.

Pemphigoid

D: An autoimmune subepidermal blistering (bullous) disease of the skin.

A: Caused by antibodies against skin basement membrane hemidesmosomal proteins. The trigger is unknown.

A/R: Possibly associated with malignancy.

E: Common (particularly in > 60-year-olds), more common than pemphigus, slightly more common in women.

H: Acute onset. The tense blisters are tender and can be very itchy.
New blisters can keep developing without adequate treatment.

E: Primary lesions are often erythematous and eczematous plaques, generalized on trunk and limbs. Large tense blisters then develop on these sites. ('Cicatricial' pemphigoid: heals with scarring and may affect the eye and orogenital mucous membranes.)

P: **Micro:** Subepidermal inflammation with polymorph and eosinophil infiltrate under the epidermis. The epidermis may separate from the dermis. Direct immunofluorescence will show linear IgG and C3 staining on the basement membrane zone.

I: **Skin biopsy:** Shows subepidermal blister and inflammation.
Blood: Circulating antibasement membrane IgG: ~85–90 % of patients (indirect immunofluorescence).

M: **Medical:** Potent topical corticosteroids supplemented with oral prednisolone 20–80 mg/day until there are no new blisters. Immunosuppressants such as azathioprine or methotrexate can be used instead. The blisters should be treated with wet dressings. In severe cases, monitor fluid balance as in severe burns.
Treat secondary infections and provide analgesia.

C: Fluid and electrolyte loss, secondary infections, complications of steroids (diabetes mellitus, hypertension, gastric ulceration, osteoporosis).

P: Good. Control of pemphigoid is easier than that of pemphigus. Complete remission after 1 year is common.

D: Autoimmune intraepidermal blistering disease.

A: Believed to be caused by autoimmunity against the proteins attaching the epidermal cells to each other (desmosomal proteins, desmoglein 1 and 3). The trigger is unknown. Rarely, it may be caused by penicillamine or captopril.

A/R: Possibly associated with malignancies, ↑ incidence in patients with thymoma and myasthenia gravis.

E: Rare, usually 45–60 years, ♂ = ♀.
Affects all racial groups, more common in Ashkenazi Jews and those from the Indian Subcontinent.

H: Acute onset of sore blisters (see Examination).

E: Primary lesions may be confined to the oral mucosa and throat (oral pemphigus). The flaccid blisters rupture readily and leave raw erosions. Oral involvement may be followed by thin-roofed blisters (e.g. axilla or trunk). Denuding of these blisters produce very tender red exuding areas.
New lesions appear at the site of lateral sheering forces (Nikolsky's sign*). Rarely, large moist verrucous plaques studded with pustules in flexural and intertriginous zones may be seen (pemphigus vegetans).

P: **Micro:** Intraepidermal split and blister formation with separation of individual cells (acantholysis), split may be just above the basal layer (suprabasal blister) leaving an intact layer of basal cells ('row of tombstones'): pemphigus vulgaris. In pemphigus foliaceus, there is a superficial epidermal split (only stratum granulosum is involved.) Direct/indirect immunofluorescence will show IgG and C3 localized intercellularly in the epidermis.

I: **Skin biopsy:** (see Pathology).
Blood: Antidesmosome IgG: positive in ~90 % of patients (indirect immunofluorescence), useful for monitoring disease activity.
Monitor FBC and LFT if azathioprine is used (see Complications).

M: **Medical:** High-dose prednisolone (60–120 mg/day orally, smaller doses may have to be continued lifelong). Methotrexate, azathioprine, ciclosporin or cyclophosphamide can be used to avoid steroids. Potent topical steroids can be used for mucocutaneous lesions. Resistant cases may require IV immunoglobulins.
Treat patient as if they had severe burns, thus requiring inpatient care, fluid replacements and wet dressings.
Nasogastric tube feeding may be required with mouth involvement.
Treat secondary infections, analgesia.

C: Fluid and electrolyte loss, death, secondary infection, complications of treatment (e.g. prednisolone: osteoporosis, diabetes, hypertension), slight ↑ risk of skin cancer and other malignancies with other immunosuppressants.

P: High mortality if untreated.

*Also positive in toxic epidermal necrolysis (see Erythema multiforme).

Peptic ulcer

D: Ulceration of areas of the gastrointestinal tract caused by exposure to gastric acid and pepsin, most commonly gastric and duodenal, also in oesophagus and Meckel's diverticulum.

A: Cause is an imbalance between damaging action of acid and pepsin and mucosal protective mechanisms.
Common: Very strong association with *Helicobacter pylori* (present in 95 % duodenal and 70–80 % of gastric ulcers), NSAIDs use.
Rare: Zollinger–Ellison syndrome.

A/R: Weak association with smoking, alcohol, genetic susceptibility, blood group O.

E: Common. Annual incidence of ulcers is about 1–4 in 1000. More common in males. Gastric ulcers have a mean age in the thirties, while gastric ulcers have a mean age n the fifties. *H. pylori* is usually acquired in childhood and the prevalence is roughly equivalent to age in years.

H: **Epigastric abdominal pain:** Relieved by antacids.
Symptoms have a variable relationship to food (e.g. if worse soon after eating, more likely to be gastric ulcers; if worse several hours later, more likely to be duodenal).
May present with complications (e.g. haematemesis or melaena or severe pain caused by perforation).

E: May be no physical findings.
Epigastric tenderness.
Signs of complications (anaemia, succession splash in pyloric stenosis, peritonism if perforation occurs).

P: **Pathogenesis:** There is a strong correlation with *H. pylori* infection, but it is unclear how the organism causes formation of ulcers.
Macro: Ulceration (usually < 3 cm) with well-defined edges and a grey-white floor. There may be surrounding erythema or a visible bleeding vessel.
Micro: Four layers (Askanazy's zones).
Layer 1 Thin exudate of fibrin and inflammatory cells.
Layer 2 Necrotic tissue layer.
Layer 3 Inflammatory granulation tissue.
Layer 4 Layer of dense fibrous tissue.

I: **Blood:** FBC (for anaemia), amylase (excludes pancreatitis), U&E, clotting screen (if GI bleeding), LFT, cross-match if actively bleeding.
Endoscopy: Four quadrant gastric ulcer biopsies to rule out malignancy, duodenal ulcers need not be biopsied.
Rockall scoring for severity after a GI bleed based on age, systolic BP, heart rate, comorbidity, underlying diagnosis and stigmata of recent haemorrhage.
Testing for *H. pylori*:
^{13}C –urea breath test: Radiolabelled urea given orally and detection of ^{13}C in the expired air. Useful for confirming eradication after treatment.
Serology: IgG antibody against *H. pylori*, confirms exposure but not eradication, as IgG may remain positive.
Campylobacter-*like organism test:* Gastric biopsy is placed with a substrate of urea and a pH indicator, if *H. pylori* is present, ammonia is produced from the urea and there is a colour change (yellow to red).
Histology of biopsies: Difficult to visualize *H. pylori*.

M: **Acute:** Resuscitation if perforated or bleeding, and proceeding to treatment by endoscopy or surgery.

Endoscopy: Treatment of bleeding by injection sclerotherapy, laser or electrocoagulation.

Surgical: If perforated, ulcer can be oversewn or an omental patch can be placed over it. Haemorrhage is controlled by tying off the affected vessels (usually gastroduodenal artery). In chronic cases where ulcer-related bleeding cannot be controlled, partial gastrectomy and/or vagotomy can be attempted.

Medical: *H. pylori:* Eradication with 'triple therapy' for 1–2 weeks. Various combinations are recommended made up of:

- 1 proton pump inhibitor/ranitidine bismuth sulphate.
- 2 antibiotics (e.g. clarithromycin + amoxicillin, metronidazole + tetracycline).

If not associated with H. pylori: Treat with proton pump inhibitors (e.g. lansoprazole) or H_2-antagonists. Stop NSAID use (especially diclofenac), use misoprostol (prostaglandin E_1 analogue), if NSAID use necessary.

C: **Major complication rate:** 1 % per year including haemorrhage (haematemesis, melaena, iron-deficiency anaemia), perforation, obstruction/pyloric stenosis (caused by scarring, penetration, pancreatitis).

P: Overall lifetime risk ~10 %. Good, as peptic ulcers associated with *H. pylori* can be cured by eradication.

Pericarditis

D: Inflammation of the pericardium, may be acute, subacute or chronic.

A: Idiopathic.
Infective (commonly, coxsackie B, echovirus, mumps virus, streptococci, fungi, staphylococci, TB).
Connective tissue disease (e.g. rheumatoid arthritis, sarcoid, SLE, scleroderma).
Postmyocardial infarction (24–72h) in up to 20% of patients.
Dressler's syndrome: Weeks to months after acute MI.
Malignancy (carcinoma of bronchus, breast, lymphoma, leukaemia, melanoma).
Metabolic: Myxoedema, uraemia.
Radiotherapy, thoracic surgery, drugs (e.g. hydralazine, isoniazid).

A/R: May be associated with a pericardial effusion.

E: Uncommon. The clinical incidence is < 1 in 100 hospital admissions. More common in males.

H: **Chest pain:** Sharp and central which may radiate to neck or shoulders. Aggravated by coughing, deep inspiration and lying flat. Relieved by sitting forward.
Dyspnoea, nausea.

E: Fever, pericardial friction rub (best heard lower left sternal edge, with patient leaning forward in expiration), heart sounds may be faint in the presence of an effusion.
Cardiac tamponade: ↑ JVP, ↓ BP and muffled heart sounds (Beck's triad). Tachycardia, pulsus paradoxus (reduced systolic BP by > 10 mmHg on inspiration).
Constrictive pericarditis (chronic): ↑ JVP with inspiration (Kussmaul's sign), pulsus paradoxus, hepatomegaly, ascites, oedema, pericardial knock (rapid ventricular filling), atrial fibrillation.

P: Acute inflammatory infiltration with increased vascularity and serous, fibrinous, haemorrhagic or purulent exudates (classical 'bread and butter' appearance in fibrinous pericarditis).

I: **ECG:** Widespread ST elevation that is saddle-shaped.
Echocardiogram: For assessment of pericardial effusion and cardiac function.
Blood: FBC, U&E, ESR, CRP, cardiac enzymes (usually normal). Where appropriate: blood cultures, ASO titres, ANA, rheumatoid factor, TFT, Mantoux test, viral serology.
CXR: Usually normal (globular heart shadow if > 250 mL effusion). Pericardial calcification can be seen in constrictive pericarditis (best seen on lateral CXR or CT).

M: **Acute:** Cardiac tamponade treated by emergency pericardiocentesis.
Medical: Treat the underlying cause, NSAIDs for relief of pain and fever.
Recurrent: Low-dose steroids, immunosuppressants or colchicine.
Surgical: Surgical excision of the pericardium (pericardiectomy) in constrictive pericarditis.

C: Pericardial effusion, cardiac tamponade, cardiac arrythmias.

P: Depends on underlying cause. Good prognosis in viral cases (recovery within ~2 weeks), poor in malignant pericarditis. Pericarditis can become recurrent (particularly in those caused by thoracic surgery).

Phaeochromocytoma

D: Rare catecholamine-secreting tumour of chromaffin cells of the adrenals.

A: Cause of sporadic cases unknown, reflection of genetic tendency to tumour development in familial forms.

A/R: Can occur in the background of multiple endocrine neoplasia (MEN type II), neurofibromatosis and von Hippel–Lindau syndrome.

E: Rare. $< 0.1\,\%$ of hypertensive patients.

H: Paroxysmal episodes of headache (80 %).
Palpitations, sweating, anxiety, pallor, weakness, heat intolerance, dyspnoea, nausea, tremor (70 %). Epigastric pain or chest pain (20–40 %).
Episodes may be triggered by physical exertion or emotional stress.
Occasionally preceded by sensation of 'impending doom'.

E: Hypertension (50–70 %): two-thirds of cases sustained, one-third paroxysmal. Postural hypotension: secondary to ↓ plasma volume.
Irregular pulse, fever, weight loss.

P: 10 % are extra-adrenal, malignant, multiple, familial, in children.
Macro: Grey or tan in cross-section. Most common extra-adrenal sites are para-aortic areas (75 %), bladder (10 %), thorax (10 %) and remainder occur in neck or pelvis.
Micro: Chromogranin-staining cells in cords or nests with pleomorphic nuclei and granules that secrete catecholamines (85 % noradrenaline (norepinephrine)) either continuously or intermittently. Malignant phaeochromocytomas appear histologically similar to benign.

I: **24-h urine collection** (in acid-containing bottle): Catecholamines, metanephrines and vanillylmandelic acid. Vanilla ingestion interferes with results.
Clonidine suppression test (not in hypovolaemic patients).
Blood: Blood glucose, Ca^{2+} (↑ in MEN or malignant forms).
Tumour localization: CT or MRI scan, ^{123}I-MIBG (meta-iodobenzyguanidine) scintigraphy.

M: **Medical:** Normalization of blood pressure:
α-blockade: phenoxybenzamine, phentolamine is short-acting for intraoperative BP control; and
β -blockade: never start before α-blockers as hypertension may be worsened.
Surgery: Open or laparoscopic, postoperative hypotension and hypoglycaemia common. After tumour removal, catecholamine levels should fall to normal in approximately 1 week.
Metastatic disease: Metastatic lesions should be resected if possible, therapeutic doses of ^{131}I-MIBG, combination chemotherapy, radiotherapy, α- and β-blockade, methyl-tyrosine (inhibits tyrosine hydroxylase, the enzyme catalysing the rate-limiting step in catecholamine synthesis).
Screening: For associated syndromes.

C: Atrial or ventricular fibrillation, MI, dilated cardiomyopathy, diabetes mellitus, hypertensive encephalopathy, cerebrovascular accident.

P: For localized and benign disease, complete resection has normal life expectancy. 5-year survival in metastatic disease is 35 %.

Pneumoconiosis

D: Fibrosing interstitial lung disease caused by chronic inhalation of mineral dusts.

Simple: Coalworker's pneumoconiosis or silicosis is not associated with symptoms.

Complicated: Pneumoconiosis (progressive massive fibrosis) results in loss of lung function.

Asbestosis: A pneumoconiosis in which diffuse parenchymal lung fibrosis occurs as a result of prolonged exposure to asbestos.

A: Caused by inhalation of particles of coal dust, silica or asbestos (two main types of fibre: white asbestos and blue asbestos or crocidolite, the latter the more dangerous).

A/R: **Occupational exposure:** In coal mining, quarrying, iron and steel foundries, stone cutting, sandblasting, insulation industry, plumbers, ship builders. Risk depends on extent of exposure, size and shape of particles and individual susceptibility, as well as co-factors such as smoking and TB.

E: Incidence ↑ in developing countries, disability and mortality from asbestosis will ↑ for the next 20–30 years.

H: Occupational history is important, there may be a long latency between disease exposure and expression.

Asymptomatic: Picked up on routine CXR (simple coal or silica pneumoconiosis).

Symptomatic: There is usually insidious onset of shortness of breath and a dry cough. Occasionally, black sputum (melanoptysis) is produced in coalworker's pneumoconiosis. Workers exposed to asbestos may develop pleuritic chest pain many years after first exposure as a result of acute asbestos pleurisy.

E: Examination may be normal.
Decreased breath sounds in coalworker's pneumoconiosis or silicosis.
End-inspiratory crepitations and clubbing in asbestosis.
Signs of a pleural effusion or right heart failure (cor pulmonale).

P: **Complicated disease:** There are large nodules in the lung, consisting of dust particles (coal or silica) surrounded by layers of collagen and dying macrophages. Mechanisms of damage include:

1. direct cytotoxicity by particles;
2. particle ingestion by macrophages results in activation and excessive free radical production causing lipid peroxidation and cell injury; and
3. proinflammatory cytokines and growth factors from macrophages and epithelial cells stimulate fibroblast proliferation and eventual scarring.

Asbestosis: Asbestos bodies consisting of fibres coated with an iron-containing protein are seen in regions of fibrosis, especially in the lung bases.

I: **CXR:**

Simple: Micronodular mottling is present.

Complicated: Nodular opacities in the upper lobes, micronodular shadowing, eggshell calcification of hilar lymph nodes is characteristic of silicosis. In asbestosis, there is often bilateral lower zone reticulonodular shadowing and pleural plaques, visible as white lines when calcified, often most obvious on the diaphragmatic pleura or as 'holly leaf' patterns.

CT scan: Fibrotic changes can be visualized before they are evident on CXR.

Bronchoscopy: Visualizes changes. Allows for bronchoalveolar lavage.
Lung function tests: Restrictive ventilatory defect, impaired gas diffusion.

M: **General:** Prevention of exposure. Avoidance of further exposure.
Medical: No specific treatment other than supportive care, e.g. oxygen or trial of inhaled steroids, and the treatment of complications.
Note: Patients are entitled to compensation for occupational lung diseases.

C: Progressive massive fibrosis, emphysema, cor pulmonale, Caplan's syndrome, end-stage respiratory failure, benign and malignant pleural effusions, lung carcinoma and mesothelioma (malignancy of pleura, seen especially with blue asbestos, crocidolite, exposure).

P: Not curable. Lifespan shortened with complicated disease. Prognosis is poor if malignancy develops.

Pneumonia

D: Infection of distal lung parenchyma. Several ways of categorization:

1 Community-acquired, hospital-acquired or nosocomial.
2 Aspiration pneumonia, pneumonia in the immunocompromised.
3 Typical and atypical (*Mycoplasma*, *Chlamydia*, *Legionella*).

A: **Community-acquired:** *Streptococcus pneumoniae* (70 %), *Haemophilus influenzae* and *Moraxella catarrhalis* (COPD), *Chlamydia pneumonia* and *C. psittaci* (birds/parrots), *Mycoplasma pneumonia* (occurs in epidemics, 4-yearly), *Legionella* (anywhere with air conditioning), *Staphylococcus aureus* (recent influenza infection, IV drug users), *Coxiella burnetii* (Q fever, rare), TB (may present as pneumonia; see Tuberculosis).

Hospital-acquired: Gram-negative enterobacteria (*Pseudomonas*, *Klebsiella*), anaerobes (aspiration pneumonia).

A/R: (see Aetiology). Age, smoking, alcohol, pre-existing lung disease, immunodeficiency, contact with pneumonia.

E: Incidence ~5–11 in 1000 (25–44 in 1000 in elderly). Community-acquired causes >60 000 deaths/year in the UK.

H: Fever, rigors, sweating, malaise, cough, sputum (yellow, green or rusty in *S. pneumoniae*), breathlessness and pleuritic chest pain, confusion (severe cases, elderly, *Legionella*).

Atypical pneumonia: headache, myalgia, diarrhoea/abdominal pain.

E: Pyrexia, respiratory distress, tachypnoea, tachycardia, hypotension, cyanosis.

↓ Chest expansion, dullness to percussion, ↑ tactile vocal fremitus, bronchial breathing (inspiration phase lasts as long as expiration phase), inspiratory crepitations on affected side.

Chronic suppurative lung disease (empyema, abscess): clubbing.

P: **Lobar pneumonia stages:**

1 *Congestion* with vascular engorgement, intra-alveolar bacteria.
2 *Red hepatization:* alveolar spaces filled with neutrophils, fibrin and RBC.
3 *Grey hepatization:* RBC disintegration, with fibrin and suppurative inflammation.
4 *Resolution:* exudate in alveolar spaces is degraded removed by macrophages.

Bronchopneumonia:

Macro: Patchy areas of consolidation with grey–yellowish appearance throughout lung.

Micro: Neutrophil inflammatory infiltrate in bronchi, bronchioles and adjacent alveoli.

I: **CXR:** Lobar or patchy shadowing, may lag behind clinical signs, pleural effusion, *Klebsiella* often affects upper lobes, repeat 6–8 weeks (if abnormal suspect underlying pathology, e.g. lung cancer). May detect complications: abscess (cavitation and air-fluid level).

Blood: FBC (abnormal WCC), U&E (↓ Na^+, especially with *Legionella*), LFT, blood cultures (sensitivity 10–20 %), ABG (assess pulmonary function), blood film (RBC agglutination by *Mycoplasma* caused by cold agglutinins; see Anaemia, haemolytic).

Sputum/pleural fluid: Microscopy, culture and sensitivity, Ziehl–Neelsen stain.

Urine: *Pneumococcus*, *Legionella* or *Chlamydia* antigens.-

Atypical viral serology: ↑ Antibody titres between acute and convalescent samples (>2 weeks post-onset).

Bronchoscopy (and bronchoalveolar lavage): Test for *Pneumocystis carinii*.

M: **Medical:** (Refer to British Thoracic Society Guidelines 2001)

Assess severity: (see Prognosis; if ≥1 feature present, manage in hospital).

Start empirical antibiotics:

- Oral amoxicillin (0 markers).
- Oral or IV amoxicillin and erythromycin (1 marker).
- IV cefuroxime/cefotaxime/co-amoxiclav and erythromycin (>1 marker).
- Add metronidazole, if aspiration, lung abscess or empyema suspected.
- Switch to appropriate antibiotic as per sensitivity.

Supportive treatment:

- Oxygen (maintain PO_2 >8 kPa, start with 28 % O_2 in COPD to avoid hypercapnia).
- Parenteral fluids for dehydration or shock, analgesia, chest physiotherapy.
- CPAP, BiPAP or ITU care for respiratory failure.
- Surgical drainage may be needed for empyema/abscesses.

Prevention: Pneumococcal, *Haemophilus influenzae* type B vaccination in vulnerable groups (e.g. elderly, splenectomized).

C: Pleural effusion, empyema (pus in the pleural cavity), localized suppuration → lung abscess* (especially staphylococcal, *Klebsiella* pneumonia, presenting with swinging fever, persistent pneumonia, copious/foul-smelling sputum), septic shock, ARDS, acute renal failure.

***Mycoplasma* pneumonia:** Erythema multiforme, myocarditis, haemolytic anaemia, meningoencephalitis, transverse myelitis, Guillain–Barré syndrome.

P: Most resolve with treatment (1–3 weeks), high mortality of severe pneumonia (community-acquired 5–10 %; hospital-acquired 30 %, 50 % in those in ITU). Markers of severe pneumonia:

- **C**onfusion.
- **U**rea > 7 mmol/L.
- **R**espiratory rate >30/min.
- **B**P (diastolic < 60 mmHg).

Other markers are hypoxia < 8 kPa, WCC < 4 or > 20 × 10^9/mm^3, age > 50 years.

*May also be secondary to obstruction (e.g. malignancies), infarction or septic emboli (staphylococcal).

Pneumothorax

D: Air in the pleural space (the potential space between visceral and parietal pleura). Other variants depend on the substance in the pleural space (e.g. blood: haemothorax; lymph: chylothorax).
Tension pneumothorax: Emergency when a functional valve lets air enter the pleural space during inspiration, but not leave during expiration.

A: **Spontaneous** (in individuals with previously normal lungs): Probably caused by rupture of a subpleural bleb.
Secondary: Pre-existing lung disease (COPD, asthma, TB, pneumonia, lung carcinoma, cystic fibrosis, diffuse lung disease).
Traumatic: Caused by penetrating injury to chest, often iatrogenic causes, e.g. during subclavian or jugular venous cannulation, thoracocentesis, pleural or lung biopsy, or positive pressure-assisted ventilation.

A/R: Spontaneous, particularly in tall thin habitus, Marfan's disease and Ehlers–Danlos syndrome.

E: Annual incidence of spontaneous pneumothorax is 9 in 100 000. Mainly affects 20–40 year olds. Four times more common in males.

H: May be asymptomatic if pneumothorax is small.
Sudden onset breathlessness or chest pain, especially on inspiration.
Distress with rapid shallow breathing if tension pneumothorax.

E: Signs may be absent if small.
Signs of respiratory distress with reduced expansion, hyper-resonance to percussion, ↓ breath sounds.
Tension: Severe respiratory distress, tachycardia, hypotension, cyanosis, distended neck veins, tracheal deviation away from side of pneumothorax.

P: Air is drawn into the negative intrapleural space equalizing pressures and resulting in chest wall expansion, lung collapse, alveolar compression and atelectasis. Mediastinal shift and great vein compression in a tension pneumothorax compromise cardiac function.

I: **CXR:** A pneumothorax is seen as a dark area of film where lung markings do not extend to. Fluid level may be seen if there is blood present. In small pneumothoraces, expiratory films may make it more prominent.

M: **Tension pneumothorax (emergency):** Maximum O_2, insert large-bore needle into second intercostal space, midclavicular line, on side of pneumothorax to relieve pressure, insert chest drain soon after.
Small pneumothorax (<15–20 %): If there is no underlying lung disease, pleural fluid or clinical compromise, give reassurance, analgesia if required and advice on avoiding air travel for at least 6 weeks.
Moderate pneumothorax (>20 %): Aspiration, under local anaesthesia, using a large-bore cannula inserted into the second intercostal space in the midclavicular line, with a three-way tap. Up to 2.5 L of air can be aspirated (stop if patient repeatedly coughs or resistance is felt). Follow-up CXR should be performed just after, 2 h and 1 week later. Chest drain should be inserted if aspiration fails, there is fluid in the pleural cavity or after decompression of a tension pneumothorax. It is inserted into the 4–6th intercostal space in midaxillary line.
Recurrent pneumothoraces (> 1): Pleurodesis (visceral and parietal pleura fusion with tetracycline or talc).

C: Recurrent pneumothoraces, persistant pneumothorax, development of a bronchopleural fistula.

P: After one spontaneous pneumothorax, at least 20 % will have another, with the frequency increasing with repeated pneumothoraces.

D: Infection of the meninges and motor neurones of the spinal cord and brainstem, with poliovirus.

A: Polio (an RNA picornavirus) is highly infectious and is spread by the faecal–oral or respiratory route. Live attenuated oral vaccine has, on rare occasions, been reverted to neurotropic form and caused vaccine-associated paralytic polio.

A/R: Risk groups: children < 3 years; non-immunized.

E: Rare in industrialized world because of immunization. Remaining cases are confined to Indian Subcontinent, east Mediterranean and Africa.

H: **Incubation:** Asymptomatic (6–10 days).
Prodrome: Non-specific 'flu-like illness (headache, fever, vomiting) for 7–14 days. ≥90 % recover; ≤10 % progress to CNS disease.
Non-paralytic (4–8 %): Fever, tachycardia, meningism (headache, stiff neck).
Paralytic (1 %): Myalgia, muscle weakness/paralysis, swallowing difficulty.

E: Moderate pyrexia.
Meningism (neck stiffness, photophobia, Kernig's sign).
LMN signs (fasciculation, wasting, flaccid weakness, ↓ reflexes) with variable patchy asymmetrical muscle involvement (**spinal polio**, paraparesis; **bulbar polio**, facial and bulbar palsy).
Hyperaesthesia (↑ sensitivity to stimuli).
Deformities, e.g. pes cavus (later).

P: **Macro:** Poliovirus multiplies in the gut lymphatic tissue (e.g. tonsils and appendix) and eventually infects the spinal cord and meninges. The virus has a 'tropism' for the anterior horn cells of the spinal cord and equivalent cells in the brainstem.

I: **Stool/throat culture:** Virus persists in the stool for up to 6 weeks. PCR differentiates between types.
Polio serology: ↑ IgM.
Lumbar puncture: ↑ Lymphocytes, protein (↑ or normal), virus detection by PCR.

M: **Medical:** No specific treatment. If paralysis involves the respiratory musculature, ITU care is recommended with ventilatory support. Analgesia and heat pads used to treat myalgia. Physiotherapy is needed to restore muscle bulk and prevent contractures.
Public health: Polio is a notifiable disease. In the UK, Sabin live attenuated vaccine is given orally at 2, 3, 4 months, and before entering and leaving school (boosters). This oral polio vaccine gives gut immunity (resulting from virus-specific IgA in the gut). The killed Salk vaccine is administered to immunocompromised children by subcutaneous injection. This vaccine gives good blood antibody levels but does not produce gut immunity.

C: Bulbar and respiratory failure, myocarditis, hypertension/shock (secondary to bulbar damage), diaphragmatic involvement predisposing to rupture. 'Post-polio syndrome' is a late deterioration (progressive weakness, muscle pain) caused by the added effects of other illnesses (controversial).

P: Small improvement usually seen at the end of the paralytic stage; however, some are left with permanent weakness. Few need long-term ventilatory support. 15–30 % mortality in adults mainly as a result of paralysis of respiratory muscles and myocarditis.

Polycystic kidney disease (PKD)

D: Autosomal dominant inherited disorder characterized by the development of multiple renal cysts that gradually expand and replace normal kidney substance, variably associated with extrarenal (liver and cardiovascular) abnormalities.

A: 85 % are mutations in PKD1 (polycystin-1) on chromosome 16, a membrane-bound multidomain protein involved in cell–cell and cell–matrix interactions; 15 % are mutations in PKD2 (polycystin-2) on chromosome 4, a Ca^{2+} permeable cation channel.

A/R: Associated with intracranial (Berry aneurysms) and aortic aneurysms, liver cysts, diverticular disease, hernias and aortic valve disease.

E: Most commonly inherited kidney disorder affecting 1 in 800, responsible for nearly 10 % of end-stage renal failure in adults.

H: Usually present at 30–40 years. 20 % have no family history.
May be asymptomatic.
Pain in flanks as a result of cyst enlargement/bleeding, stone, blood clot migration, infection.
Haematuria (may be gross).
Hypertension.
Headaches.

E: Abdominal distension, enlarged cystic kidneys and liver palpable, hypertensive, signs of chronic renal failure at late stage.

P: Pathological process considered a proliferative/hyperplastic abnormality of the tubular epithelium. In early stages, cysts are connected to the tubules from which they arise and the fluid content is glomerular filtrate. When cyst diameter >2 mm, most detach from the patent tubule and the fluid content is derived from secretions of the lining epithelium. With time, cysts enlarge and cause progressive damage to adjacent functioning nephrons.

I: **Ultrasound or CT imaging:** Multiple cysts observed bilaterally in enlarged kidneys, sensitivity of detection poor for those < 20 years.

M: **Medical:** *Blood pressure:* Closely controlled.
Haematuria: Managed conservatively.
Infections: Prompt treatment with non-nephrotoxic antibiotics (ciprofloxacin or co-trimoxazole). Avoid the use of NSAIDs.
End-stage renal failure: (see Renal failure, chronic).
Screening for intracranial aneurysm if family history of aneurysm.
Surgery: Cyst decompression reserved for selected cases, occasionally required for stone management. Liver cyst aspiration, marsupialization or resection if gives rise to pain.
Genetic counselling.

C: Chronic renal failure, renal stones (20 %).
1–2 % suffer subarachnoid haemorrhage/intracerebral bleed.
Cysts develop in the liver (70 %) and pancreas (10 %) but these rarely cause organ dysfunction. Mitral valve prolapse, diverticulosis of the colon.

P: 50 % develop end-stage renal failure by age 60 years. Renal replacement therapy prolongs life by 15 years (mean).

Polycystic ovary syndrome (PCOS)

D: A syndrome of hyperandrogenism and anovulation associated with polycystic ovaries and the metabolic consequences of insulin resistance.

A: Unknown. Postulated that raised insulin levels may precipitate hyperandrogenaemia in genetically susceptible individuals by unmasking latent abnormalities in the regulation of steroidogenesis.

A/R: Genetic susceptibility (loci such as CYP11a and insulin gene *VNTR* implicated), obesity, hyperlipidaemia, hypertension and progression to diabetes mellitus Type II (metabolic syndrome or syndrome X).

E: Affects 5–10 % of premenopausal women (20 % of women have polycystic ovaries on ultrasound). Onset usually aged around 15–30 years.

H: Menstrual irregularities (oligomenorrhoea or amenorrhoea).
Infertility.
Hirsutism or alopecia.
Acne.

E: Obesity (in 30–50 %), increased waist : hip ratio.
Hypertension.
Hirsutism, male pattern balding and acne.
Acanthosis nigricans: Velvety thickening and hyperpigmentation of the skin of axillae, neck and intertriginous areas (a marker for severe insulin resistance).

P: **Macro:** >8 subcapsular follicular cysts of <10 mm in diameter and increased ovarian stroma.
Micro: Thickened capsule, scarcity of corpora lutea or albicans, hyperplasia and fibrosis of stroma, follicular cysts with decreased granulosa cell layer and increased theca cell layer thickness.

I: **Blood:** ↑ LH but normal FSH. Oestrone : oestradiol ratio is increased. ↑ Testosterone, androstenedione and DHEAS. ↓ SHBG. Glucose and HbA1c.
Thyroid function tests and prolactin levels: Often performed to rule out other causes of symptoms.
Ultrasound of pelvis: To image ovaries.
Oral glucose tolerance test.
Fasting lipids.

M: **Advice:** Reduce weight, exercise and stop smoking.
Medical:
Oligomenorrhoea: Oral contraceptive pill to improve menstrual regularity.
Hirsuitism: Oral contraceptive pill with cyproterone acetate or spironolactone, flutamide (non-steroidal androgen receptor antagonist), cosmetic measures (e.g. electrolysis).
Insulin resistance: Metformin (also normalizes menstrual irregularities). Thiazoledinediones (e.g. rosiglitazone) may ↓ peripheral insulin resistance and are under assessment.
Infertility: Clomifene citrate (induces gonadotrophin release by occupying hypothalamic oestrogen receptors and interferes with feedback mechanisms). Gonadotrophins. *In vitro* fertilization techniques (increased risk of hyperstimulation ovary syndrome and multiple pregnancy).
Surgery: For infertility, laparoscopic ovarian diathermy.

C: Infertility, recurrent miscarriage, gestational diabetes, endometrial carcinoma, diabetes mellitus, MI, stroke.

P: Wide spectrum of severity, lifestyle and medical interventions are generally successful.

Polycythaemia

D: An increase in haemoglobin concentration above the upper limit of normal for a person's age and sex. Classified into relative polycythaemia (normal red cell mass but ↓ plasma volume) or true/absolute polycythaemia (↑ red cell mass).

A: **True primary:**
Polycythaemia rubra vera: Neoplastic disorder of erythroid progenitor cells.
True secondary:
Appropriate ↑ erythropoietin: Caused by chronic hypoxia (e.g. high altitude, chronic lung disease) leading to upregulation of erythrogenesis.
Inappropriate ↑ erythropoietin: Renal (carcinoma, cysts, hydronephrosis), hepatocellular carcinoma, fibroids, cerebellar haemangioblastoma.
Relative: Dehydration (e.g. diuretics, burns, enteropathy), Gaisböck's syndrome (characterized by young male smokers with increased vasomotor tone and hypertension).

A/R: Polycythaemia rubra vera is associated with other myeloproliferative disorders (e.g. myelofibrosis, essential thrombocythaemia and chronic myeloid leukaemia). Secondary polycythaemia may be a feature of erythropoietin abuse amongst athletes.

E: Annual UK incidence of polycythaemia rubra vera is 1.5 in 100 000. Peak age is 45–60 years.

H: Headaches, dyspnoea, tinnitus, blurred vision as a result of hyperviscosity.
Pruritus after hot bath, night sweats.
Thrombosis (DVT, stroke), pain resulting from peptic ulcer disease, angina, gout, choreiform movements.

E: Ruddy, plethoric complexion.
Scratch marks as a result of itching, conjunctival suffusion and retinal venous engorgement.
Hypertension.
Splenomegaly (present in 75 % of polycythaemia rubra vera).
Signs of underlying aetiology in secondary causes.

P: Polycythaemia rubra vera results from clonal expansion of a transformed haemopoietic stem cell. Increased red cell mass results in hyperviscosity and vascular stasis, combined with a frequently raised platelet count results in increased risk of thrombosis.

I: **Required for diagnosis:** FBC (↑ Hb, ↑ haematocrit, ↑ red cell count, ↑ red cell mass, ↑ packed cell volume).
In polycythaemia rubra vera, there is ↑ WCC and ↑ platelets, ↑ neutrophil alkaline phosphatase, ↑ vitamin B_{12}, ↑ vitamin B_{12}-binding capacity, ↑ urate.
To distinguish between relative and absolute polycythaemia: Isotope dilution techniques using radiolabelled albumin (^{131}I) and RBCs (^{51}Cr) allows confirmation of actual red cell mass.
If absolute:
To diagnose polycythaemia rubra vera: Bone marrow trephine and biopsy would show erythroid hyperplasia and ↑ megakaryoctyes.
In those secondary to hypoxia: Sat O_2 levels, ABG, CXR.
In those secondary to ↑ erythropoietin: Serum erythropoietin, abdominal ultrasound or CT.

M: **Polycythaemia rubra vera:** Regular venesection to reduce packed red cell volume to <0.45. Aspirin to reduce risk of thrombosis. Chemotherapy is useful in reducing risk of malignancy (e.g. with hydroxyurea, interferon-α, busulfan). Symptomatic treatment of complications (e.g. allopurinol for hyperuricaemia, H_2-antagonists for peptic ulcers).
Secondary or relative: Treat underlying disorder.

C: Thrombosis is a major complication (stroke, MI), haemorrhage (resulting from defective platelet function), gout and renal calculi (hyperuricaemia), peptic ulceration occurs in 5–10 % of patients with polycythaemia rubra vera.

P: Good prognosis with management. In polycythaemia rubra vera, the mean survival is 16 years. Without treatment median survival ~1–2 years. 30 % develop myelofibrosis and 5 % acute leukaemia.

Polymyositis and dermatomyositis

D: Idiopathic primary inflammatory myopathies characterized by chronic inflammation of striated muscle (polymyositis) and skin (dermatomyositis).

A: Unknown. Proposed autoimmune aetiology, possibly infective or malignancy trigger in genetically predisposed individual.

A/R: Polymyositis may be associated with autoimmune connective tissue diseases (e.g. scleroderma).
Dermatomyositis may be associated with bronchial, stomach, testicular, breast and ovarian malignancy specially in older age groups, autoantibodies anti-Jo-1, anti-PM-Scl, anti-Mi2, HLA linkage to *DRW52*.

E: Rare. Annual incidence is 0.2–1 in 100 000. Peaks at childhood (5–15 years) and adult (40–60 years). ♂ : ♀ (1 : 1 in association with malignancy, 1 : 10 with connective tissue disease). More common in Afro-Caribbeans than white people.

H: Gradual onset (3–6 months) of progressive painless proximal muscle weakness (difficulty raising objects above head, rising from chair, climbing stairs), skin rash, fatigue, malaise, dyspnoea.
There may also be dysphagia (pharyngeal muscle involvement), myalgia, arthralgia, Raynaud's phenomenon and symptoms of associated conditions.

E: Upper and lower limb proximal muscle weakness.
Hoarseness, dysphonia, waddling gait.
Skin lesions in dermatomyositis: Macular 'lilac' heliotrope rash on upper eyelids with periorbital oedema, rash on chest wall, neck, elbows or knees. Gottren's papules (scaly erythematous raised plaques on finger joints, periungal telangiecstasia, ragged cuticles), 'mechanics' hands' (fissuring dermatitis of finger pads).

P: **Polymyositis:** Evidence of cell-mediated immune mechanisms with ↑ cytotoxic $CD8^+$ T cells which appear to recognize an antigen on muscle fibre surface. Cellular infiltrate is mainly within the fascicle. Abnormal muscle fibres are scattered throughout the fascicle. No signs of vasculopathy or immune complex deposition.
Dermatomyositis: Evidence of humorally mediated disorder and the primary lesion in the muscle is located in the blood vessels. Cellular infiltrate is predominantly perifascicular and often perivascular. The terminal complement C5b-9 membrane attack complex is detectable in vessel walls before the appearance of inflammatory cell infiltrate. Inflammatory infiltrate is composed of B cells and a high ratio of $CD4^+$: $CD8^+$ T cells. Abnormal muscle fibres are usually grouped in one portion of the fascicle.

I: Careful evaluation for underlying malignancy.
Blood: FBC (↓ Hb of chronic disease), ↑ESR (normal in one-third), CK (↑ in 95 % of cases), autoantibody titres.
EMG: Shows ↑ insertional activity, ↑ spontaneous fibrillations; abnormal myopathic low-amplitude short-duration polyphasic motor potentials and bizarre high-frequency discharges.
Muscle biopsy: Required for definitive diagnosis.
CT or MRI: To look for malignancies.

M: **Medical:** Corticosteroids are mainstay of therapy (e.g. prednisolone, monitoring response by CK levels). Steroid-sparing therapies (e.g. methotrexate, azathioprine, cyclophosphamide, IV immunoglobulin).
Other: Physiotherapy and occupational therapy aids.

C: The risk of malignancy is greatest in the first 2 years after dermatomyositis has been diagnosed. Interstitial pneumonitis and cardiac involvement can occur. Children may develop necrotizing vasculitis involving gut. Severe muscle weakness may result in aspiration pneumonia or respiratory failure.

P: Long remissions are possible, especially in children. The majority of patients experience multiple remissions and exacerbations.

Note: inclusion body myositis: rare idiopathic inflammatory myopathy with clinicopathological manifestations that are distinct from polymyositis and dermatomyositis. Mean age at onset is ~60 years. Characterized by insidious onset, variable distribution of weakness. May be primarily distal. Muscle biopsy shows inflammation, rimmed vacuoles and inclusion bodies. It responds poorly to treatment.

Porphyria

D: Heterogeneous group of inherited disorders of haem biosynthesis. A clinical classification is as follows.

Acute attacks: Autonomic dysfunction and neuropsychiatric features (e.g. acute intermittent porphyria).

Cutaneous: Skin lesions and photosensitivity (e.g. porphyria cutanea tarda, erythropoietic protoporphyria).

Mixed: Combination of the above (e.g. variegate porphyria, hereditary coproporphyria).

A: Partial deficiency of any of the enzymes in haem biosynthesis pathway results in seven different types of porphyrias. For example, the most common one is acute intermittent prophyria which is an autosomal dominant disorder caused by ↓ porphobilinogen (PBG) deaminase.

A/R: Precipitating factors: drugs (e.g. carbamazepine, oral contraceptives, cocaine), fasting, smoking, alcohol, infection, relapses in pregnancy, premenstrually.

Cutaneous porphyria may be associated with hepatitis C virus infection, iron overload, liver cell damage and diabetes mellitus.

E: Rare. Prevalence varies widely between countries and different type of porphyrias.

Acute attacks are more common in the thirties. More common in women.

H: May remain latent. Clinically classified into the following.

Acute attacks:

GI: Abdominal pain, nausea, vomiting, constipation.

Neurological: Sensory neuropathies (e.g. paraesthesias), motor neuropathy (e.g. muscle weakness, quadriplegia), seizures (secondary to hyponatraemia).

Psychiatric: Agitation, depression, mania, schizophrenia-like symptoms.

Cutaneous lesions:

Photosensitivity: Burning, itching and erythema on exposure to sunlight. Vesicles and bullae (e.g. on the back of the hands) that heal with scarring.

Hyperpigmentation.

Hypertrichosis.

Fragile skin.

E: *GI:* Abdominal tenderness.

Autonomic dysfunction: ↑ BP, tachycardia, pyrexia, sweating, pallor.

Neuropsychiatric signs.

Cutaneous lesions (see History).

P: Porphyrin overproduction may occur in liver, bone marrow, or both, depending on different porphyrias.

Acute porphyrias: ↑ Porphyrins and porphyrin precursors (e.g. PBG, ALA) proximal to the enzyme defect.

Cutaneous: ↑ Porphyrins only.

Pathogenesis: Neurotoxicity of porphyrin precursors (e.g. ALA), ↓ haem in nervous tissue. It has been postulated that free radical damage may also contribute.

I: **Acute attacks:** FBC (neutrophilia), U&E (↑ urea, ↓ Na^+ as a result of SIADH), LFT abnormalities (also seen in cutaneous porphyria), clotting screen (avoid haem arginate treatment if there is evidence of coagulopathy).

Urine: Turns dark red or brown on standing because of polymerization of porphyrin precursors. (Addition of Ehrlich's aldehyde reagent also turns urine red.)

Porphyrin and porphyrin precursor analysis: Can be measured in urine (↑ ALA and PBG during acute attacks), erythrocytes and faeces (to determine the type of pororphyria). Samples must be protected from light.

M: **Advice:** Avoid precipitating factors, Medicalert bracelet. Encourage family screening.

Acute attacks: Remove the precipitating factor, IV infusion of haem arginate (inhibits ALA synthase and reduces porphyrin precursor synthesis), 10 % glucose infusion or glucose polymer drink (e.g. Hycal) to maintain high energy intake.

Analgesia: Opiates and chlorpromazine (pain ↓ in sleep).

Seizures: Strict fluid restriction. Vigabatrin or gabapentin.

Hypertension: Propranolol.

Cutaneous: Barrier creams. Avoid sunlight, alcohol and oestrogens. Venesection for iron overload, oral chloroquine (↑ urinary porphyrin excretion), β-carotene (quenches active oxygen species). Screen for hepatitis C virus.

C: Respiratory paralysis, chronic hypertension, chronic renal failure (rare).

P: 1 % fatality in acute attacks. Minority (mainly females) have recurrent attacks with no precipitants.

Primary biliary cirrhosis

D: Primary biliary cirrhosis is a chronic inflammatory liver disease involving progressive destruction of intrahepatic bile ducts, leading to cholestasis and, ultimately, cirrhosis.

A: Unknown. Autoimmune aetiology is likely, but genetic and environmental factors have also been proposed.

A/R: Associated with autoimmune diseases (e.g. autoimmune thyroid disease, rheumatoid arthritis, Sjögren's syndrome and ulcerative colitis).

E: Prevalence is 10–20 in 100 000 in UK. Much less common cause of cirrhosis than alcoholic cirrhosis. Usually affects middle-aged women (♀ : ♂ ratio is 9 : 1).

H: May be an incidental finding on blood tests (e.g. ↑ AlkPhos, ↑ cholesterol).
Insidious onset.
Lethargy and itching (pruritus).
Skin pigmentation or discomfort in the RUQ of the abdomen (rarely).
May present with a complication of liver decompensation (e.g. jaundice, ascites, variceal haemorrhage).
Symptoms of associated conditions (see Associations/Risk factors).

E: **Early:** May be no signs.
Late: Jaundice, scratch marks, xanthomas (secondary to hypercholesterolaemia), hepatomegaly, ascites and other signs of liver disease may be present.
Signs of chronic liver disease (palmar erythema, clubbing and spider naevi are rare).

P: **Micro:** Chronic inflammatory cells and granulomas can be seen around the intrahepatic bile ducts. Destruction of bile ducts is followed by inflammation extending beyond the portal tracts, with fibrosis and regenerating nodules of hepatocytes. Eventually, this leads to cirrhosis. ? Staining of copper-binding protein as a result of cholestasis.

I: **Blood:** LFT (↑ AlkPhos, γ-GT. Bilirubin may be normal or ↑ in later stages. Transaminases usually normal or ↑, with disease progression and development of cirrhosis), clotting (prolongation of PT). Antimitochondrial antibodies, ↑ IgM and ↑ cholesterol are typical.
Ultrasound: To exclude extrahepatic biliary obstruction (e.g. by gallstones or strictures).
Liver biopsy: (see Pathology).

M: **Symptomatic:** Itching can be treated with colestyramine (binds bile acids in the GI tract), rifampicin (may work by upregulating liver enzymes that metabolize factors which cause pruritus) or naloxone.
Medical: Ursodeoxycholic acid is most commonly used. It is a hydrophilic bile acid which may decrease the toxicity or improve elimination of retained bile acids. It improves the biochemical markers and may improve symptoms and survival.
Treatment of complications:
Osteoporosis: With calcium supplementation and bisphosphonates.
Vitamin replacement (A, D, E and K).
Portal hypertension: β-Blockers and endoscopic banding of varices if present.
TIPS: A radiological procedure whereby a vascular tract is created in the liver from hepatic to portal veins allowing decompression of the portal hypertension. Increases risk of hepatic encephalopathy.

Surgical: Liver transplantation for intractable symptoms or end-stage liver disease.

C: Liver cirrhosis and all associated complications (e.g. jaundice, encephalopathy, ascites, variceal bleeding, hepatocellular carcinoma, osteoporosis, hyperlipidaemia and malabsorption of fat-soluble vitamins).

P: Rate of disease progression can be variable. Prognostic scores have been developed (e.g. Mayo score), and the most important factor is the serum bilirubin level. Median survival time from diagnosis ~10 years. The 5-year survival rate after liver transplantation is >70 %. Primary biliary cirrhosis can recur in the transplanted liver.

Primary sclerosing cholangitis

D: Chronic cholestatic liver disease characterized by progressive inflammatory fibrosis and obliteration of intrahepatic and extrahepatic bile ducts.

A: Unknown. Postulated immune and genetic predisposition and toxic or infective triggers.

A/R: Close association with IBD, especially UC (present in 70 %). About 5 % of those with UC will develop PSC.

E: Prevalence 2–7 in 100 000. Usually presents between 25 and 40 years.

H: May be asymptomatic and diagnosed after persistently ↑ AlkPhos.
May present with intermittent jaundice, pruritus, RUQ pain, weight loss and fatigue.
Episodes of fever and rigors caused by acute cholangitis are less common.
History of ulcerative colitis.
Symptoms of complications.

E: May have no signs or have evidence of jaundice, hepatosplenomegaly, spider naevi, palmar erythema or ascites.

P: **Micro:** Periductal inflammation with periductal concentric fibrosis ('onion skin'), portal oedema, bile duct proliferation and expansion of portal tracts, progressive fibrosis and development of biliary cirrhosis.
Liver biopsy staging:
1 Portal changes. **3** Septum formation.
2 Periportal extension. **4** Cirrhosis.

I: **Blood:** LFT (↑ AlkPhos, ↑ γ-GT, mild ↑ transaminases). In later stages, ↓ albumin and ↑ bilirubin.
Serology: Immunoglobulin levels (↑ IgG in children, ↑ IgM in adults), ASM and ANA (present in ~30 %), antimitochondrial antibodies (usually absent), pANCA (present in ~70 %).
ERCP: Stricturing and interspersed dilation (beading) of intrahepatic and, occasionally, extrahepatic bile ducts, small diverticula on the common bile duct may be seen.
MRCP: Enables non-invasive imaging of the biliary tree.
Liver biopsy: Confirms diagnosis and allows staging of disease.

M: **Acute cholangitis:** Resuscitation (particularly fluid), antibiotics (e.g. cephalosporin and metronidazole).
Medical: No curative treatment with management concentrating on symptom control. Colestyramine for pruritus, fat-soluble vitamins for deficiency, adequate dietary Ca^{2+}. Endoscopic or percutaneous transhepatic stenting or balloon dilation of major extrahepatic bile duct strictures to relieve biliary obstruction.
Surgical: Liver transplantation for end-stage disease. Very few recurrences reported. Surgery for ulcerative colitis has no effect on the course.

C: Recurrent cholangitis, biliary cirrhosis, cholangiocarcinoma (bile duct carcinoma, ~15 % of cases), portal hypertension (encephalopathy, ascites/oedema, variceal bleeding), metabolic bone disease.

P: Variable. Prognostic factors at presentation (Mayo model): age, bilirubin, biopsy stage (histology), enlarged spleen. Median survival from presentation to liver transplantation or death is about 10 years. 4-year survival after liver transplantation is about 85 %.

Pseudogout

D: Arthritis associated with deposition of calcium pyrophosphate dihydrate crystals in joint cartilage.

A: Unknown (possibly an age-related phenomenon). Familial cases and associations with metabolic diseases have been described.

A/R: Most causes of joint damage predispose to pseudogout (e.g. osteoarthritis, trauma), More rarely, conditions such as haemochromatosis, hyperparathyroidism, hypomagnesaemia, hypophosphatasia* can predispose to pseudogout. Provoking factors: intercurrent illness, surgery, local trauma.

E: ♀ : ♂ ratio is ~2:1. More common in elderly (> 60 years).

H: **Acute arthritis:** Painful, swollen joint (e.g. knee, ankle, shoulder, elbow, wrist).
Chronic arthropathy: Pain, stiffness, functional impairment.
Uncommon presentations: tendonitis (e.g. Achilles), tenosynovitis (tendons of the hand), bursitis (e.g. olecranon bursitis).

E: **Acute arthritis:** Red, hot, tender, restricted range of movement, fever.
Chronic arthropathy (similar to osteoarthritis): Bony swelling, crepitus, deformity, e.g. varus in knees, restriction of movement.

P: Calcium pyrophosphate crystals are deposited in joints. Chondrocalcinosis, a form of cartilage calcification, also occurs (e.g. fibrocartilage, menisci in knee joint, triangular cartilage in wrist joint) and hyaline cartilage (e.g. knee joint). Shedding of crystals into the joint cavity precipitates acute arthritis.

I: **Blood:** FBC (may show ↑ WCC in acute attack), ESR (may be ↑), blood culture (excludes infective arthritis).
Joint aspiration: Microscopy shows short rhomboid brick-shaped crystals, with weak positive birefringence under polarized light. Culture or Gram staining (exclude infective arthritis).
Plain radiograph of the joint: Chondrocalcinosis (linear calcification of cartilage), or signs of osteoarthritis: loss of joint space, osteophytes, subchondral cysts, sclerosis.
Investigation for any associated conditions or differential diagnoses (e.g. gout, haemarthroses).

M: **Acute:** Joint aspiration, intra-articular steroids (florid cases), simple analgesia: NSAIDs (with caution in elderly), rest and mobilization after acute attack has settled.
Chronic: Similar to osteoarthritis (e.g. lose weight, walking aids), physiotherapy, simple analgesics (e.g. paracetamol). Surgery may be necessary for severe cases.

C: Chronic pyrophosphate arthropathy, GI haemorrhage (secondary to NSAID use).

P: Acute attacks resolve in 1–3 weeks. Chronic pyrophosphate arthropathy has good outcome.
Rarely, a destructive arthropathy (with Charcot's joint features), recurrent haemarthrosis and joint capsular rupture occur in very elderly women.

*Hypophosphatasia is an autosomal recessive disease, characterized by reduced bone mineralization, ↓ serum AlkPhos, which can lead to rickets and recurrent fractures.

Pseudomembranous colitis

D: Large bowel inflammation with mucosal destruction and inflammatory exudates forming pseudomembranes on the bowel wall associated with toxin-releasing *Clostridium difficile* bacilli.

A: The organism responsible is *C. difficile*, a Gram-positive anaerobic bacilli. Colonic overgrowth of these toxin-forming bacteria is associated with disturbance of gut microflora, nearly always brought about by antibiotic use. In rare cases, it may occur without antibiotic use.

A/R: Associated with antibiotic use, especially clindamycin, ureidopenicillins, ampicillin and broad-spectrum cephalosporins.

E: *C. difficile* is commonly carried asymptomatically (2 % of the population). Pseudomembranous colitis is common in hospitals, where there is both increased carriage of *C. difficile* and antibiotic use.

H: History of antibiotic use.
Onset of watery diarrhoea, which may become bloody in nature, associated with crampy abdominal pain.
Often a low-grade fever.

E: Pyrexia, abdominal tenderness.
In severe cases, toxic megacolon or perforation may occur.

P: *C. difficile* releases two potent toxins. Toxin A is an enterotoxin that inactivates Rho-GTPase (epithelial cytoplasmic protein) causing intestinal hypersecretion, disaggregation of epithelial actin microfilaments and cell death.
Macro: Colon wall appears to form raised pale plaques with intervening reddened mucosa. Mucous and fibrin adheres to these plaques, giving a superficial appearance of a 'pseudomembrane'.
Micro: Denuded necrotic surface epithelium with dense infiltrate of polymorphs. Crypts are distended and filled with thick mucopurulent discharge, coalescing on the surface forming a pseudomembrane.

I: **Blood:** FBC (↑ WCC), ↑ CRP, blood culture (excludes other organisms), U&E (electrolyte status).
Stools: Demonstration of *C. difficile* toxin by ELISA. (Note: Stool culture is only useful in excluding other enteric infections.)
Sigmoidoscopy/colonoscopy: Visualizes colitis and pseudomembranes.

M: **Medical:** Oral metronidazole or vancomycin for 7–10 days, or longer if diarrhoea persists. Discontinue other antibiotics. Supportive treatment to replenish fluid and electrolyte loss. Isolate and barrier nurse.

C: Toxic megacolon (see Ulcerative colitis). Intestinal perforation. Septic shock.

P: Recovery is prompt with treatment. 25 % relapse on stopping treatment.

D: A chronic inflammatory skin disease which has characteristic lesions and may be complicated by arthritis.

A: Unknown. Genetic, environmental factors and drugs (e.g. may be triggered by *Streptococci* infections, antimalarial agents, β-blockers, lithium).

A/R: Associated with *HLA-CW6*. 5 % are associated with IBD.
Guttate psoriasis: *Streptococci* sore throat.
Palmoplantar pustulosis: Smoking, middle-aged women, autoimmune thyroid disease, SAPHO (synovitis, acne, palmoplantar pustulosis, hyperostosis seen on radiographs, osteitis: chronic recurrent multifocal inflammation of bones, e.g. sternoclavicular, sacroiliac joint).
Generalized pustular: Hypoparathyroidism.

E: Affects 1–2 % of the population. Peak age of onset ~20 years, ♂ : ♀ ~ 1:1.

H: Itching or occasionally tender skin.
Pinpoint bleeding with removing scales (Auspitz phenomenon).
Skin lesions may develop at the site of trauma/scars (Koebner phenomenon).

E: **Discoid/nummular psoriasis:** Symmetrical well-demarcated erythematous plaques with silvery scales over extensor surface (knee, elbows, scalp, sacrum).
Flexural psoriasis: Less scaly plaques in axilla, groins, perianal/genital skin.
Guttate: Small (~1 cm) drop-like lesions over trunk, limbs.
Palmoplantar: Erythematous plaques with pustules on palms and soles of feet.
Generalized pustular psoriasis: Pustules distributed over limbs and torso.
Nail: Pitting, onycholysis (lifting off of the nail-plate from the nail-bed), subungual hyperkeratosis, 'salmon patch' on the nail.
Joints: Seronegative arthritis with six possible presentations:
- monoarthritis;
- distal asymmetrical oligoarthritis (distal interphalangeal joints);
- dactylitis (interphalangeal arthritis and flexor tenosynovitis);
- rheumatoid arthritis-like (symmetrical polyarthritis);
- arthritis mutilans (telescoping of the digits); and
- ankylosing spondylitis.

Poor correlation between joint and skin involvement.

P: **Micro:** Excess proliferation of epidermal cells (rapid cell turnover possibly mediated by cytokines released by lymphocytes in the dermis) and accelerated upward migration of immature keratinocytes.
Parakeratotic layer (covering epidermis): Abnormal keratin, fragments of keratinocyte nuclei cover the epidermis, microabscesses of Munro (neutrophil aggregations, dominant feature in palmoplantar psoriasis and pustular psoriasis).
Epidermis: Rete ridge elongation, epidermal thinning over dermal papillae.
Dermis: Dermal papillae contain dilated capillaries. Dermis contains inflammatory infiltrates.

I: Majority of patients do not need any investigations.
Guttate psoriasis: Anti-streptolysin O titre, throat swab.
Flexural lesions: Skin swabs (exclude candidiasis).

Nail: Analyse nail clippings to exclude onychomycosis (fungal infection).
Joint involvement: Rheumatoid factor (negative), radiographs (distal interphalangeal joints): erosions, periarticular osteoporosis, 'pencil-in-cup' deformity (whittling and cupping of the phalanges); sacroiliitis.

M: **Skin:** Emollients for moisturizing skin, moderately potent topical steroids (e.g. Eumovate), dithranol (can irritate/burn the skin), coal tar (↓ DNA synthesis), vitamin D_3 analogue (calcipotriol), topical retinoids, PUVA (oral psoralen followed by ultraviolet A light), ultraviolet B (shorter wavelength).
Systemic (severe cases): methotrexate (teratogenic in males and females), retinoids (for pustular psoriasis, avoid in pregnant women), ciclosporin, anti-TNF-α drugs (infliximab and etanercept) may be promising.
Joints: NSAIDs, intra-articular steroids. Severe cases: methotrexate, ciclosporin (alone or in combination).
Advice: Avoid exacerbating factors for the patient, e.g. smoking, alcohol, etc.

C: Arthritis (7 % of cases), anterior uveitis, erythroderma, social complications of the disease if disfiguring.

P: Chronic disease, which relapses and remits over years. Mortality of generalized pustular psoriasis is improving.

Pulmonary embolism

D: Occlusion of pulmonary vessels, most commonly by thrombus that has travelled in the vascular system from another site.

A: Thrombus (>95 % originating from DVT of the lower limbs and rarely from right atrium in patients with atrial fibrillation). Other agents that can embolize to pulmonary vessels include amniotic fluid embolus, air embolus, fat emboli, tumour emboli and mycotic emboli from right-sided endocarditis.

A/R: Risk factors for DVT (Virchow's triad*) e.g. surgical patients, immobility, obesity, oral contraceptive pill, heart failure, malignancy.

E: Relatively common, especially in hospitalized patients, they occur in 10–20 % of those with a confirmed proximal DVT.

H: Depends on the size and site of the pulmonary embolus:
Small: May be asymptomatic.
Moderate: Sudden onset breathlessness, cough, haemoptysis and pleuritic chest pain.
Large (or proximal): All of the above, plus severe central pleuritic chest pain, shock, collapse, acute right heart failure or sudden death.
Multiple small recurrent: Symptoms of pulmonary hypertension and right heart failure.

E: **Small:** Signs may be absent. Low-grade pyrexia and tachycardia. Low sat O_2.
Moderate: Tachypnoea, tachycardia (may be atrial fibrillation), pleural rub, low sat O_2 (despite oxygen), signs of DVT (see Deep vein thrombosis).
Massive pulmonary embolism: Shock, cyanosis, signs of right heart strain (↑ JVP, left parasternal heave, accentuated S_2).
Multiple recurrent pulmonary embolism: Signs of pulmonary hypertension and right heart failure.

P: **Moderate pulmonary embolism:** Occlusion of pulmonary artery branches causing pulmonary infarction and a peripheral wedge-shaped haemorrhagic area, usually when there is coexisting compromised collateral bronchial artery circulation.
Massive pulmonary embolism: Large emboli may wedge at the pulmonary artery bifurcation (saddle embolus).

I: **Blood:** ABG, D-dimer (tests for cross-linked fibrin degradation products released into the circulation following fibrin breakdown, it is not very specific—especially if postoperative—but negative result makes pulmonary embolism very unlikely), FBC (to exclude other diagnoses), thrombophilia screen.
ECG: Usually normal or sinus tachycardia. Classical S_I, Q_{III}, T_{III} pattern and right ventricular strain.
CXR: Often normal. May show a wedge-shaped peripheral opacity, pulmonary oligaemia (↓ vascular markings), linear atelectasis or a small pleural effusion. Mainly to exclude other differential diagnoses.
VQ scan: IV administration of ^{99m}Tc macro-aggregated albumin and inhalation of ^{81}krypton gas. This identifies any areas of ventilation and perfusion mismatch which would indicate areas of infarcted lung. May be difficult to interpret if there is coexisting lung disease.

*Virchow's triad are disorders of blood flow (e.g. venous stasis), disorders of the vessel wall (e.g. endothelial injury) and disorders of blood composition (e.g. thrombophilia).

Spiral CT pulmonary angiogram: Non-invasive. Poor sensitivity for small emboli, but very sensitive for medium to large emboli.

Pulmonary angiography: Gold standard, but invasive. May be performed prior to surgery for massive emboli.

Doppler ultrasound of the lower limb: To examine for venous thrombosis.

Echocardiogram: May show thrombus in heart or pulmonary artery.

M: **Primary prevention:** Graded pressure stockings and heparin prophylaxis in those at risk (e.g. undergoing surgery). Early mobilization and adequate hydration postoperatively.

If haemodynamically stable: Anticoagulation with heparin or LMW heparin for 5–6 days, until the INR > 2. Start oral warfarin therapy as soon as diagnosis is confirmed, continue for a minimum of 3 months (INR 2–3). Analgesia for pain.

If haemodynamically unstable: Resuscitate and give oxygen (60 %), IV fluid resuscitation, thrombolysis with tissue-plasminogen activator (tPA). Analgesia, followed by prevention of further thrombi (see above).

Surgical/radiological: Embolectomy (when thrombolysis is contraindicated). Inferior vena cava filters (Greenfield filter) may be used when there are recurrent pulmonary emboli despite adequate anticoagulation or when anticoagulation is contraindicated.

C: Death, pulmonary infarction, pulmonary hypertension, right heart failure (cor pulmonale).

P: 30 % untreated mortality, 8 % with treatment (as a result of recurrent emboli or underlying disease).

Patients have ↑ risk of future thromboembolic disease.

D: A consistently increased pulmonary arterial pressure (>20 mmHg) under resting conditions.

A: **Primary:** Idiopathic.
Secondary: Left heart disease (mitral valve disease, left ventricular failure, left atrial myxoma/thrombosis), chronic lung disease (COPD), recurrent pulmonary emboli, ↑ pulmonary blood flow (ASD, VSD, patent ductus arteriosus), connective tissue disease (e.g. SLE, systemic sclerosis), drugs (e.g. amiodarone).

A/R: (see Aetiology).

E: Primary pulmonary hypertension is usually seen in young females.

H: Dyspnoea (on exertion), chest pain, syncope, tiredness.
Symptoms of the underlying cause (e.g. chronic cough).

E: ↑ JVP (prominent *a* wave in the JVP).
Palpation: Left parasternal heave (right ventricular hypertrophy).
Auscultation: Loud pulmonary component of S2 (S3/S4 may be heard), an early diastolic murmur (Graham-Steell murmur) caused by pulmonary regurgitation may be present, if tricuspid regurgitation develops (large cv wave and pansystolic murmur).
Signs of the underlying condition, or right heart failure in severe cases.

P: Pulmonary hypertension → enlarged proximal pulmonary arteries → right ventricular hypertrophy → right atrial dilation.
Vascular changes: medial hypertrophy, intimal proliferation and thrombosis.

I: **CXR:** Cardiomegaly (right ventricular enlargement, right atrial dilation), prominent main pulmonary arteries (which taper rapidly), signs of the cause (e.g. COPD, calcified mitral valves).
ECG: Right ventricular hypertrophy (right axis deviation, prominent R wave in V1, T inversion in V1, V2), right atrial enlargement (peaked P wave in II, called 'P pulmonale'), limb leads exhibit low voltage (R <5 mm) in COPD.
Echocardiography or Doppler echo: To visualize right ventricular hypertrophy or dilation and possible underlying cause. Doppler echo can measure right heart ejection fraction.
Lung function tests: To assess for chronic lung disease.
VQ scan: To assess for pulmonary embolism.
Cardiac catheterization: To assess severity, right heart pressures and response to vasodilators.
Spiral CT: Images pulmonary arteries and to diagnose lung disease.
Lung biopsy: Assesses structural lung changes.

M: **Medical:** Treat secondary conditions. For primary pulmonary hypertension, anticoagulation (warfarin), oral calcium-channel antagonists (e.g. verapamil), continuous IV prostacycline analogues (e.g. iloprost) may improve symptoms.
Surgical: Heart and lung transplantation may be an option for younger patients.

C: Right heart failure, arrhythmias (atrial fibrillation, ventricular tachycardia, ventricular fibrillation), sudden death.

P: Chronic and incurable with unpredictable survival rate. Length of survival has improved to up to 15–20 years.

Raynaud's phenomenon

D: Episodic condition characterized by pallor, cyanosis and erythema affecting fingers, toes and occasionally other parts of the body.

A: Reversible spasm of peripheral arterioles (e.g. those supplying fingers and toes).
May be precipitated by cold or stress.

A/R: May be associated with the following.
- Occupation (e.g. vibrating tools).
- Medication (e.g. β-blockers).
- Connective tissue disease (e.g. systemic sclerosis, SLE, rheumatoid arthritis, Sjögren's syndrome).
- Hyperviscosity syndromes (e.g. Waldenström's macroglobulinaemia, cryoglobulinaemia).
- Cervical rib or band of fibrous tissue compressing the brachial plexus at the thoracic outlet.

E: Common, up to 10 % of the adult population, less common in males.

H: Attacks lasting minutes to hours.
Affects fingers of both hands but also may affect toes, ears, nose, jaw or tongue.
Acute changes of skin colour: Pallor (as a result of vasoconstriction) followed by cyanosis (↓ blood flow) and then erythema (reactive hyperaemia). Remember the colours: white → blue → crimson. May not be in that order.
Numbness, burning or pain in the fingers.

E: During acute attacks: changes in skin colour (see History).
Gangrene, trophic changes in severe cases.
Finger and toe ulcers.
Symptoms of associated connective tissue diseases (e.g. in systemic sclerosis look out for sclerodactyly, calcinosis, digital ulcers, hard skin).

P: Patients may have baseline ischaemia and ↓ blood flow under normal conditions (e.g. hyperviscosity or narrowing of vessels in systemic sclerosis). Vasospasm may be superimposed on background hypoxia. In systemic sclerosis, ↑ endothelin-1 (a vasoconstrictor substance) may play a part.

I: **Blood:** FBC (to exclude polycythaemia).
Investigate for other associated disease if there are clinical suspicions (e.g. antinuclear antibodies).
Nail-fold capillary examination (using microscopy or ophthalmoscopy): The normal regular pattern of capillary loops is replaced with abnormally large loops with areas without any capillaries in early scleroderma.
Thermography.

M: **Advice:** Avoid cold weather, keep hands warm, stop smoking. Warming gloves are available.
Medical: Severe cases, calcium-channel antagonists: (nifedipine), prostaglandin analogues (IV iloprost infusion). Avoid β-blockers.
Surgery: Rarely, sympathectomy may be used for severe cases involving the lower limb, digital sympathectomy for acute finger ulcers, lumbar sympathectomy for feet problems.

C: 1 % may develop a connective tissue disease (most commonly systemic sclerosis), necrosis of affected organ, gangrene and ulceration.

P: Prognosis generally good if no underlying disorder, but symptoms may be troublesome, especially in winter.

Reactive arthritis (Reiter's syndrome)

D: Condition characterized by a sterile arthritis occurring after an infection at a distant site (commonly gastrointestinal or urogenital). Reiter's syndrome is defined by a triad of arthritis, urethritis and conjunctivitis.

A: Associated with infections of gastrointestinal tract (e.g. *Salmonella, Shigella, Yersinia, Campylobacter*) and urogenital origin (*Chlamydia* in ~60 %).

A/R: Associated with *HLA-B27*, see also Aetiology.

E: ♂ : ♀ ratio is about 20:1 in Reiter's syndrome. Age of onset 20–40 years, seen in 2 % of patients with non-specific urethritis and 0.2 % of those with dysentery.

H: Symptoms may develop 3–30 days after the infection.
Symptoms of burning or stinging on passing water (urethritis), arthritis, low back pain (sacroiliitis), painful heels (plantar fasciitis), conjunctivitis.

E: *Signs of arthritis:* Asymmetrical, oligoarticular (e.g. sausage-shaped digits).
Signs of conjunctivitis: Red eye, anterior uveitis (10 % of patients).
Signs of oral ulceration: Usually painless.
Circinate balanitis: Scaling red patches, which may evolve, encircling the glans penis.
Keratoderma blenorrhagica (10 % of patients): Brownish-red macules, vesicopustules and yellowish brown scales on soles or palms.
Other: Fever. Nail dystrophy, hyperkeratosis or onycholysis.

P: Precise pathophysiology is not understood. Serum IgA levels ↑ during active disease. Bacterial cell wall fragments and complement have been shown in the synovial fluid in arthropathy associated with some infections. Lymphocytes in the synovial fluid are mainly CD4.

I: **Blood:** FBC (anaemia may be an indication of severity and extent of systemic illness), ↑ ESR or CRP, serum agglutinin tests for known causes (high or increasing titres, which fall in the following months).
Stool or urethral swabs and cultures: May be negative by the time arthritis develops.
Plain X-ray radiographs (chronic cases): Erosions at MTPs and at insertions of Achilles tendon (entheses), plantar spurs, sacroiliitis, spinal disease with asymmetrical syndesmophytes.

M: **Medical:** *Arthritis:* Initially rest, NSAIDs for pain, aspiration of effusions. When intra-articular infection has been excluded, intra-articular injection of steroids may be given, mobilize/exercise. In uncommon cases of chronic inflammatory joint disease, sulfasalazine can be used.
Conjunctivitis: Antibiotic for secondary infection, artificial tear substitute, management of anterior uveitis by ophthalmologists (see Uveitis, anterior).
Treatment of active gastrointestinal or chlamydial infection: If still present.
Oral ulcers: Antiseptics, local anaesthetic mouthwash.
Balanitis: 1 % hydrocortisone ointment, local hygiene.

C: Psoriatic arthritis, chronic inflammatory joint disease, cardiac complications similar to ankylosing spondylitis.

P: Active arthritis may last 3–6 months. May resolve after few weeks or may last >6 months with risk of erosive disease. About 80 % have evidence of disease activity after 5 years. More severe in those with HIV.

Renal calculi

D: Different types include calcium oxalate (65 %), calcium phosphate (15 %) magnesium ammonium phosphate (10–15 %), uric acid (2–5 %), cystine (1 %).

A: **Dehydration.**
Urinary tract infection.
Changes in urinary pH: Calcium oxalate, calcium phosphate and magnesium ammonium phosphate stones arise in alkaline urine (e.g. renal tubular acidosis, urease-producing UTIs, e.g. *Proteus*, *Klebsiella*, *Pseudomonas* spp.), Cystine and uric acid stones arise in acid urine (e.g. ileostomies and loss of bicarbonate from GI secretions).
Hypercalciuria: Idiopathic possibly dietary, ↑ in urinary calcium excretion.
Hypercalcaemia: Causes include:
Renal tubular acidosis (see Renal tubular acidosis).
Endocrine: Hyperparathyroidism, ↑↑ vitamin D (self-administration, sarcoid, TB, lymphoma), hyperthyroidism, phaeochromocytoma, acromegaly, Addison's.
Malignancy: Myeloma, bone metastasis: prostate, kidney, thyroid, breast, bronchus.
Drugs (lithium, thiazides): Immobility, ↑ calcium intake ('milk-alkali syndrome').
Hyperoxaluria: Causes: ↑ intake (in rhubarb, spinach, strawberries, tea, tomatoes, beetroots, beans, chocolate, nuts), ↑ colonic absorption in patients with small bowel disease or resection, autosomally recessive inherited enzyme deficiency → ↑ oxalate production and excretion.
Hyperuricaemia: (see Gout). Tumour lysis syndrome, high cell turnover states (e.g. malignancy).
Cystinuria: Autosomal recessive, defect of renal tubular transport of cystine and dibasic amino acids.
↑ Prevalence in primary renal diseases (e.g. polycystic kidney disease, medullary sponge kidney).
Bladder stones are caused by outflow obstruction (urethral strictures, prostatic enlargement, etc.) and foreign bodies (catheter, non-absorbable sutures).

A/R: (see Aetiology).

E: UK prevalence 2 %, lifetime incidence up to 12 %. Peak age of presentation 20–50 years. ♂ : ♀ ~2:1.

H: May be asymptomatic.
Pain: *Kidney stones:* Loin pain.
Ureteric stones: Renal colic radiating from loin → groin, scrotum, labium. Nausea and vomiting.
Bladder stones: Dysuria, frequency, strangury, penile tip pain.
Urethral stones: Obstructive symptoms, urinary retention and bladder distension.
Haematuria: Symptoms of urinary tract **infection** and **obstruction**.

E: Signs of above.

P: *Calcium oxalate:* 'Mulberry' stones with spiky surface, dark (covered by blood from the mucosa of the renal pelvis injured by the sharp projections).
Calcium phosphate and magnesium ammonium phosphate: Smooth, may be large and take the shape of calyces. 'Staghorn' calculi, dirty white.

Uric acid: Hard, smooth, faceted, yellow/light brown. These are radiolucent.
Cystine: Translucent, white.

I: **Blood:** U&E, calcium, phosphate, albumin (to calculate corrected calcium).
PTH, vitamin D, urate, bicarbonate, serum ACE, thyroid function.
Urine: Urinalysis (blood, protein, nitrites), microscopy and culture (? UTI). 24-h collection: creatinine clearance, calcium, phosphate, oxalate and urate. Random urine for cystine, glyoxolate, citrate.
Imaging: Plain radiography ('KUB film') showing radio-opaque stones (90 %): all stones except urate stones are radio-opaque, cystine stones are semi-opaque, renal ultrasound (exclude hydronephrosis or hydroureter), intravenous urography (filling defect, delayed nephrogram, dilated collecting system).
Chemical analysis of the stone (if passed).

M: **Medical:** Analgesics (opiates/NSAIDs), treat the cause, e.g. antibiotics for UTI, oral fluids (stones <5 mm usually pass spontaneously).
Surgical: Indications include failure of medical treatment, persistent pain or infection proximal to obstruction.
Renal stones: Percutaneous nephrolithotomy, extracorporeal shockwave lithotripsy.
Ureter/bladder stones: Cystoscopic removal.
Large stones: Cystoscopic removal.
Prevention: ↑ Fluid intake (e.g. >3 L/day avoiding high Ca^{2+} water).
Calcium stones: ↓ Calcium (milk/cheese, white bread) and vitamin D intake.
Oxalate stones: ↓ Oxalate-containing foods and vitamin C intake.
Uric acid stones: Allopurinol (inhibits xanthine oxidase and uric acid synthesis), urinary alkalization (oral sodium bicarbonate).
Cystine stones: D-penicillamine, urinary alkalinization.

C: Obstruction and hydronephrosis, infection, complications of the cause, e.g. renal failure in primary hyperoxaluria.

P: Up to 50 % of patients may have recurrence within 5 years.

Renal failure, acute

D: Impairment of renal function over days or weeks, which often results in ↑ plasma urea/creatinine and oliguria (<400 mL/day) and is usually reversible.

A: **Prerenal (↓ renal perfusion):** Shock (hypovolaemic, sepsis, cardiogenic), hepatorenal syndrome (liver failure).
Renal:
Acute tubular necrosis: Ischaemia, drugs and toxins (paracetamol, aminoglycosides, amphotericin B, NSAIDs, ACE-inhibtors, Li^+).
Acute glomerulonephritis.
Acute interstitial nephritis: NSAIDs, penicillins, sulphonamides, leptospirosis.
Small or large vessel obstruction: Renal artery/vein thrombosis, cholesterol emboli, vasculitis, haemolytic microangipathy (e.g. HUS or TTP).
Others: Light-chain (myeloma), urate (lympho- or myeloproliferative disorders), pigment (haemolysis, malaria, rhabdomyolysis) nephropathy, accelerated phase hypertension (e.g. in pre-eclampsia).
Postrenal: Stone, tumour (pelvic, prostate, bladder), blood clots, retroperitoneal fibrosis.

A/R: Acute illnesses, multiorgan failure (e.g. MI, pancreatitis), multisystem diseases (e.g. vasculitis, thrombotic microangiopathy).

E: Annual incidence of acute renal failure requiring dialysis is 5 in 1 000 000.

H: Malaise, anorexia, nausea, vomiting, pruritus, drowsiness, convulsions, coma (caused by uraemia).
Symptoms of the cause or complications usually dominate.

E: Oedema, signs of the cause and complications.

P: **ATN:** Biphasic recovery starting with oliguria then leading to polyuria (resulting from regeneration of the tubular cells).
Macro: Enlarged kidneys with pale cortex.
Micro: Swelling and necrosis of the tubular cells, interstitial oedema with macrophage and plasma cell infiltration (see Glomerulonephritis).

I: **Blood:** ABG, FBC, U&E (urea, creatinine, Na^+, K^+), LFT, ESR/CRP, Ca^{2+}, clotting, culture, blood film: red cell fragmentation in HUS/TTP.
Other blood tests: CK (for rhabdomyolysis), urate, serum electrophoresis and autoantibodies.
Urine: *Stick testing:* Haematuria, proteinuria (e.g. glomerulonephritis).
Phase contrast microscopy: Casts in glomerulonephritis.
Culture:

- *Renal ARF:* ↓ Urine osmolality/specific gravity as a result of ↓ renal concentrating ability, ↑ urine Na^+ (as a result of ↓ reabsorptive ability), ↑ fractional excretion of Na ($P_{Cr}.U_{Na}/P_{Na}.U_{Cr}$).
- *Prerenal ARF:* ↑ Urine osmolality, ↓ urine Na^+ and fractional excretion of Na^+.

CXR: To monitor for fluid overload.
ECG: Check for hyperkalaemia (tented T waves).
Renal ultrasound: To exclude an obstructive cause.
Renal biopsy (e.g. acute tubulointerstitial nephritis: tubulitis and intense interstitial cellular infiltrate including eosinophils).

M: **Resuscitate:** According to ABC; consult nephrologists.
Monitor: U&E, temperature, pulse, respiratory rate, BP, sat O_2, urinary output, CVP, weight.

Treat complications:

Hyperkalaemia:

1 *Protect the myocardium:* 10 mL 10 % calcium gluconate and ECG monitoring.

2 *Drive K^+ into cells:* 10 units insulin and 50 mL 50 % IV dextrose. Salbutamol nebulizers can also lower K^+. Monitor blood glucose and K^+ closely.

3 *Reduce bowel absorption:* Ca^{2+}/Na^+ resonium (PO/PR).

4 *Dialysis* (see below).

Acidosis (pH <7.25): IV 1.26 % bicarbonate.

Pulmonary oedema: (see Cardiac failure).

Gastric ulcer (prevention: H_2-blockers).

Treat cause:

Sepsis: Antibiotics.

Hypovolaemia: IV fluids. If hypovolaemia is corrected (normal CVP) but urinary output not improving, consider giving diuretics (furosemide (frusemide)) and dopamine.

Pigment/light-chain/urate nephropathy: Forced alkaline diuresis (give allopurinol if ↑ urate).

Haemofiltration (continuous arteriovenous or venous–venous): Removal of plasma filtrate from the patient and infusion of replacement solution, necessary if urine output not improving despite fluid resuscitation.

Dialysis: Intermittent haemodialysis or peritoneal dialysis for mobile patients.

Nutrition: Enteral/parenteral nutrition (if necessary). A controversial step is to restrict daily dietary Na^+, K^+ and protein.

Avoid potential causative drugs, postrenal: catheters, stents, nephrostomy or surgery.

C: **Common and life-threatening:** Hyperkalaemia, sepsis, metabolic acidosis, hypertension, pulmonary oedema.

Less common: Gastric ulceration, bleeding (platelet dysfunction), muscle wasting (hypercatabolic state), uraemic pericarditis, uraemic encephalopathy, acute cortical necrosis.

P: Depends on the number of other organs involved, e.g. heart, lung. Many of those with acute tubular necrosis recover. Acute cortical necrosis may cause hypertension and CRF.

Renal failure, chronic

D: Characterized by ↓ GFR and persistently high urea and creatinine concentrations:
Mild: GFR ~30–50 mL/min.
Moderate: GFR ~10–30 mL/min.
Severe: GFR <10 mL/min.
End-stage: GFR <5 mL/min.

A: Diabetes mellitus and hypertension are the two most common causes.
Glomerular disease: Glomerulonephritis, diabetes, amyloid, SLE.
Vascular disease: Hypertension, renal artery atheromatous disease, vasculitis.
Tubulointerstitial disease: Pyelonephritis/interstitial nephritis, nephrocalcinosis, tuberculosis.
Obstruction and others: Myeloma, HIV nephropathy, scleroderma, gout, renal tumour, inborn errors of metabolism (e.g. Fabry's disease).
Congenital/inherited: Polycystic kidney disease, Alport's syndrome, congenital hypoplasia.

A/R: See above.

E: Incidence of end-stage CRF in England >110 per million population per year. Higher incidence in Asian immigrants than native British population.

H: Anorexia, nausea, malaise, pruritus. Later: diarrhoea, drowsiness, convulsions, coma.
Symptoms of the cause and other complications.

E: Systemic: Kussmaul's breathing (acidosis), signs of anaemia, oedema, pigmentation, scratch marks.
Hands: leuconychia, brown line at distal end of nail.
There may be an arteriovenous fistula (buzzing lump in wrist or forearm).
Signs of complications (e.g. neuropathy, renal bone disease).

P: Progressive fibrosis of the remaining glomeruli, tubules and small vessels leading to renal scarring.

I: **Blood:** FBC (↓ Hb: normochromic, normocytic), U&E (↓ urea and creat) ↓ Ca^{2+}, ↑ phosphate, AlkPhos, PTH.
Investigate for suspected aetiology.
24-h urine collection: Protein, creatinine clearance (which is a rough estimate of GFR).
Imaging: Signs of osteomalacia and hyperparathyroidism. CXR may show pericardial effusion or pulmonary oedema.
Renal ultrasound: Measure size, exclude obstruction and visualize structure.
Renal biopsy: For changes specific to the underlying disease, contraindicated for small kidneys.

M: Treat the underlying cause. Treat:
Anaemia: Correct iron stores. Regular IV or SC erythropoietin (usually monthly).
BP control: ACE inhibitors (caution with renal artery stenosis).
Ca^{2+}: Maintain serum levels with 1-hydroxylated vitamin D analogues, e.g. alfacalcidol.
Diet: High-energy intake, potassium intake restriction (in hyperkalaemia or acidosis, oral $NaHCO_3$ may be required), restriction of protein and phosphate intake (using phosphate binders, e.g. calcium bicarbonate or aluminum hydroxide to ↓ phosphate absorption).

Drugs: Avoid nephrotoxic drugs and NSAIDs. Adjust doses of other drugs.
Oedema: Diuretics, e.g. furosemide (frusemide), metolazone.
CAPD: Dialysate is introduced and exchanged through a 'Tenkoff' catheter, inserted via a subcutaneous tunnel into the peritoneum.
Haemodialysis: Blood is removed via an arteriovenous fistula surgically constructed in the wrist or forearm to provide high flow. Uraemic toxins are removed by diffusion across a semipermeable membrane in an extracorporeal circuit (this may activate coagulation so patients are heparinized).
Transplantation and long-term immunosuppressants to ↓ rejection (e.g. steroids, ciclosporin A, tacrolimus, azathioprine, antilymphocyte globulin).

C: **Haematological:** Anaemia (↓ erythropoietin production, ↓ marrow activity, ↓ RBC survival, ↓ dietary Fe/folate, ↑ blood loss: haemodialysis/sampling), abnormal platelet activity (bruising, epistaxis).
CVS: Accelerated atherosclerosis, ↑ BP, pericarditis.
Neuromuscular: Peripheral and autonomic neuropathy, proximal myopathy.
Renal osteodystrophy: Osteoporosis, osteomalacia (↓ 1α-hydroxylation of vitamin D), secondary or tertiary hyperparathyroidism, osteosclerosis.
Endocrine: Amenorrhoea, erectile impotence, infertility.
Peritoneal dialysis: Peritonitis (e.g. *Staphylococcus epidermidis*).
Haemodialysis:
Acute: Hypotension (excessive removal of extracellular fluid).
Long-term:

- Atherosclerosis.
- Sepsis (secondary to peritonitis, *Staph. aureus* infection).
- Amyloidosis: failure of removal of β_2-microglobulin (component of HLA molecules) by dialysis membranes → periarticular deposition → arthralgia (e.g. shoulder) and carpal tunnel syndrome.
- Aluminum toxicity: accumulation of aluminum from the dialysis fluid and phosphate binders → dementia, osteodystrophy, microcytic anaemia (less common now).

Transplantation/immunosuppression: ↑ BP, opportunistic infections (e.g. CMV), malignancies (lymphomas and skin), recurrence of renal disease (e.g. Goodpasture's syndrome), side-effects of drugs (e.g. steroids: features of iatrogenic Cushing's syndrome; ciclosporin: gum hyperplasia).

P: Depends on complications. Timely dialysis/transplantation ↑ survival.

Renal tubular acidosis

D: Metabolic acidosis caused by impaired renal H^+ secretion or bicarbonate reabsorption.

A: **Type 1** (↓ distal H^+ secretion):
Autoimmune: Sjögren's syndrome, SLE, primary biliary cirrhosis and other hypergammaglobulinaemic state.
Nephrocalcinosis: Hypercalcaemia, medullary sponge kidney.*
Toxic: Amphotericin, lithium.
Transplanted kidney: Rejection.
Sickle cell anaemia.
Type 2 (↓ proximal bicarbonate reabsorption):
Hereditary: As part of Fanconi's syndrome (glycosuria, phosphaturia, amino aciduria), fructose intolerance, cystinosis, Wilson's disease, tyrosinaemia.
Acquired: Myeloma, hyperparathyroidism, vitamin D deficiency.
Drugs: Acetazolamide, heavy metals.
Type 4: (↓ renin and aldosterone):
Diabetes: Pyelonephritis (tubulo-interstitial disease), ↓ prostaglandin synthesis required for renin production (NSAIDs), potassium-sparing diuretics, urinary obstruction, sickle cell disease, obstructive uropathy.

A/R: (see Aetiology).

E: Type 4 is the most common. Type 1 and 2 are rare.

H: Often asymptomatic.
Type 1 and 2: Symptoms of hypokalaemia, symptoms of osteomalacia/rickets, failure to thrive/grow (children) in type 2. Type 1 are also more prone to renal stones.
Type 4: Symptoms of associated condition, e.g. diabetes mellitus.

E: *Type 1:* Weakness.
Type 4: Signs of the underlying cause, e.g. diabetes mellitus.

P: *Type 1 and 2:* ↓ H^+ secretion or HCO_3^- reabsorption is accompanied by ↓ Na^+ reabsorption. This results in ↑ aldosterone and consequently ↓ K^+.
Type 4: ↓ Renin/aldosterone results in ↓ Na and ↑ K^+.

I: **ABG:** Hyperchloraemic metabolic acidosis: ↓ pH, ↓ HCO_3^-, ↓ $P\text{CO}_2$.
U&E: ↓ K^+ (type 1 and 2), calculate anion gap.† In RTA the anion gap is normal and differentiating it from acidosis with high anion gap (e.g. diabetic ketoacidosis, lactic acidosis, renal failure and salicylate poisoning).
Urine pH: >5.5 in the presence of metabolic acidosis.
Ammonium chloride loading test: Urine pH > 5.5 indicates type 1.
Bicarbonate loading test: Urine pH < 5.5 = indicates type 2, ↑ urine Na^+, ↑ HCO_3^-.
Tests to determine the underlying cause, e.g. ↑ PTH.
Imaging: Abdominal film of kidney–ureters–bladder (may show nephrocalcinosis).

M: **Medical:** Treatment of underlying condition, e.g. stop causative drug.

*Characterized by dilation of the collecting ducts in the medulla, causing cysts in the papillae containing calculi (may present with renal colic/haematuria).
†Anion gap = $(Na^+ + K^+)-(HCO_3^- + Cl^-)$.

Type 1 and 2: Hypokalaemia (correct with K^+) before correcting acidosis. Oral sodium bicarbonate (higher dose in type 2, hydrochlorothiazide may be given to ↓ bicarbonate requirements), vitamin D supplements.
Type 4: Fludrocortisone, diuretics/ion exchange resins to ↓ serum K^+, oral sodium bicarbonate.

C: *Type 1:* Nephrocalcinosis, nephrolithiasis (↓ urinary citrate prevents calcium phosphate precipitation, leading to hypercalciuria and alkaline urine) and UTI.
Type 2: Osteomalacia/rickets: from vitamin D deficiency, the buffering of H^+ by Ca^{2+} in bone and loss of phosphate in urine. Complications of the associated disease (e.g. diabetes mellitus in type 4).

P: Depends on the associated conditions. Type 1 renal tubular acidosis may progress to renal failure.

Retinal vein and artery occlusion

D: **Retinal vein occlusion (RVO):** Occlusion of central or a branch retinal vein.

Retinal artery occlusion (RAO): Occlusion of central or a branch retinal artery.

A: **RVO** may be caused by:

Changes in blood constituents: ↑ Stickiness of the cells (e.g. diabetes mellitus), hyperviscosity syndromes (e.g. multiple myeloma, hyperlipidaemia).

Changes in vessel wall: ↑ Intraocular pressure (glaucoma), hypertension causing arteriosclerosis (veins have a common sheath with arteries in the eye and may be compressed by them), primary inflammation (e.g. vasculitis: primary vasculitides, Behçet's syndrome, sarcoidosis).

The most common causes are diabetes mellitus, hypertension and glaucoma.

RAO: Emboli from carotids arteries (fibrin–platelet or cholesterol emboli) or heart valves (calcific emboli), thrombosis, arteritis.

A/R: (see Aetiology).

E: Common causes of sudden painless loss of vision (RVO >RAO).
More common in the middle-aged and elderly.

H: Sudden painless loss of vision.

RAO may be described as a 'descending curtain'. It may be temporary (*amaurosis fugax*) when the embolus gets dislodged.

E: ↓ **Visual acuity** (when macula is affected), **visual field loss** and relative afferent pupillary defect (RAPD) may be present in both RAO and RVO.

Fundoscopy:

RVO: Flame haemorrhages, cotton wool spots, swollen optic disc (in central RVO).

RAO: Pale oedematous retina with cherry red spot (see below), narrow truncated arteries, emboli may be seen (white: calcium; yellow: cholesterol).

Tonometry: To measure intraocular pressure (↑ intraocular pressure may be the cause or complication of central RVO).

Signs of the underlying cause: Hypertension, diabetes mellitus.

P: **RVO:** Venous occlusion raises intravascular pressure, rupturing veins to produce flame haemorrhages.

Cotton wool spots are accumulation of mitochondria caused by disruption of their transport from the cell body across the axons to the nerve endings.

RAO: ↓ Arterial blood supply causes retinal infarction, oedema and swelling of the retina. This masks the vascularized choroid except at the macula, which is very thin. This is the 'cherry red spot'.

I: Exclude other causes of sudden loss of vision (vitreous haemorrhage, retinal detachment, giant cell arteritis, ischaemic optic neuropathy).

Tests to identify the cause/risk factors:

RVO: Blood glucose, ESR, exclude hyperviscosity syndromes and vasculitides, lipid profile and intraocular pressure.

RAO: Carotid Doppler ultrasonography, ECG, echocardiogram, lipid profile.

Fluorescein angiography: Sequential photographs of the fundus are taken following IV injection of fluorescein to identify areas of leakage and poor perfusion to assess risk of rubeosis.

M: **RVO:** Treat the underlying condition. Laser may be used to ↓ macular oedema, treat ischaemic areas and prevent neovascularization.
RAO: Lie patient flat, ocular massage, CO_2 rebreathing (may cause arterial dilatation), IV acetazolamide, anterior chamber paracentesis.

C: Loss of vision.
RVO: Macular oedema, neovascularization of the retina and iris (rubeosis) and glaucoma.
RAO: Neovascularization and glaucoma can occur, although uncommon.

P: **RVO:** Poor prognosis with cotton wool spots and RAPD (indicators of ischaemic retinal damage).
RAO: Very poor prognosis even with immediate treatment.

Rheumatic fever

D: An inflammatory multisystem disorder, occurring following group A β-haemolytic *Streptococci* infection.

A: Thought to be secondary to antistreptococcal antibodies which are cross-reactive to host antigens.

A/R: Contact with patients with streptococcal upper respiratory tract infection. Poverty and overcrowding.

E: Peak incidence is between 5 and 15 years. More common in the Far East, Middle East, eastern Europe and South America. ↓ Incidence in the West because of antibiotics and improved sanitation.

H: 1–5 weeks after group A streptococcal infection.
General: Sudden onset, fever, malaise, anorexia.
Joints: Painful, swollen joints, ↓ movement/function.
Cardiac: Breathlessness, chest pain, palpitations.

E: **Duckett Jones criteria:** Positive diagnosis if at least two major criteria, or one major plus two minor criteria are present.
Major criteria:

- *Arthritis:* migratory or fleeting polyarthritis with swelling, redness and tenderness of large joints.
- *Carditis:* murmurs (new murmur or Carey Coombs murmur of aortic regurgitation). Pericarditis, pericardia effusion or rub, cardiomegaly, cardiac failure, ECG changes (see Investigations).
- *Chorea* (Sydenham's): rapid, involuntary, irregular movements with flowing or dancing quality. May be accompanied by slurred speech. More common in females.
- *Nodules:* small firm painless subcutaneous nodules seen on extensor surfaces, joints and tendons.
- *Erythema marginatum* (20 % cases): transient erythematous rash with raised edges, seen on trunk and proximal limbs. They may form crescent- or ring-shaped patches.

Minor criteria:

- Pyrexia.
- Previous rheumatic fever.
- Arthralgia (only if arthritis is not present as major criteria).
- Recent streptococcal infection (supported by positive throat cultures or ↑ antistreptolysin O titre).
- ↑ Inflammatory markers (ESR, CRP or WCC).
- ↑ PR and QT intervals on ECG (only if carditis not present as major criteria).

P: **Heart:** Inflammation of all three layers (pancarditis) can be seen, characterized by pericarditis with serofibrinous effusion, Aschoff bodies (granulomatous lesions with central necrosis) in the myocardium, and warty aseptic vegetations on the valves.
Chronic rheumatic heart disease: Valvular scarring, deformation and dysfunction. Fibrous thickening of leaflets and calcification, bridging fibrosis and fusion of commisures and stenosis. There may also be thickened, shortened and fused mitral valve chordae.
Skin: Granulomatous lesions clinically seen as subcutaneous nodules.
Joints: Acute inflammation of the synovial membranes.

I: **Blood:** FBC (↑ WCC), ESR or CRP (↑), antistreptolysin O titre or antistreptokinase titre.
Throat swab and culture: Group A *Streptococcus*.

ECG: Saddle-shaped ST elevation and PR segment depression (pericarditis), arrhythmias.

Echocardiogram: Pericardial effusion, myocardial thickening or dysfunction, valvular dysfunction.

M: *Strict bed rest:* (~4 weeks) Gradual mobilization with clinical improvement.

Antibiotics: Eradicate residual streptococcal infection using oral penicillin V. Prevention of recurrence may be necessary in those 5–18 years of age, with long-term oral penicillin V.

Anti-inflammatory drugs: High-dose aspirin or, for more severe carditis, consider corticosteroids.

Chorea: May be controlled with diazepam or haloperidol.

C: Recurrence, may be precipitated by streptococcal infection, more common in patients with residual cardiac damage. Chronic rheumatic valvular disease (usually mitral or aortic) after 10–20 years, more common in those with carditis as part of acute rheumatic fever.

P: Acute rheumatic fever may last up to 3 months if untreated. ♀ more likely to develop mitral stenosis. Patients with valvular disease may later require surgical intervention.

Rheumatoid arthritis

D: Chronic inflammatory systemic disease characterized by symmetrical deforming polyarthritis and extra-articular manifestations.

A: Autoimmune disease of unknown cause. Probably multifactorial, including immunogenetic susceptibility, environmental factors and sex hormones.

A/R: More common in those with *HLA DR-1* and *DR-4*. Associated with other autoimmune phenomenon (e.g. Raynaud's phenomenon, Sjögren's syndrome). Felty's syndrome is the combination of rheumatoid arthritis, splenomegaly, neutropenia and lower limb pigmentation.

E: Common. Prevalence is 1 % of general population. Worldwide distribution. Three times more common in females, peak incidence at 30–50 years.

H: Gradual (occasionally rapid) onset.
Joint pain, swelling, morning stiffness, impaired function.
Usually affects **peripheral joints symmetrically** (occasionally monoarticular involvement, e.g. knee).
Systemic: Fatigue, fever, weight loss.

E: **Arthritis:** Most common sites are in the hands.
Early: Spindling of fingers, swelling at MCP and PIP joints, Warm, tender joints, ↓ range of movement.
Late:

- Symmetrical deforming arthropathy.
- Ulnar deviation of fingers as a result of subluxation (partial dislocation) at MCP joints.
- Radial deviation of the wrist.
- Swan neck deformity (fixed flexion of MCP and DIP, hyperextension of PIP).
- Boutonnière deformity (extension of MCP and DIP joint, flexion of PIP).
- Z deformity of the thumb.
- Trigger finger (unable to straighten finger, tendon sheath nodule palpable), tendon rupture.
- Wasting of the small muscles of the hand, palmar erythema.

Rheumatoid nodules: Firm subcutaneous nodules (e.g. on elbows, palms, over extensor tendons).

P: **Micro:** Synovium is infiltrated by lymphocytes, plasma cells and macrophages, and undergoes hyperplasia and hypertrophy (forming villi). Synovium grows over the articular cartilage (known as a 'pannus') and erodes the cartilage and adjacent bone. CD4 T-cells and cytokines (IL-1 and TNF-α) may play a part.
Rheumatoid nodules: Central necrosis with surrounding fibroblasts and macrophages at pressure points; similar lesions may be seen in other tissues, e.g. lung, heart.

I: **Blood:** FBC (↓Hb, ↑platelets), ↑ ESR and CRP, rheumatoid factor (monoclonal IgM against Fc portion of IgG, present in 70 % of patients and 5 % normal population, associated with subcutaneous nodules and extra-articular manifestations), antinuclear antibodies (30 %).
Acutely: Exclude septic arthritis with joint aspiration and blood cultures.
Joint X-ray radiography: Soft tissue swelling, angular deformity, periarticular erosions and osteoporosis.

M: **Medical:**

Immunosuppressants: Disease-modifying drugs such as methotrexate (a first-line agent combined with folic acid), sulfasalazine, penicillamine, azathioprine, gold, hydroxychloroquine and cyclophosphamide. May take months to work, reduce complications and slow the disease progression. Careful monitoring is needed for side-effects, e.g. FBC (for bone marrow suppression), LFT (for hepatitis), U&E (for renal failure), urinalysis (for nephrotic syndrome), eye examination (for retinopathy and corneal deposits).

NSAIDs: For treating pain and stiffness.

Steroids: Use limited by side-effects. Only used in severe extra-articular disease or with rapid or widespread arthritis. Intra-articular long-acting steroids may ↓ pain and joint effusions.

Etanercept, infliximab: Newer immunomodulatory anti-TNF-α agents are extremely promising.

Physiotherapy and occupational therapy: Essential to maintain joint function and quality of life.

Surgery: Synovectomy, arthrodesis, arthroplasty, tendon repair or joint replacement.

C: Numerous organs can be involved.

Vasculitis (of skin): Nail-fold infarcts, digital gangrene, ulcers, pyoderma gangrenosum, purpuric rash.

Lung: Pleural effusion, fibrosis, rheumatoid nodules in parenchyma, obliterative bronchioloitis.

Heart: Pericarditis, pericardial rub, myocarditis, conduction abnormalities, valvular regurgitation.

Haematological:

Anaemia of chronic disease.

Megaloblastic anaemia (↑ demand for folic acid).

Aplastic anaemia (from drugs).

Haemolytic anaemia (in Felty's syndrome).

Neuromuscular: Mononeuritis multiplex, peripheral neuropathy, carpal tunnel syndrome, atlantoaxial subluxation and spinal cord compression.

Renal: Analgesic nephropathy, amyloidosis.

Eyes: Scleritis, episcleritis, scleromalacia and scleromalacia perforans.

P: Variable. 10 % severely affected after 10 years and ~20 % have minimal disease. Poor prognostic factors are ♀, persistent ↑ inflammatory markers, high-titre rheumatoid factor, extra-articular manifestations.

Rosacea

D: Persistent non-comedonal inflammation of the facial skin.

A: Unknown.

A/R: Associated with photosensitivity, may coexist with acne vulgaris.

E: Common. 1 % of dermatology outpatients, ♀ > ♂, middle-aged to elderly.

H: Erythema, papules, telangiectasia and pustules on face.
Symptoms of conjunctivits and blepharitis (sore, gritty eyes/eyelids).

E: Erythema on forehead, nose and cheeks, involving the nasolabial folds. Papules and pustules may be visible. On the nose, it can cause disfiguring rhinophyma. No comedones. Conjunctivitis and blepharitis (inflamed lid margins with crusts).

P: **Micro:** Dermal vascular ectasia, oedema and a variable degree of lymphocytic inflammatory cell infiltrate which can become granulomatous in severe cases.

I: Normally none required.
Blood: Antinuclear antibodies (e.g. anti-dsDNA) to exclude lupus, particularly in females.
Swab of pustules may detect infections (rarely necessary).

M: **Medical:** Papules and pustules may respond to topical metronidazole. Avoid topical steroids as they have minimal effect and may cause rebound erythema.
Oral oxytetracycline, erythromycin.
Isotretinoin in refractory cases (by specialist prescription only; side-effects: teratogenic, hyperlipidaemia). Cosmetics may be required for the redness/flushing.
Surgery: Plastic surgery possible for severe rhinophyma involving excision of excessive soft tissue. Carbon dioxide laser may also be used for rhinophyma. Pulsed dye laser for telangiectasia and erythema.
Advice: Avoidance of spicy food and alcohol may be helpful.

C: Facial scarring (particularly the nose), persisting facial erythema.

P: Improves spontaneously over a period of months to years, but may relapse and remit.

D: Sarcoidosis is a multisystem granulomatous inflammatory disorder.

A: Unknown. Transmissible agents (e.g. viruses or atypical mycobacterium), environmental and genetic factors have all been suggested.

A/R: No identified risk factors.

E: Uncommon. More common in 20–40-year-olds, Africans and females. The prevalence is very variable worldwide. Prevalence in UK is 16 in 100 000 (highest in Irish women).

H & E: **General:** Fever, malaise, weight loss, bilateral parotid swelling, lymphadenopathy, hepatosplenomegaly.
Lungs: Breathlessness, cough (usually unproductive), chest discomfort. Minimal clinical signs (e.g. fine inspiratory crepitations).
Symptoms of multiorgan involvement:
Musculoskeletal: Bone cysts (e.g. 'dactylitis' in phalanges), polyarthralgia, myopathy.
Eyes: Keratoconjunctivitis sicca (dry eyes), uveitis, papilloedema.
Skin: Lupus pernio (red–blue infiltrations of nose, cheek, ears, terminal phalanges), erythema nodosum, maculopapular eruptions.
Neurological: Lymphocytic meningitis, space-occupying lesions, pituitary infiltration, cerebellar ataxia, cranial nerve palsies (e.g. bilateral facial nerve palsy), peripheral neuropathy.
Heart: Arrhythmia, bundle branch block, percarditis, cardiomyopathy, congestive cardiac failure.

P: The unknown antigen is presented on the MHC Class II complex of macrophages to CD4 (TH1) lymphocytes, which accumulate and release cytokines (e.g. IL-1/IL-2). This results in formation of non-caseating granulomas (in a variety of organs) composed of epithelioid cells (activated macrophages), multinucleate Langhans cells and mononuclear cells (lymphocytes).

I: **Blood:** ↑ Serum ACE, ↑ Ca^{2+}, ↑ ESR, FBC (↓ WCC because of lymphocyte sequestration in the lungs), immunoglobulins (polyclonal hyperglobulinaemia), LFT.
24-h urine collection: Hypercalciuria.
CXR:
Stage 0 May be clear.
Stage 1 Bilateral hilar lymphadenopathy.
Stage 2 Stage 1 with pulmonary infiltration and paratracheal node enlargement.
Stage 3 Pulmonary infiltration and fibrosis.
High-resolution CT scan: For diffuse lung involvement.
^{67}Gallium scan: Shows areas of inflammation (classically parotids and around eyes).
Pulmonary function tests: ↓ FEV_1, *FVC* and gas transfer (showing restrictive picture).
Bronchoscopy and bronchoalveolar lavage: ↑ Lymphocytes with ↑CD4 : CD8 ratio.
Transbronchial lung biopsy (or lymph node biopsy): (see Pathology).

M: **Medical:** Corticosteroids for symptomatic disease (e.g. oral prednisolone reducing slowly).
Symptomatic:
Musculoskeletal: NSAIDs.
Ocular sarcoid: Topical corticosteroids and a mydriatic (atropine).
Skin: Chloroquine or methotrexate may be used for lupus pernio.

Arrhythmias: Pacemakers.

C: Multiple organ involvement (see above), nephrocalcinosis and interstitial nephritis.

P: Two-thirds of white patients and one-third of black patients remit without treatment.
Mortality (e.g. as a result of respiratory failure) is up to 10 % in Afro-Caribbean and < 5 % in white people.
Best prognosis is in white people with Stage 1 disease.

D: **Systemic inflammatory response syndrome (SIRS):** Defined as the body's response to severe clinical insults and is manifest by two or more of:

Temperature: <36°C or >38°C.

Heart rate: >90 beats/min.

Respiratory rate: >20/min or $Paco_2$ < 32 mmHg.

WCC: < 4 or > 12 × 10^9/L.

Sepsis: Defined as SIRS with a demonstrated source of infection.

Severe sepsis or sepsis syndrome: Sepsis and evidence of organ dysfunction.

Septic shock: When in sepsis there is hypotension refractory to adequate fluid replacement.

Multiple organ dysfunction syndrome (MODS): Describes a state where dysfunction is seen in several organs such that homoeostasis cannot be maintained without intervention.

A: The systemic response of the body to infection or other injuries including trauma, tissue ischaemia, burns, hypovolaemia or acute pancreatitis.

A/R: (see Aetiology).

E: Sepsis occurs in 1–2 % of hospital admissions in the UK.

H: Presentation depends on site of infection or injury.

General symptoms of infection include fever, sweating, chills or rigors.

The patient may complain of pain, headache, nausea, vomiting or be confused (especially in the elderly).

E: Initially, BP is maintained despite reduced systemic vascular resistance by increased cardiac output evident as tachycardia, warm peripheries and a bounding pulse.

Later, hypotension develops.

Other features mentioned above include pyrexia, hypoxia and tachypnoea and oliguria.

Focal signs may point to the site of infection.

P: SIRS is part of the normal response to injury or infection. Local production of cytokines and inflammatory mediators enter the systemic circulation and activate the acute phase response, influencing the thermoregulatory centre of the hypothalamus and mobilizing of cells from bone marrow. An excess of inflammatory mediators such as TNF-α, IL-1, IL-6 and PAF floods the circulation, resulting in systemic activation of inflammatory cells, endothelial damage and organ dysfunction. In Gram-negative sepsis, bacterial endotoxin (lipopolysaccharides) induce release of cytokines and cellular dysfunction. In Gram-positive sepsis, lipo-oligosaccharides and bacterial superantigen toxins have a similar effect.

The mechanisms of organ injury are thought to involve endothelial dysfunction, impaired perfusion, free radical and enzymatic damage.

I: **Blood:** FBC, U&E, blood cultures, clotting studies, LFT, CRP, lactate, ABG (metabolic acidosis).

Culture: Blood, sputum, urine, line-tips, wound swabs, throat swab, CSF (if indicated).

Imaging: To locate focus of sepsis or inflammation.

M: **Resuscitation:** Airway, Breathing, Circulation. Essential to restore and maintain optimal tissue perfusion and oxygenation with aggressive fluid resuscitation. Appropriate antibiotics should be started to treat infection. Patients in shock require ventilatory support, CVP monitoring and inotropic support on high-dependency facilities with multidisciplinary care.
Role of corticosteroids: High-dose steroids may be used in very severe cases, even in cases of infection.
Surgical: Operative intervention, where appropriate, for drainage or débridement of infected tissue.

C: Organ failure involving the lungs (ARDS), kidneys (acute renal failure), CNS (confusion), GI tract (liver failure, stress ulceration) and the cardiovascular system (cardiac depression and DIC).

P: Septic shock carries a mortality of 40–60 %. In cases of organ failure, mortality is higher, often 80–90 %.

D: A chronic condition with sickling of red blood cells caused by inheritance of haemoglobin S (Hb S).
Sickle cell anaemia: Homozygosity for Hb S, *Sickle cell trait*: carry one copy of Hb S.
Sickle cell disease: Includes compound heterozygosity for Hb S and C and for Hb S and β-thalassaemia.

A: Autosomally recessive inherited point mutation in the β-globin gene resulting in valine substituting glutamic acid on position 6, producing the abnormal protein, haemoglobin S.

A/R: Factors precipitating sickling are infection, dehydration, hypoxia and acidosis.

E: Rarely presents before 4–6 months (because of continuous production of fetal haemoglobin). Common in Africa, Caribbean, Middle East and areas with high prevalence of malaria (carrier frequency in Afro-Caribbeans ~8 %).

H: **Symptoms secondary to vaso-occlusion or infarction** (see Pathology):
Autosplenectomy (splenic atrophy or infarction) leading to increased risk of infections with encapsulated organisms (e.g. pneumococcus, *Haemophilus influenzae*, meningococcus, *Salmonella*).
Abdominal pain.
Bones: Painful crises affecting small bones of hands or feet (dactylitis) in children and ribs, spine, pelvis and long bones in adults. Chronic hip or shoulder pain (avascular necrosis). Myalgia and arthralgia.
CNS: Can cause fits or strokes (e.g. hemiplegia).
Retina: Visual loss (proliferative retinopathy).
Symptoms of sequestration crises (red cell pooling in various organs):
Spleen, liver: Exacerbation of anaemia.
Lungs: 'Acute chest syndrome': breathlessness, cough, pain, fever.
Corpora cavernosa: Persistent erection (pripiasm) and impotence.

E: **Signs secondary to vaso-occlusion, ischaemia or infarction** (see History):
Bone, joint or muscle tenderness or swelling: Caused by avascular necrosis.
Short digits: caused by infarction in small bones.
Retina: Cotton wool spots from areas of ischaemic retina.
Signs secondary to sequestration crises: (see History):
Organomegaly: Spleen is enlarged in early disease but later reduces in size because of splenic atrophy.
Priapism.
Signs of anaemia

P: Deoxygenation of Hb S alters the conformation with resulting hydrophobic interactions between adjacent Hb S and formation of insoluble polymers, resulting in sickling (formation of a crescent shape) of red cells with ↑ fragility and inflexibility. They are prone to:

1. Sequestration and destruction, leading to ↓ RBC survival (~20 days).
2. Occlusion small blood vessels causing hypoxia which, in turn, causes further sickling and occlusion.

I: **Blood:** FBC (anaemia, reticulocytes are ↑ in haemolytic crises and ↓ in aplastic crises), U&E.
Blood film: Sickle cells, anisocytosis, features of hyposplenism (target cells, Howell–Jolly bodies).
Sickle solubility test: Dithionate added to blood causes ↑ turbidity.

Haemoglobin electrophoresis: Shows Hb S, absence of Hb A (in Hb SS) and ↑ levels of Hb F.
Hip X-ray: Common site for avascular necrosis of the femoral head.
MRI or CT head: If there are neurological complications.

M: **Acute:** (painful crises): oxygen, IV fluids, strong analgesia, antibiotics.
Medical: *Infection prophylaxis:* Penicillin V. Regular vaccinations (e.g. against pneumococcus).
Folic acid: In severe haemolysis or in pregnancy.
Hydroxyurea: Increases Hb F levels and ↓ frequency and duration of sickle cell crisis.
Red cell transfusion: For severe anaemia. Repeated transfusions with iron chelators may be necessary for those with frequent crises or after CNS crisis.
Exchange transfusion: In severe crises, before surgery, pregnancy.
Advice: Avoid precipitating factors, good hygiene and nutrition, genetic counselling, prenatal screening.
Surgical: Bone marrow transplantation in selected patients, joint replacement for avascular necrosis.

C: Complications of vaso-occlusion and sequestration (see History).
Aplastic crises (infection with B19 parvovirus, temporary cessation of erythropoiesis), haemolytic crises, pigment gallstones, cholecystitis, renal papillary necrosis, leg ulcers (local ischaemia), cardiomyopathy.

P: Most of those with sickle cell disease, with good care, survive to ~50 years. Major mortality is usually a result of pulmonary or neurological complications (adults) or infection (children).

D: Characterized by inflammation and destruction of exocrine glands (mainly salivary and lacrimal glands). When associated with other autoimmune diseases, Sjögren's syndrome is said to be secondary.

A: Unknown. An interaction between genetic and environmental factors (e.g. viral infection) resulting in autoimmunity has been suggested.

A/R: Associated with rheumatoid arthritis, scleroderma, SLE, polymyositis.
Organ-specific autoimmune diseases: primary biliary cirrhosis, autoimmune hepatitis, autoimmune thyroid disease, myasthenia gravis.
Linked to *HLA-B8, DR3*.

E: Onset usually between 15 and 65 years. ♂ : ♀ ~ 1 : 9.

H: **General:** Fatigue, fever, weight loss, depression.
Dry eyes (keratoconjunctivitis sicca): Gritty, sore eyes, photophobia, heaviness of lids.
Dry mouth (xerostomia): Dysphagia may result secondarily.
Dry upper airways: Dry cough, recurrent sinusitis.
Dry skin or hair (less commonly).
Dry vagina: can cause dyspareunia (less commonly).
↓ Gastrointestinal mucus secretion causing symptoms of reflux oesophagitis, gastritis, constipation.
Symptoms of associated diseases and their systemic complications (see Associations/Risk factors).

E: Parotid or salivary gland enlargement.
Dry eyes.
Dry mouth or tongue.
Signs of the associated conditions.

P: **Micro:** Periductal infiltration of CD4 lymphocytes, ductal epithelial hyperplasia, acinar atrophy and fibrosis within salivary or lacrimal glands.

I: **Blood:** ↑ ESR.
Autoantibodies: Rheumatoid factor, ANA (60 %), anti-La (50 % of primary Sjögren's), anti-Ro.
FBC: Anaemia.
Amylase: Raised if salivary glands involved.
Schirmer's test: Filter paper strip under eyelid. Positive if < 10 mm of the strip is wet in 5 min.
Fluorescein/rose bengal stains: Punctate or filamentary keratitis (clumps of mucus on the cornea).
Others: ↓ Parotid salivary flow rate, ↓ uptake or clearance on isotope scan.
Biopsy: Salivary or labial glands (lower lip) (see Pathology).

M: **Dry mouth:** Saliva substitutes, good oral hygiene, treatment of oral candidiasis.
Dry eyes: Shielded spectacles, artificial tears (hypromellose eye drops), simple ointment (at night), topical acetylcysteine (mucolytic), treatment of secondary bacterial conjunctivitis. Lacrimal punctol occlusion (temporary/permanent) or tarsorrhaphy may rarely be required.
Systemic disease: Steroids or immunosuppressants. Treatment of the accompanying diseases.

C: **Mouth:** Chronic oral candidiasis, caries.
Eyes: Conjunctivitis (bacterial), corneal epithelial, thinning (melt), filamentary keratitis.

Vasculitis: Occurs in < 10 % of patients. Associated with myositis, mononeuritis multiplex, axonal neuropathy, immune complex glomerulonephritis and purpura.
Kidney: Interstitial nephritis.
Lymphoma: 40 times increased risk. Usually B-cell non-Hodgkin type.
Complications of the associated diseases.
Pregnancy: Anti-Ro and anti-La (can cross placenta and cause congenital heart block, 1 % risk).

P: Good for primary Sjögren's. Depends on accompanying autoimmune disorder in secondary Sjögren's.

D: Slow-growing malignancy of the squamous cells in the epidermis.

A: The main aetiological risk factor is ultraviolet radiation from sunlight exposure. Can also develop in areas of skin damage in burns, radiation or from chronic skin disease (e.g. lupus, leukoplakia).

A/R: Exposure to carcinogens (e.g. tar derivatives, cigarette smoke, soot, industrial oils and arsenic), radiation exposure, patients on long-term immunosuppression (e.g. transplant recipients, HIV patients).

E: Second most common cutaneous malignancy. Often occurring in middle-aged and elderly light-skinned individuals. Annual incidence is about 1 in 4000.

H: (see Examination).

E: Non-healing pink ulcerated lesion with hard indurated edges extending beyond visible superficial border. Variable appearance: ulcerated, hyperkeratotic, crusted or scaly.
Can occur on sun-exposed sites (face, temples, cheeks) or on mucous membranes.
It can often arise from long-standing lesions (e.g. solar keratoses, leg ulcers).
Bowen's disease (intraepidermal carcinoma *in situ*): Solitary or multiple red–brown scaly patch often resembling psoriasis, dermatitis or dermatophyte infection.

P: **Micro:** The abnormal squamous epithelial cells often extend directly down through into the dermis, through the basement membrane. In Bowen's disease, the basement membrane is intact.

I: **Skin biopsy:** Confirms the malignancy and distinguishes it from other skin lesions.
Lymph node biopsy: Only necessary if there is suspicion of metastasis (e.g. on lips).

M: **Surgery:** For Bowen's disease, curettage and cryotherapy or cauterization is sufficient to eradicate lesion. Invasive SCCs should be excised with wide margin and through into subcutaneous fat and histology is needed to confirm adequate clearance at margins.
Mohs' micrographic surgery: Excision with close margins and histological examination during surgery. Can be used in areas where large excisions are difficult (e.g. lips, near eyes).
Local radiotherapy: For larger lesions or if surgery is difficult. Usually lighter scar, forming a depression.
Medical: Topical 5-fluorouracil for Bowen's disease or intralesional interferons if other options are difficult.
Follow-up should be arranged to check for recurrence.

C: Sun-exposed skin SCCs are usually local at the time of diagnosis, but one-third of those on lips or lingual membranes have metastasized by time of diagnosis.

P: Good, as it is easily treatable. High cure rate.

Stroke

D: Focal or global impairment of CNS function developing rapidly and lasting > 24 h (see Transient ischaemic attack).

A: **Infarction (90 %):**
Emboli: Usually from either atheromatous plaques in the carotid or vertebrobasilar arteries or from the heart (e.g. atrial fibrillation, recent MI).
Thrombosis: Atherosclerosis affecting mainly the small cerebral vessels.
Hypotension: If below the autoregulatory range maintaining cerebral blood flow, infarction results in the 'watershed' zones between different cerebral artery territories.
Others: Carotid or vertebral artery dissection, vasculitis, syphilis.
Haemorrhage (10 %): Hypertension, Charcot–Bouchard microaneurysm rupture, Alzheimer's disease. Less commonly, trauma, tumours, arteriovenous malformations, vasculitis.

A/R: Diabetes, family history, hypertension, hyperlipidaemia, smoking, ↑ age, ↑↑ alcohol, anticoagulants.

E: Common. Annual incidence is 2 in 1000. Third most common cause of death in industrialized countries.

H: Rapid onset.
Weakness, sensory or visual impairment, impaired coordination, loss of cognitive function or consciousness. May gradually improve over weeks or months.
Head or neck pain (in carotid or vertebral artery dissection).
Enquire if history of atrial fibrillation, MI, valvular heart disease, carotid artery stenosis.

E: Examine for underlying cause (e.g. atrial fibrillation, heart murmurs, carotid bruit, fundoscopy).
Infarction:
Cerebral cortex: Depending on cerebral artery affected:

- *Middle (most common):* facial weakness, hemiparesis (motor cortex), hemisensory loss (somatosensory cortex), apraxia, hemineglect (parietal lobe), receptive or expressive dysphasia (language centres), quadrantanopia (superior or inferior optic radiations).
- *Posterior:* hemianopia or cortical blindness (visual cortex).
- *Anterior:* lower limb weakness (motor cortex), confusion (frontal lobe).
- *Gerstmann syndrome* (acalculia, finger agnosia, agraphia, left–right disorientation, mild hemineglect). Caused by non-dominant parietal lobe infarct.

Small vessels (lacunar): Degenerative small-vessel disease in the deep perforating arteries:

- *Internal capsule or pons:* pure sensory or motor deficit (or combination of both).
- *Thalamus:* loss of consciousness, hemisensory deficit.
- *Basal ganglia:* hemichorea, hemiballismus, movement disorders.
- *Multiple lacunar infarcts:* vascular dementia, gait apraxia (difficulty to start walking and '*marche à petits pas*', shuffling small-stepped gait).

Note: landmark trials include IST and CAST (role of aspirin in ischaemic stroke), NINDS (benefit of tPA if < 3 h in ischaemic stroke), IST3 (the role of tPA < 6 h in ischaemic stroke) is ongoing.

Brainstem: Any combination of cranial nerves and spinal tracts. A classic syndrome is:

- *Lateral medullary syndrome* (occlusion of posterior inferior cerebellar artery): vomiting, vertigo, ipsilateral Horner's syndrome, dysphagia, dysarthria, cerebellar signs, loss of pain and temperature sensation on contralateral body and ipsilateral face.

Haemorrhage:
Intracerebral: Headache, focal neurological signs, nausea and vomiting, signs of raised ICP, seizures.
Subarachnoid: (see Subarachnoid haemorrhage).
Acute: Initially, ↓ tone and reflexes. Later, UMN signs develop (↑ tone, reflexes and extensor plantars).

P: **Non-haemorrhagic ('anaemic'):**
24 h: Blurring of white and grey matter junction.
48 h: Pale, soft, swollen (because of intracellular swelling and vasogenic oedema from breakdown of blood –brain barrier).
Days: Macrophages phagocytose lipid-rich myelin. Infarcted tissue liquefies producing a fluid-filled cavity with surrounding proliferating astrocytes ('gliosis').
Months: Penumbra around infarcted area gradually recovers function.
Haemorrhagic: Resulting from reflow of blood back into capillaries damaged by ischaemia.

I: **Blood:** FBC, U&E, ESR, glucose, lipids (occasionally: homocysteine levels, lupus anticoagulant, anticardiolipin antibodies, syphilis serology), blood cultures (if infective endocarditis suspected).
ECG: Identifies any arrhythmias which predispose to embolism.
Echocardiogram: Identifies cardiac thrombus, valvular endocarditis or other sources of embolism.
Carotid Doppler ultrasound: Important to exclude carotid atherosclerosis as source of emboli.
Brain CT/MRI: Detects ischaemia or haemorrhages. Excludes tumours and subdural haemorrhage.
SPECT: Measures perfusion of brain. Rarely available routinely.

M: **Acute ischaemic stroke:** Supportive. Aspirin (300 mg) to prevent further thrombosis. If known to be ischaemic cause and < 3 h of onset, tPA thrombolysis is beneficial. Heparin anticoagulation is only beneficial in certain subgroups where there is a high risk of emboli recurrence or stroke progression. Assess if patient can eat or drink (nasogastric tube may be required). Close nursing to prevent pressure sores.
Prevention: Low-dose aspirin, warfarin anticoagulation (if atrial fibrillation), stop smoking, control hypertension and hyperlipidaemia.
Multidisciplinary rehabilitation (best managed by specialist stroke unit): Speech and language therapy. Occupational therapy. Physiotherapy.
Intracerebral haemorrhage: Control hypertension and seizures. IV mannitol and hyperventilation helps lower intracranial pressure. Evacuation of haematoma or ventricular drainage may be required.
Surgical: Carotid endartectomy is indicated if stenosis > 70 %.

C: Cerebral oedema (↑ ICP and local compression), immobility, infections (e.g. pneumonia, UTI, from pressure sores), DVT, cardiovascular events (arrhythmias, MI, cardiac failure), death.

P: **Stroke:** 10 % mortality in first month. Up to 50 % of those who survive remain dependent. 10 % have a recurrence in 1 year. Generally, worse for haemorrhages than for infarction.

Subarachnoid haemorrhage

D: Arterial haemorrhage into the subarachnoid space.

A: Rupture of a saccular aneurysm at the base of the brain (usually at Circle of Willis): 85 %.
Perimesencephalic haemorrhage (e.g. parenchymal haemorrhages tracking onto surface of brain): 10 %.
Arteriovenous malformations, bleeding diatheses, vertebral or carotid artery dissection with intracranial extension, mycotic aneurysms, drug abuse (e.g. cocaine, amphetamines): 5 %.

A/R: Hypertension, smoking, excess alcohol intake, saccular aneurysms are associated with polycystic kidney disease, Marfan's syndrome, pseudoxanthoma elasticum and Ehlers–Danlos syndrome.

E: Annual incidence is 10 in 100 000. Peak age of incidence in the fifth decade.

H: Sudden onset severe headache (classically described 'as if hit at the back of the head').
Nausea, vomiting, neck stiffness, photophobia.
↓ Level of consciousness.

E: **Meningism:** Neck stiffness, Kernig's sign (resistance or pain on knee extension when hip is flexed) because of irritation of the meninges by blood. Pyrexia may also occur.
Glasgow Coma Scale: *Assess and regularly monitor for deterioration.
Signs of increased intracranial pressure: Papilloedema, IV or III cranial nerve palsy. Hypertension and bradycardia.
Fundoscopy: Subhyaloid haemorrhage (between retina and vitreous membrane).
Focal neurological signs: Usually develop on second day and are caused by ischaemia from vasospasm and reduced brain perfusion.

P: Aneurysms are abnormal localized dilation of blood vessels.
Berry aneurysms: Macroscopically, saccular aneurysms are usually seen at the site of bifurcation of arteries in the circle of Willis. The mechanism by which the aneurysms form is controversial; may result from congenital weaknesses in the vessel wall.
Subarachnoid haemorrhage: Blood subarachnoid space may be diffuse or localized to the site of the bleed.

I: **Blood:** FBC, U&E, ESR/CRP, clotting (? bleeding diathesis).

*The Glasgow Coma Scale is a rapid measure of consciousness. Made up of three components, totalling 15.

Eye opening	Verbal response	Motor response
Spontaneously (4)	Oriented (5)	Obeys commands (6)
To speech (3)	Confused (4)	Localizing pain (5)
To pain (2)	Inappropriate (3)	Flexion to pain (4)
None (1)	Incomprehensible (2)	Abnormal flexion to pain (3)
	None (1)	Extending to pain (2)
		None (1)

CT scan: Hyperdense areas in the basal regions of the skull (caused by blood in the subarachnoid space). Identifies any intraparenchymal or intraventricular haemorrhages as well.

Angiography (MRI, CT or intra-arterial): To detect the source of bleeding if the patient is a candidate for surgery or endovascular treatment.

Lumbar puncture: ↑ Opening pressure, ↑ red cells, few white cells, xanthochromia (straw-coloured CSF) because of breakdown of Hb, confirmed by spectrophotometry of CSF supernatant after centrifugation.

M: **Acute:** Resuscitate, bed-rest, analgesia and obtain neurosurgical review. IV fluids (to maintain a degree of hypertension to keep brain perfused). Nimodipine (calcium-channel antagonist) should be given to reduce vasospasm.

Surgical: Clipping or wrapping the aneurysm.

Interventional neuroradiology: Coiling (usually with platinum) of the aneurysm.

Arteriovenous malformations: May be managed by interventional radiology, radiotherapy and/or surgery.

C: Obstructive hydrocephalus (CSF flow blocked in the ventricles by blood clot), communicating hydrocephalus (as meninges and arachnoid villi are damaged by the haemorrhage). Major neurological deficits depending on the site of haemorrhage.

P: High, with $>30\%$ mortality in the first few days. Significant risk of a severe rebleed in the first 2 months. Worse prognosis with subsequent episodes of rebleeding. Lower mortality in cases of perimesencephalic subarachnoid haemorrhage and arteriovenous malformations than bleeding from aneurysms.

Syndrome of inappropriate ADH (SIADH)

D: Syndrome of inappropriate antidiuretic hormone (SIADH) is characterized by continued secretion of ADH, despite the absence of normal stimuli for secretion (↑ serum osmolality or ↓ blood volume).

A: **Brain:** Haemorrhage/thrombosis, meningitis, abscess, trauma, tumour, Guillain–Barré syndrome.
Lung: Pneumonia, TB, abscess, aspergillosis, small cell carcinoma.
Tumours: Small cell lung cancer, lymphoma, leukaemia, pancreas, prostate, mesothelioma, sarcoma, thymoma, etc. It may be caused by ectopic ADH secretion.
Drugs: Vincristine, opiates, carbamazepine, chlorpropamide.
Metabolic: Porphyria, alcohol withdrawal.

A/R: see Aetiology for associated conditions.

E: Hyponatraemia is the most common electrolyte imbalance seen in hospitals. <50% of all severe hyponatraemia are a result of SIADH.

H: **Mild hyponatraemia** (Na^+: 125–135 mmol/L): May be asymptomatic.
Severe hyponatraemia ($Na^+ < 115$ mmol/L): Headache, nausea/vomiting, muscle cramp/weakness, irritability, confusion, drowsiness, convulsions and coma.
Symptoms of the underlying cause.

E: **Mild hyponatraemia:** No signs.
Severe hyponatraemia: ↓ Reflexes, extensor plantar reflexes.
Signs of the underlying cause.

P: Excess ADH ↑→↑ water reabsorption → plasma dilution, ↓ plasma osmolality and ↑ urine osmolality (urine is inappropriately concentrated).
The hyponatraemia in SIADH is dilutional from ↑ body water (antidiuresis) and not ↓ total body Na^+.

I: **Blood:** U&E (↓ Na^+) is the key blood test. Other tests are creatinine (renal function), glucose, serum protein and lipids (to exclude pseudohyponatraemia seen with ↑ protein or lipids).
Urine: ↑ Na^+ and ↑ osmolality are the two key diagnostic features.
Adrenal function: (short Synacthen test to exclude Addison's, pituitary function test: exclude ↓ ACTH), thyroid function tests (exclude hypothyroidism).
Tests for identifying the cause, e.g. CXR.
SIADH diagnosis: ↓ Plasma osmolality: <270 mOsm/kg and ↓ [Na^+] (<125 mmol/L: hyponatraemia). ↑ Urine osmolality (inappropriately higher than serum osmolality) and ↑ Na^+ (>30 mmol/L).
The presence of the above and absence of hypovolaemia/hypotension, oedema, renal, adrenal and thyroid dysfunction can lead to a diagnosis of SIADH.

M: **Mild cases:** Treat the underlying cause.
Symptomatic cases: Water restriction (0.5–1 L/day); if ineffective, give demeclocycline (blocks the renal tubular effect of ADH).
In severe cases, slow IV hypertonic saline (300 mmol/L) and furosemide (frusemide) to inhibit circulatory overload.

C: Convulsions, coma, death. Central pontine myelinosis (quadreparesis, respiratory arrest, fits) occurs with rapid correction of hyponatraemia.

P: Depends on the underlying cause. High morbidity and mortality with [Na^+] < 110 mmol/L. Up to 50 % mortality with central pontine myelinolysis.

D: Syringomyelia is the progressive cavitation of the central parts of the spinal cord usually starting at the cervical level. Also known as hydromyelia.

A: For the majority, the aetiology is unknown although possibly linked with Arnold–Chiari malformation or obstruction at the foramen magnum. A few cases are caused by spinal cord tumours, trauma or arachnoiditis.

A/R: Arnold–Chiari malformation (protrusion of cerebellar tonsils through foramen magnum), Dandy–Walker syndrome (failure of cerebellar vermis development and outflow obstruction to the fourth ventricle), intramedullary tumours (e.g. von Hippel–Lindau disease).

E: Rare and sporadic epidemiology. Usually presents at 25–45 years.

H: Insidious onset.
Weakness in arms and legs.
Loss of pain and temperature sensation in arms and shoulders.
Pain (boring or lancinating) may be present.

E: **Loss of pain and temperature sensation:** 'Dissociated anaesthesia' in a 'cape' distribution of neck, shoulders, upper arms and torso. Posterior columns are usually spared.
Motor: LMN signs (flaccid, wasted with fasciculations) in upper limbs. UMN signs (spastic and hyper-reflexia) in lower limbs.
Horner's syndrome: May be present (if C8, T1 or T2 are affected).
Syringobulbia (when syrinx extends into the medulla): Horner's syndrome and bilateral lower cranial nerve palsies in addition to signs of syringomyelia.

P: **Pathogenesis:** The main (unproven) theory is that there is obstruction of the normal CSF flow from the fourth ventricle out through the foramen of Luschka and Magendie, leading to transmission of a CSF pulse pressure wave which opens the central canal and dissects the grey matter along it.
Macro: The syrinx (CSF-filled cavity) starts in the central grey matter of the cervical cord interrupting decussating pathways, gradually enlarging into the posterior and anterior horns. It may be asymmetrical and is usually paramedian and longitudinal.
Micro: The syrinx cavity is lined with astrocytic glia and a few thick-walled blood vessels and contains low-protein CSF (unless associated with tumour).

I: **MRI scan with gadolinium:** Gold standard. Allows assessment of severity of syringomyelia and the presence of any cervical malformations or tumours. Delayed CT scans can also detect the changes.
Myelogram: Invasive. Largely superceded by MRI.

M: **Medical:** Only supportive measures for symptoms are available.
Surgical: Foramen magnum decompression. Syringostomy (drainage of the syrinx).

C: Extension upwards into bulbar region or downwards into thoracic region.
Kyphoscoliosis.

P: Variable. Some patients have the same level of symptoms for years, but more often there is very slow intermittent worsening of symptoms.

Systemic lupus erythematosus (SLE)

D: A systemic autoimmune disorder associated with the presence of anti-nuclear antibodies.
Four out of 11 criteria of the American Rheumatism Association (ARA) are required to diagnose SLE:

1 Malar rash	2 Discoid rash	3 Photosensitivity
4 Serositis (pericarditis, pleuritis)	5 Arthritis (non-erosive)	6 Oral ulcers
7 Renal involvement (casts or proteinuria > 0.5 g/24 h)	8 Seizures or psychosis	9 Haematological (see Investigations)
10 Immunological (e.g. anti-dsDNA, anti-Sm, anti-Ro, lupus anticoagulant, anticardiolipin)	11 Antinuclear antibodies	

A: Unknown. Combination of hormonal, genetic (↑ concordance in monozygotic twins, HLA clustering) and exogenous factors (e.g. drugs such as hydralazine and procainamide can cause a reversible SLE-like disorder).

A/R: Associated with other autoimmune diseases.

E: Common. Prevalence is 2 in 1000. More common in young (20–40-year-olds. 15 % cases > 60 years), Afro-Caribbean and Chinese. Nine times more common in females.

H & E: **General:** Fever, fatigue, weight loss, lymphadenopathy, splenomegaly.
Raynaud's phenomenon: Common, seen in 30 %.
Oral ulcers.
Skin rash:
Malar (butterfly) rash: Primarily affects the cheeks and the bridge of the nose. Discoid rash, photosensitivity, vasculitic (digital infarcts), urticaria, purpura, bullae, livedo reticularis, atypical erythema multiforme-like rash (Rowell's syndrome), hair loss.
Discoid lupus: Red and scaly patches (e.g. face), which later heal with scarring and pigmentation.
Systemic involvement:
Musculoskeletal: Arthritis, tendonitis, myopathy, avascular necrosis of femoral head.
Heart: Pericarditis, myocarditis, arrhythmias, Libman–Sacks endocarditis (non-infective, involving the mitral valve), aortic valve lesions.
Lung: Symptoms of pleuritis, pleural effusions, basal atelectasis, restrictive lung defects.
Neurological: Headache, stroke, cranial nerve palsies, confusion, chorea, fits, peripheral neuropathy.
Psychiatric: Depression, psychosis, depersonalization (feeling 'distant').
Renal: Symptoms of glomerulonephritis.

P: Tissue damage may be mediated by vascular immune complex deposition (e.g. glomerulonephritis: can be minimal change, mesangial, focal proliferative, diffuse proliferative, membranous or interstitial forms).

I: **Blood:** FBC, U&E, LFT, ↑ ESR with normal CRP, clotting, complement (↓ C3/C4).
Autoantibodies:
60 % of cases: anti-dsDNA
30–50 % of cases: rheumatoid factor
30 % of cases: anti-RNP
30 % of cases: anti-Ro
30 % of cases: anti-Sm
15 % of cases: anti-La
Anticardiolipin and lupus anticoagulant (see Antiphospholipid syndrome).
Antihistone antibody in drug-induced lupus.
Coombs test: For haemolytic anaemia.
Urine: Haematuria, proteinuria, microscopy (for casts).
Joints: Plain X-ray radiographs.
Heart and lung: CXR, ECG, echocardiogram, CT scan.
Kidney: Renal biopsy (if glomerulonephritis suspected).
CNS: CT or MRI scan.

M: **Medical:** Oral corticosteroids. Immunosuppressants (e.g. cyclophosphamide, azathioprine) may be added in renal or cerebral involvement.
Joints: NSAIDs for pain. Local steroid injection.
Skin rash: Hydroxychloroquine (ophthalmic monitoring).
Discoid lupus: Topical steroids and avoid sunlight.
Resistant thrombocytopenia: Danazol or IV immunoglobulins.

C: Vasculitis affecting any organ. Large vessel thrombosis. Anti-Ro can cross the placenta and cause congenital heart block in the fetus.

P: 10-year survival rate is ~90 %. Mortality is usually a result of infection (e.g. streptococcal sepsis) or renal failure. Prognosis worse if onset with renal involvement during pregnancy.

Systemic sclerosis

D: Rare connective tissue disease characterized by widespread small blood vessel damage and fibrosis in skin and internal organs. Also known as scleroderma. Spectrum of disease includes the following.

Prescleroderma: Raynaud's phenomenon, nail-fold capillary changes and antinuclear antibodies.

Diffuse cutaneous systemic sclerosis (40 %): Raynaud's phenomenon followed by skin changes with sacral and truncal involvement, tendon friction and joint contractures, early lung, heart, GI and renal disease, nail-fold capillary dilation.

Limited cutaneous systemic sclerosis (60 %): Previously known as CREST (calcinosis, Raynaud's, oesophageal dysmotility, sclerodactyly, telangiecstasia).

Scleroderma sine scleroderma (1 %): Internal organ disease with no skin changes.

A: Unknown. Genetic and environmental factors (e.g. vinyl chloride, epoxy resins) have been suggested.

A/R: Overlap syndromes with polymyositis and SLE.

E: Age of onset 30–60 years. Three times more common in females. Annual incidence is 1 in 10 000.

H & E: Symptoms of the following.

Skin: *Raynaud's phenomenon* (see Raynaud's phenomenon).

Hands: Initially swollen oedematous painful fingers. Later they become thickened, tight, shiny and bound to underlying structures. Changes in pigmentation and finger ulcers.

Face: Microstomia (puckering and furrowing of perioral skin), telangiecstasia.

Lung: Pulmonary fibrosis leading on to pulmonary hypertension.

Heart: Pericarditis or pericardial effusion, myocardial fibrosis, heart failure or arrhythmias.

GI: Dry mouth, oesophageal dysmotility (dysphagia), reflux oesophagitis, gastric paresis (nausea, vomiting, anorexia), watermelon stomach, bacterial overgrowth, small bowel pseudo-obstruction, colonic hypomotility (constipation), anal incontinence, angiodysplasia.

Kidney: Hypertensive renal crisis and eventually chronic renal failure.

Neuromuscular: Trigeminal neuralgia, muscular wasting or weakness.

Other: Hypothyroidism, impotence, dryness of mucus membranes can cause dyspareunia.

P: Exact pathogenesis unclear, but specific antibodies (humoral immunity) and activated monocytes and macrophages and lymphocytes (cellular immunity) may interact with:

- Endothelial cells → endothelial cell damage, platelet activation, myointimal cell proliferation and narrowing of blood vessels.
- Fibroblasts → lay down collagen in the dermis.

I: **Blood:** *Antinuclear antibodies:*

- Anti-centromere (70 % positive in limited cutaneous systemic sclerosis).
- Anti-topoisomerase (30% positive in diffuse cutaneous systemic sclerosis).
- Anti-nucleolar antibodies.
- PmScl (associated with myositis).
- RNA-polymerase antibody (associated with renal crisis).

Nail-fold capillary ophthalmoscopy or microscopy: To detect fine nail-fold changes.

Investigations for complications:

Lung: CXR, pulmonary function tests, high-resolution CT scan.

Heart: ECG, echocardiography.

GI: Endoscopy, barium studies, oesophageal scintigraphy.

Kidney: U&E and measurement of creatinine clearance.

Neuromuscular: Electromyography, nerve conduction studies, biopsy.

Joints: Radiography (for subcutaneous calcification, acro-osteolysis, flexion deformities).

Skin: Biopsy (to exclude fasciitis, rarely necessary), muscle biopsy for associated myositis.

M: **Treatment of affected organs:**

Skin: Moisturizers and anti-thymocyte globulin help treat skin sclerosis. Laser therapy for telangiectasia (see Raynaud's phenomenon for treatment of symptoms in hands).

Lung: IV prostacyclin for pulmonary hypertension. Prostacyclin prolongs life expectancy. Bosentan (endothelin-receptor antagonist) and warfarin.

GI: Proton pump inhibitors for reflux disease, promotility drugs, pancreatic supplements, PEG feeding or parenteral nutrition may all be necessary at some stage.

Neuromuscular: Methotrexate for associated myositis.

Renal: ACE-inhibitors reduce incidence of renal crisis. In renal crisis, IV prostacyclin or peritoneal dialysis may be used.

C: (see History).

P: Variable (5-year survival rate is 35–75 %). Poor prognostic factors: male sex, age, ↑ extent of skin involvement with heart, lung and renal disease. More severe in non-white patients.

Thalassaemias

D: Group of genetic disorders characterized by reduced globin chain synthesis.

A: Autosomal recessive inheritance.
α-Thalassaemia: ↓ α-Globin chain synthesis. There are four α-globin genes on chromosome 16.
Deletion of all four genes: Hb Barts (γ_4) and intrauterine death (hydrops fetalis).
Deletion of three of four genes: Microcytic hypochromic anaemia and splenomegaly, 4–10 % Hb H (β_4).
Deletion of onr or two of four genes: Microcytic hypochromic red cells, usually no anaemia, ↑ red cell count.
β-Thalassaemia major or Cooley's anaemia (homozygous β-thalassaemia): β-Globin gene mutations on chromosome 11 causes no or minimal β-chain synthesis (β^0 or β^+).
β-Thalassaemia intermedia: Mild defect in β-chain synthesis causing microcytic anaemia, ↓ α-chain synthesis or ↑ γ-chains.
β-Thalassaemia trait (heterozygous carrier): Asymptomatic, mild microcytic anaemia, ↑ red cell count.

A/R: A thalasaemic allele may be associated with Hb S allele (sickle-β-thalassaemia, 'compound heterozygote').

E: Worldwide, but more common in Mediterranean and areas of the Middle East. Equal gender distribution.

H: **β-Thalassaemia major:** Anaemia presenting at 3–6 months (when γ-chain synthesis switches to β-chain synthesis). Failure to thrive and prone to infections.
α- or β-thalassaemia trait: May be asymptomatic. Detected on routine blood tests or from a family history.

E: **β-Thalassaemia major:** Signs of anaemia (pallor, malaise, dyspnoea), mild jaundice.
Frontal bossing and thalassaemic facies (marrow hyperplasia).
Hepatosplenomegaly (erythrocyte pooling, extramedullary haemopoiesis).
Signs of complications (see Complications).
Note that patients with β-thalassaemia intermedia may also have the above signs.

P: The genetic defects result in an imbalance of globin chain production and deposition in erythroblasts and erythrocytes causing ineffective erythropoiesis, haemolysis, anaemia and extramedullary haemopoiesis.

I: **Blood:** FBC (↓Hb, ↓ MCV, ↓ MCH).
Blood film: Hypochromic, microcytic anaemia, target cells, nucleated red cells and ↑ reticulocyte count.
Hb electrophoresis: Absent or ↓ levels of Hb A and ↑ levels of Hb F (fetal Hb, $\alpha_2\gamma_2$).
Bone marrow: Hypercellular with erythroid hyperplasia.
DNA analysis: For specific mutations.
SXR: 'Hair-on-end' appearance (caused by expansion of marrow into cortex) in β-thalassaemia major.

M: α- or β-thalassaemia trait do not usually require treatment.

β-Thalassaemia major: Regular blood transfusions together with SC desferrioxamine or oral deferiprone (for iron chlelation to prevent of iron overload) 5–7 nights weekly.
Surgical: Splenectomy (if requirements for blood transfusion are very high, but delay operation until 5–6 years old). Bone marrow transplant from an HLA-matched donor in selected individuals.
Prophylaxis:
Before splenectomy: Vaccination against encapsulated organisms (e.g. pneumococcus, meningococcus and *H. influenzae*) and hepatitis B.
After splenectomy: Penicillin V daily, low-dose aspirin for persistent post-splenectomy thrombocytosis to ↓ risk of thromboembolism.
Treatment of complications.

C: Severe thalassamias can cause the following complications.
Iron overload:
Skin: 'Slate-grey' skin pigmentation.
Liver: Secondary haemochromatosis leading to liver damage.
Endocrine organs: Short stature, delayed puberty, diabetes mellitus, hypothyroidism.
Heart: Cardiac failure or arrhythmias.
Infections: Prone to encapsulated organisms (e.g. meningococcal and pneumococcus) after splenectomy. *Yersinia entercolitica* and *Rhizopus* (rare fungal infection) in those taking desferrioxamine.
Osteoporosis: Secondary to marrow expansion and endocrinological complications, fractures.
Hypersplenism (↓Hb, ↓platelets, ↓neutrophils) secondary to splenomegaly.

P: Normal life expectancy in those with thalassemia trait.
In β-thalassaemia major, regular transfusions and iron chelation improves prognosis. Mortality is mainly caused by heart failure (from iron overload) and infections. Bone marrow transplantation has 90 % success rate.

Transient ischaemic attack (TIA)

D: Impairment of CNS (or retinal) dysfunction developing rapidly and lasting <24 h. TIAs lasting >24 h but with full recovery are called reversible ischaemic neurological deficits (see Stroke).

A: *Emboli:* Usually from either atheromatous plaques of carotid or vertebrobasilar arteries, or from the heart (e.g. in atrial fibrillation, recent MI).
Thrombosis: Atherosclerosis affecting small intracerebral vessels.
Compression: Compression of vertebrobasilar arteries in particular neck postures (e.g. by osteophytes).
Hypotension: If below the autoregulatory range that normally maintains cerebral blood flow.

A/R: Diabetes, family history, hypertension, hyperlipidaemia, smoking, ↑ age, ↑↑ alcohol, anticoagulants.

E: Common.

H: Rapid onset that resolves within 24 h, by definition.
Weakness, sensory or visual impairment, dysphasia, diplopia, impaired coordination.
Loss of cognitive function or consciousness, syncope.
Enquire if history of atrial fibrillation, MI, valvular heart disease, carotid artery stenosis.

E: Examine for underlying cause (e.g. atrial fibrillation, heart murmurs, carotid bruit, fundoscopy).

Circulation	Clinical signs
Carotid	Hemiparesis, hemianopia, hemisensory loss, dysphasia
Ophthalmic	Amaurosis fugax (transient mono-ocular visual loss like a 'falling curtain')
Vertebrobasilar	Vertigo, vomiting, diplopia, dysarthria, dysphagia, ataxia, uni- or bilateral vision loss, bilateral or alternating sensorimotor loss

P: No lasting structural damage occurs.

I: **Blood:** FBC, U&E, ESR, glucose, lipids (occasionally, homocysteine levels).
ECG: To exclude arrhythmias which might predispose to emboli.
Echocardiogram: To exclude the heart as source of emboli.
Carotid Doppler ultrasound: To detect any carotid stenosis.
Brain CT: Not usually necessary. Exclude tumours, arteriovenous malformations or subdural haemorrhages.

M: **Acute:** Treat any acute risk factors (e.g. anticoagulation for AF).
Prevention: Low-dose daily aspirin, encourage to stop smoking, control hypertension and hyperlipidaemia, avoid excess alcohol.
Surgical: Carotid endarterectomy is indicated if carotid stenosis detected and > 70 %.

C: Progression to stroke.

P: Annual risk of stroke ~7 % within the first 5 years. Highest risk being in the first year.

Note: 'subclavian steal' syndrome is a rare cause of vertebrobasilar TIAs. In this syndrome proximal subclavian artery stenosis causes reversal of vertebral artery flow on arm exercise. This produces focal neurological deficit which resolves spontaneously at rest. Examination reveals low BP and low pulse volume in the ipsilateral arm.

Tricuspid regurgitation

D: Tricuspid regurgitation is backflow of blood from the right ventricle to the right atrium during systole.

A: **Congenital:** Ebstein anomaly (malpositioned tricuspid valve), cleft valve in ostium primum defect.
Functional: Consequence of right ventricular dilation (e.g. in pulmonary hypertension), valve prolapse.
Rheumatic heart disease: Associated with tricuspid stenosis or other valvular disease.
Infective endocarditis: Common in IV drug users. Usually staphylococcal.
Other: Carcinoid syndrome, trauma, cirrhosis (long-standing), iatrogenic (e.g. radiotherapy to the thorax).

A/R: (see above for associated conditions and risk factors).

E: The epidemiology differs with various causes. Infective endocarditis probably most common cause.

H: Fatigue, breathlessness, palpitations, headaches, nausea, anorexia, epigastric pain made worse by exercise, jaundice, lower limb swelling.

E: **Pulse:** May be irregularly irregular due to AF (may occur with right atrial enlargement).
Inspection: ↑ JVP with giant *v* waves which may oscillate the earlobe. This is caused by transmission of right ventricular pressure to the great veins. If in sinus rhythm, there may be giant *a* wave.
Palpation: Parasternal heave.
Auscultation: Pansystolic murmur heard best at the lower left sternal edge, louder on inspiration (Carvallo sign). Loud P_2.
Chest: Pleural effusion. Causes of pulmonary hypertension (e.g. emphysema).
Abdomen: Palpable liver (tender, smooth, pulsatile), ascites.
Legs: Pitting oedema.

P: Regurgitation of the blood from the right ventricle into the right atrium gives rise to high right atrial pressure, subsequently high systemic venous pressure.

I: **Blood:** FBC, LFT, cardiac enzymes, blood cultures.
ECG: Tall P wave (right atrial hypertrophy) if in sinus rhythm. Changes indicative of other cardiac disease.
CXR: Right-sided enlargement of cardiac shadow.
Echocardiography: Extent of regurgitiation estimated by colour flow Doppler. Tricuspid valve abnormality (e.g. prolapse). Right ventricular dilation. ↑ Pulmonary artery pressure.

M: Treat the underlying condition, e.g. infective endocarditis or functional regurgitation caused by pulmonary hypertension. Diuretics may be given for fluid retention.
Surgery: Annuloplasty, plication or, rarely, replacement. Repair of the valve only in very severe tricuspid regurgitation, when the required doses of diuretics are large enough to cause metabolic consequences. Surgical removal of the valve may be required to eradicate the source of infection in IV drug users with infective endocarditis.

C: Heart failure, hepatic fibrosis.

P: Prognosis varies depending on the underlying cause.

Trigeminal neuralgia

D: Characterized by 'paroxysmal' facial pain in the distribution of the trigeminal nerve.

A: Most cases are idiopathic but occasionally may be caused by compression of the trigeminal sensory root, e.g. by tumours of the cerebellopontine angle.

A/R: Rarely associated with multiple sclerosis and demyelination of brainstem trigeminal sensory fibres, such cases occur in younger patients.

E: Less common cause of headache. Age of onset usually >50 years, ♀ : ♂ = 3:1.

H: Brief (<1 min) typically unilateral attacks of lancinating (sharp, shooting, knife-like or shock-like) pain in the distribution of one or more divisions of the trigeminal nerve on a background of dull pain.
The attacks can either be spontaneous or provoked by touching 'trigger spots' on the facial skin (e.g. shaving or washing the face, cold breeze), or movements of the skin/jaw (e.g. eating, talking).

E: Often unremarkable.
Involuntary facial spasms (*tic douloureux*) may be caused by anxiety of the palpation of trigger areas.
Look for signs of the possible underlying cause (e.g. other cranial nerve involvement in cerebellopontine angle tumours, or optic disc atrophy in multiple sclerosis).

P: Little is known about the pathology of trigeminal neuralgia.

I: MRI or CT scan to exclude any underlying causes (e.g. cerebellopontine angle tumours).

M: **Medical:** Carbamazepine is the first-line treatment. Tricyclic antidepressants, phenytoin, sodium valproate or baclofen may be tried if carbamazepine is not effective or tolerated. Radiofrequency thermocoagulation or glycerol injection of the trigeminal ganglion may also be tried if drug treatment is unsuccessful.
Surgical: Exploration of the posterior fossa and trigeminal sensory root decompression or section.

C: Depression and poor quality of life.

P: May persist lifelong in patients who are not treated. In early stages, the remissions may last for months to years. Remissions may become shorter with time.

D: A granulomatous disease caused by *Mycobacterium tuberculosis*. Commonly abbreviated as TB.

Primary: Initial infection may be pulmonary (acquired by inhalation from the cough of an infected patient) or, occasionally, gastrointestinal (e.g. terminal ileum, tonsils).

Miliary TB: Results when there is haematogenous dissemination of the bacterium.

Postprimary: Occurs after developing some immunity to mycobacteria. Caused by reinfection or reactivation.

A: *M. tuberculosis* has a lipid-rich cell wall and has the ability to survive intracellularly within macrophages.

A/R: Reactivation risk factors: ↑ age, malignancy, malnutrition, alcohol, immunodeficiency (malnutrition, diabetes, drugs, HIV).

E: Annual mortality 3 000 000 (95 % in developing countries), UK incidence 6000/year. Incidence in Asian immigrants >30 times native UK white population.

H & E: **Primary TB:** Mostly asymptomatic, may have fever, malaise, cough, wheeze, erythema nodosum and phlyctenular conjunctivitis (allergic manifestations).

Miliary TB: Fever, weight loss, meningitis, yellow caseous tubercles spread to other organs, e.g. in bone and kidney may remain dormant for years.

Postprimary TB: Fever/night sweats, malaise, weight loss, breathlessness, cough, sputum, haemoptysis, pleuritic pain, signs of pleural effusion, collapse, consolidation, fibrosis.

Non-pulmonary TB: Particularly immigrants and immunocompromised. Can affect any system.

Lymph nodes: Suppuration of cervical lymph nodes leading to abscesses or sinuses, which discharge pus and spread to skin (scrofuloderma).

CNS: Meningitis, tuberculoma.

Skin: Lupus vulgaris (jelly-like reddish/brown plaques, with glistening surfaces).

Heart: Pericardial effusion, constrictive pericarditis.

GI: Subacute obstruction, change in bowel habit, weight loss, peritonitis, ascites.

Genitourinary: Urinary tract infection symptoms, renal failure, epididymitis, endometrial or tubal involvement, infertility.

Adrenal: Insufficiency.

Bone/joints: Osteomyelitis, arthritis, paravertebral abscesses and vertebral collapse (Pott's disease), spinal cord compresson from abscesses.

P: **Primary TB:** *Primary (Ghon) focus* (usually in subpleural mid zone) showing transient acute inflammatory infiltrate, followed formation of granulomas (epithelioid macrophages, Langhans giant cells, lymphocytes, central caseating necrosis). This Ghon focus and regional lymph node granulomas is known as 'primary complex', which heals (3–8 weeks) and becomes calcified. Reaction to tuberculin test becomes positive.

I: **Sputum/pleural fluid/bronchial washings:**

Microscopy: Ziehl–Neelsen stain for acid–alcohol-fast bacilli.

Culture: Takes up to 6 weeks.

Sensitivity.

PCR: Takes ~48 h.

Tuberculin tests: Positive in previous exposure to *M. tuberculosis* or BCG. Strong positive may indicate infection.

Mantoux test: Intradermal injection of PPD, with induration and erythema after 72 h.

Heaf test: Place drop of PPD on forearm, fire spring-loaded needled gun, read after 3–7 days. Graded according to papule size and vesiculation.

CXR:

Primary infection: Peripheral consolidation, hilar lymphadenopathy.

Miliary: Fine shadowing.

Postprimary: Upper lobe shadowing, streaky fibrosis and cavitation, calcification, pleural effusion, hilar lymphadenopathy.

HIV testing (2 % may be HIV positive): Recommended by the Department of Health.

CT, lymph nodes, pleural biopsy, sampling of other affected systems: (e.g. CSF, heart, urine).

M: Needs to be treated by specialist physician. **Notifiable** disease. **Isolate** for 2 weeks if respiratory.

Antimicrobial therapy: Combined therapy necessary to prevent resistance. **D**irectly **o**bserved **t**herapy may be necessary if compliance poor. Therapy for 6 months in pulmonary, 12 months for bone or brain.

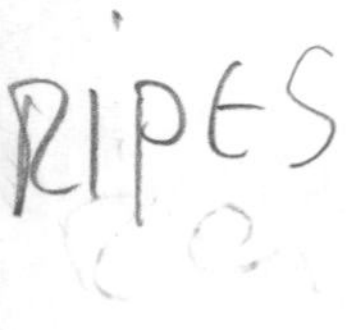

1 *Rifampicin:* side-effects: orange body fluids, enzyme-inducing, major interaction with protease inhibitors.

2 *Isoniazid:* side-effects: pyridoxine deficiency and peripheral neuropathy.

3 *Ethambutol:* side-effects: optic neuropathy, so stop if vision is affected.

4 *Pyrazinamide:* side-effects: ↑ urate/arthralgia.

5 *Streptomycin:* only for highly resistant organisms.

Steroids for pericardial, cerebral or bone involvement, monitor liver function (TB drugs are hepatotoxic).

Contact tracing: With CXR, tuberculin test, check BCG status. Consider chemoprophylaxis.

Chemoprophylaxis (e.g. isoniazid): For contacts or those with CXR evidence of TB before receiving immunosuppressants.

Advice: Explain side-effects and importance of compliance to treatment.

Prevention: BCG vaccination, a live attenuated strain derived from *M. bovis*, provides 60–80 % efficacy. It should be considered as protection against extrapulmonary TB only.

C: **Primary TB:** Lobar collapse (especially middle lobe) and bronchiectasis (Brock's syndrome), pleural effusion, pneumonic spread, miliary disease disseminated in lung or throughout body.

Postprimary TB: Pleural effusion, empyema, aspergilloma, adenocarcinoma, laryngeal disease, swelling of bronchial lymphatics and airflow obstruction, haemoptysis (invasion by an aspergilloma or breakdown of fibrous scarring), distant spread.

P: Excellent if pulmonary TB and treated. 8 % overall mortality if extrapulmonary TB, relapse because of non-adherence, resistance, cavitation, empyema, latency.

D: Tuberous sclerosis is a genetic disorder characterized by hamartoma formation in many organs. It is also called epiloia (epilepsy, low intelligence, adenoma sebaceum).

A: The inheritance is autosomal dominant. 80–90 % arise as new mutations. Genetic loci: *TSC1* (on chromosome 9 coding for hamartin), and *TSC2* (on chromosome 16 coding for tuberin with the structure of a GTPase activating protein). Hamartin and tuberin may act synergistically in the regulation of cell proliferation and differentiation.

A/R: CNS hamartomas and gliomas, rhabdomyomas, retinal phakomas, renal hamartomas or cysts (polycystic kidney), lung hamartomas.

E: Prevalence 1 in 6000–30 000. No racial or sexual predilection.

H: Patients range from showing no or few features to those who are severely affected.
CNS hamartomas: Learning disability, epilepsy.
Heart hamartomas: Palpitations (arrythmias), symptoms of congestive cardiac failure.
Kidney hamartomas: Pain or bleeding.
Lung hamartomas: Breathlessness (pulmonary fibrosis, pneumothorax, cor pulmonale).

E: **Shagreen patches:** Lumpy leathery flesh-coloured plaques over the lower back.
Hypopigmented patches: 'Ash leaf-shaped' patches over the trunk or buttocks, easier to see under ultraviolet light.
Adenoma sebaceum: Pink or skin-coloured papules with a butterfly distribution over the cheeks, also seen in the nasolabial folds and on the forehead/chin (appear < 10 years, becoming prominent after puberty).
Periungal fibromas: Pink papules growing out from the nail-beds.
Café au lait macules, intraoral fibromas and pits in dental enamel, yellow retinal phakomas.

P: Hamartomas are malformations consisting of haphazardly arranged cells normally found in an organ. CNS hamartomas consist of haphazardly arranged large distorted neurones and glia. May be calcified. Retinal phakomas are glial masses. Adenoma sebaceum are angiofibromas. Cardiac hamartomas are rhabdomyomas. Renal hamartomas are angiomyolipomas. Lung hamartomas are composed of smooth muscle cells.

I: **CNS:** CT, MRI, EEG (when initial presentation includes seizures).
Heart: ECG (arrhythmias, e.g. Wolff–Parkinson–White syndrome), echocardiography.
Kidney: Ultrasound (renal cysts/hamartomas/tumours).
Lungs: Pulmonary function test (when there are symptoms), chest CT (especially in adult females).

M: Control epilepsy (see Epilepsy). Management of learning disability and behaviour disorder.
Laser treatment for facial angiofibromas. Evaluation of family members (parents and siblings), periodic monitoring.

C: Subependymal giant cell astrocytoma may arise from subependymal hamartomas.

P: 75 % of those severely affected die at < 25 years. The prognosis for those diagnosed later in life depends on the associated internal tumours.

Turner's syndrome

D: Characterized by a phenotypic appearance caused by complete (or occasionally partial) absence of one X chromosome (karyotype: 45 XO).

A: Usually an entire X chromosome is missing. Occasionally caused either by the deletion of the small arm of the chromosome and the generation of the isochromosome of the long arm, or deletion of portions of either arm.

A/R: Associated with coarctation of the aorta (10–20 %), septal defect, aortic stenosis, small uterus, diabetes mellitus, Hashimoto's thyroiditis, horseshoe kidney and hypertension.

E: Common. 1 in 2500 live born girls.

H: Only 1 % of fetuses with 45 XO genotype are born alive.
'Syndromic' appearance.
Symptoms of hypogonadism: Primary amenorrhea, delayed/absent puberty, infertility.
Symptoms of ↓ oestrogen: Night sweats, hot flushes, vaginal dryness, dyspareunia, hair loss, thin skin.

E: **Hypogonadism:** ↓ Axillary or pubic hair.
Short stature.
Face: Hyperteloism, high-arched palate.
Neck: Short webbed neck.
Arms and hands: ↑ Carrying angle (cubitus valgus), short metacarpals (especially fourth), hypoplastic nails.
Chest: Widely spaced nipples, shield chest, signs of coarctation of aorta.
Other features: Low hairline, deafness, vertebral dysplasia, multiple naevi, lymphoedema.

P: 'Streak ovaries': devoid of ova and follicles. They appear as atrophic fibrous strands.

I: **Blood:** Oestrogen (↓), LH and FSH (↑ secondary to reduced negative feedback from ovarian oestrogen), TFT (to exclude associated thyroiditis).
Karyotype: 45 XO.
Ultrasound and MRI: Visualizes gonads and to search for cardiovascular, renal and other complications.

M: **Short stature:** Can be treated with oxandrolone (anabolic steroid) and human growth hormone.
Induce puberty: Low-dose ethinylestradiol and gradually increase the dose. Add medroxyprogesterone acetate for first 2 weeks each month. Pregnancy may be possible by ovum donation.
Prophylaxis: Female patients with 'mosaicism' (a mix of XO/XY genotype) have ↑ risk of neoplastic degeneration of the dysgenetic gonads. The gonads should be removed surgically.

C: Premature ovarian failure, osteoporosis and aging. Infertility. Complications of associated conditions.

P: Good overall diagnosis. Life expectancy is slightly shorter but can be ↑ by management of long-term complications.

Note: Noonan's syndrome affects males and females with normal (46 XY and 46 XX) genotypes. Patients show Turner's phenotype and may have right-sided cardiac lesions (e.g. pulmonary stenosis) and mental retardation. Normal ovarian function and normal fertility is seen in females. Males may have undescended testes and impaired testicular function.

D: Diseases caused by bacilli *Salmonella typhi* and *S. paratyphi* types A, B and C, respectively.

A: Transmission is via food or water contaminated by faeces or urine of a sufferer or carrier.

A/R: Recent travel to an endemic country (see Epidemiology), poor sanitation.

E: About 200 typhoid cases and 200 paratyphoid cases are seen in the UK annually (many are acquired abroad).
Endemic in the tropics, South America, the Middle East, southern and eastern Europe.

H: Incubation period: 1–4 weeks (usually 2 weeks). Rising fever, malaise, headache, dry cough, constipation, confusion, restlessness of insidious onset.
After 1 week: Diarrhoea (may be present from the onset in paratyphoid B), rash (see below).

E: Pyrexia, relative bradycardia (heart rate does not ↑ with the temperature).
Cervical lymphadenopathy, splenomegaly (>70 %), hepatomegaly (30 %), abdominal distension and pain.
Rose spots: Blanching erythematous maculopapular rash in ~30 % patients, after 1 week lasting for 2–3 days, on the upper abdomen, thorax, flanks, buttocks (rose spots are rare in paratyphoid A).
Children: Atypical presentation with high swinging fever, pneumonia, splenomegaly, few abdominal signs.
It is important to assess for dehydration and for any complications in all patients.

P: Replication of the organisms in the gut leading to invasion of bacilli into bloodstream and replication in the reticuloendothelial cells. Eventually, there is secondary bacteraemia and reinvasion of the gut (especially Peyer's patches) leading to the symptoms.

I: **Urine and stool culture:** Usually positive after first week. (Positive in faeces alone may be a result of carrier status.)
Bone marrow aspirate and culture: Very sensitive (>95 %) even during antibiotic administration.
Blood: FBC (↓ WCC), LFT (mild ↑ in transaminases), serology (Widal agglutinin test, poor sensitivity). Blood culture (in the first 2 weeks).
CXR: May show nodular/segmental pneumonitis.

M: **Medical:** Third-generation cephalosporins are the antibiotics of choice until sensitivity is known. Other options are quinolones and chloramphenicol. Growing antibiotic resistance may make treatment difficult. High-dose steroids lowers mortality in critically ill patients.
Surgical: Necessary for complications (e.g. intestinal perforation).
Chronic carriers: In up to 3 % after treatment.
Public health: Patient should be treated in isolation. Avoid high-risk food/water, Vi-polysaccharide vaccine, oral Ty21a live vaccine (not effective for all strains). Typhoid and paratyphoid fever are notifiable diseases. Note that a diagnosis has job implications for the patient.

C: Usually seen in untreated patients in week 3. Intestinal perforation or haemorrhage, pneumonia, meningitis, myocarditis, osteomyelitis, acute cholecystitis, multisystem typhoid abscesses, prolonged carrier status.

P: Untreated mortality is up to 20 % (mainly from GI complications). About 15 % relapse. This is usually less severe.

Ulcerative colitis

D: Chronic relapsing remitting inflammatory disease of the large bowel. Grouped with Crohn's disease and together they are known as inflammatory bowel disease.

A: Unknown. Suggested hypotheses include genetic susceptibility, immune response to bacterial or self-antigens, environmental factors, altered neutrophil function, abnormality in epithelial cell integrity.

A/R: Positive family history of IBD (~15 %).
Associated with ↑ serum pANCA, primary sclerosing cholangitis, other autoimmune diseases.

E: Prevalence 1 in 1500 (industrialized world). Higher prevalence in Ashkenazi Jews. Peak onset age is 20–40 years.

H: Bloody or mucous diarrhoea (stool frequency related to severity of disease).
Tenesmus and urgency.
Crampy abdominal pain before defaecation, weight loss, fever.
Symptoms of extraintestinal manifestations (see Complications).

E: Signs of iron-deficiency anaemia, dehydration.
Clubbing.
Abdominal tenderness, tachycardia.
Blood, mucous and tenderness on PR examination.
Signs of extraintestinal manifestations (see Complications).

P: **Macro:** Mucosal inflammation initially involving rectum and may extend proximally to involve the entire colon (pancolitis), red granular mucosa with superficial ulceration and pseudopolyps (islands of non-ulcerated swollen mucosa).
Micro: Acute and chronic inflammatory cells in lamina propria, inflamed areas are contiguous, crypt abscesses (neutrophils in colonic glands), cell dysplasia in those with long history.

I: **Blood:** FBC (↓ Hb, ↑ WCC), ESR/CRP (usually ↑), albumin (↓), cross-match blood if severe blood loss.
Stool: Culture (for *Escherichia coli* 0157, *Campylobacter* and *Shigella*). Detection of *Clostridium difficile* toxin.
AXR: To rule out toxic megacolon.*
Lower GI endoscopy (and biopsy): Determines severity, histological confirmation, detection of dysplasia.
Barium enema: Mucosal ulceration with granular appearance and filling defects (pseudopolyps), narrowed colon, loss of haustral pattern (lead pipe or hosepipe appearance). Colonoscopy and barium enema may be dangerous in acute exacerbations (risk of perforation).
Radiolabelled white cell scan: Highlights areas of bowel inflammation.

M: **Markers of activity:** ↓ Hb, ↓ albumin, ↑ ESR, ↑ CRP and diarrhoea frequency (<4/day mild, 4–6/day moderate, >6/day severe), bleeding, fever.
Acute exacerbation: Nil-by-mouth, IV rehydration (especially K^+), IV corticosteroids, parenteral feeding may be necessary, antibiotic prophylaxis. Monitor fluid balance and vital signs closely. Bowel resection if toxic megacolon as perforation has a mortality of 30 %.

*Toxic megacolon is characterized by inflamed dilated loops of colon (usually transverse). Radiological features include colon >5.5 cm, thickened colonic wall, 'thumb-printing' caused by stripping of inflamed mucosa. Colon needs to be resected urgently to prevent perforation.

Mild attacks: Oral or rectal 5-ASA (e.g. sulfasalazine, mesalazine) or rectal steroids.

Moderate attacks: Oral steroids and oral 5-ASA.

Maintenance of remission: 5-ASA, consider other immunosuppressants (e.g. ciclosporin, azathioprine).

Advice: Patient education and support. Treatment of complications. Regular colonoscopic surveillance.

Surgery: Indicated for failure of medical treatment, presence of complications or to prevent colonic carcinoma. Proctocolectomy with ileostomy or an ileoanal pouch formation provides good results.

C: **GI:** Haemorrhage, toxic megacolon, perforation, colonic carcinoma (in those with extensive disease for >10 years), gallstones and primary sclerosing cholangitis.

Extraintestinal manifestations (10–20 %): Uveitis, renal calculi, arthropathy, sacroiliitis, ankylosing spondylitis, erythema nodosum, pyoderma gangrenosum, osteoporosis (from steroid treatment), amyloidosis.

P: A relapsing and remitting condition, with normal life expectancy.

Poor prognostic factors (ABCDEF): **A**lbumin (<30 g/L), **B**lood PR, **C**RP raised, **D**ilated loops of bowel, **E**ight or more bowel movements per day, **F**ever (>38 °C in first 24 h).

Urinary tract infections

D: Characterized by presence of >100 000 of colony forming units per millilitre of urine.
Urinary tract infections (UTI) may affect bladder (cystitis), kidney (pyelonephritis) or prostate (prostatitis).

A: Usually transurethral ascent of normal colonic organisms. The most common organism is *Escherichia coli*, others include *Proteus mirabilis*, *Klebsiella* and *Enterococci* (more common in hospitals).
Staphylococcus saprophyticus (skin organism) is the cause in up to 30 % of sexually active women.

A/R: Females (short urethra and proximity of perianal colonic organisms to the urethra), sexual intercourse, vaginal spermicide/diaphragm contraceptive, pregnancy.
Urethral instrumentation/catheterization, urinary obstruction and stasis (stones, tumour, prostatic enlargement, congenital anatomical defects), poor bladder emptying, previous bladder epithelial damage.
Risk factors for pyelonephritis: vesicoureteric reflux, obstruction.
UTIs are potentially serious complications of diabetes mellitus, pregnancy, infection above an obstruction and infants with vesicoureteric reflux disease.

E: Common in females: >30 % of women experience UTI at some point in their lives.
UTI may be seen in 5 % of pregnant women, 2 % of young non-pregnant women, 20 % of elderly living at home and 50 % of institutionalized elderly.
UTI is rare in children and young men except homosexuals (if present, an underlying cause is suspected).

H: May be clinically silent (asymptomatic bacteruria).
Cystitis: Frequency, urgency, dysuria (pain on micturition), haematuria, suprapubic pain, smelly urine.
Pyelonephritis (acute): Fever, malaise, rigor, loin/flank pain.
Prostatitis: Fever, low back/perineal pain, irritative and obstructive symptoms (e.g. hesitancy, urgency, intermittency, poor stream, dribbling).
Elderly: Malaise, nocturia, incontinence, confusion.
Up to 30 % of women with UTI symptoms may not have bacteruria. ('urethral syndrome').

E: **Cystitis:** Fever, abdominal/suprapubic/loin tenderness, bladder distension.
Pyelonephritis: Fever, loin/flank tenderness.
Prostatitis: Tender swollen prostate.

P: Acute pyelonephritis (renal parenchymal infection with neutrophil infiltration) may be caused by ascending ureteric infection or haematogenous spread (bacteraemia).
Reflux nephropathy (or chronic pyelonephritis): back pressure from vesicoureteric reflux leads to cortical scarring and clubbing of calyces and, eventually, hypertension and chronic renal failure in children or adults.

I: **MSU:**
Dipstick test: For blood, protein, leucocyte esterase, nitrites (urinary bacteria reduce nitrates to nitrites).
Microscopy, culture and sensitivity: >10 white (pus) cells/mm^3 of urine indicates inflammation and supports—but does not confirm—UTI. Sterile pyuria (pus cells with no organisms) may be caused by TB, partially treated UTI, stones, tumour, interstitial nephritis or renal papillary necrosis. Repeat MSU if epithelial cells present, mixed growth or lower counts.

Imaging: Renal ultrasound or IVU* is necessary in:
1 women with frequent UTIs; and
2 in children and men.
This is to exclude predisposing structural/functional abnormalities.

M: **Medical:** For most cases, oral trimethoprim, nitrofurantoin or amoxicillin (3–5 days), low-dose long-term (6–12 months) antibiotics for women with frequent UTIs.
Acute pyelonephritis: IV gentamicin, cefuroxime or ciprofloxacin.
Prostatitis: Oral ciprofloxacin.
Advice: High fluid intake, wipe front to back and postcoital voiding in women, change from spermicide and diaphragm to alternative contraceptives. Regular micturation to keep bladder empty.
Surgical: Drainage of abscess, removal of any renal calculi and relief of any obstruction (prostate hypertrophy). Consider ureteric reimplantation surgery in infants with reflux disease.

C: Renal papillary necrosis (in those with underlying renal disease, e.g. diabetes mellitus or stones).
Renal/perinephric abscess (seen on renal ultrasound).
Pyonephrosis (pus in palvicalyceal system).
Gram-negative septicaemia.

P: Mostly resolve with treatment. 20 % of pregnant women develop acute pyelonephritis if not treated; however, there is a high relapse rate.

* IVU is a series of abdominal X-rays taken to visualize the full course of urinary tract following IV injection of a radio-opaque substance.

Uveitis, anterior

D: Inflammation of the iris and ciliary body (iritis or iridocyclitis).

A: It may be caused by infection, trauma or in association with systemic inflammatory conditions (see Associations/Risk factors).

A/R: **Risk factors:** Past attacks of iritis, juvenile chronic arthritis, seronegative arthropathy (ankylosing spondylitis, reactive arthritis/Reiter's syndrome, enteropathic arthropathy (IBD)) especially when associated with *HLA-B27* positivity, sarcoidosis, Behçet's disease, TB, syphilis (rare), herpes zoster ophthalmicus, Fuchs' heterochromic cyclitis.
Rarely, sympathetic ophthalmitis (bilateral ganulomatous panuveitis weeks/months after penetrating injury).

E: Incidence of uveitis is 15 in 100 000 people (75 % are anterior uveitis).

H: Pain (ciliary spasm and inflammation, pain ↑ on accommodation), photophobia, red eyes, blurred vision, lacrimation.
(Very rare: Fuchs' heterochromic cyclitis presents with floaters, cataracts and glaucoma.)

E: ↓ Visual acuity, ciliary flush (redness may be confined to the corneoscleral junction), hypopyon (see pathology), small irregular pupil and posterior synechiae (adhesions of the iris to the lens), keratic precipitates (see pathology), signs of complications (↑ intraocular pressure, cataract), fundoscopy (to exclude retinal detachment, posterior inflammation or a tumour that may give rise to anterior uveitis).

P: Proteinaceous exudate and inflammatory cells settle in the inferior angle of the anterior chamber (hypopyon). Clumps of inflammatory cells may be deposited on the corneal endothelium (seen on slit lamp examination as keratic precipitates).

I: Investigate for associated systemic conditions depending on associated symptoms, e.g. seronegative arthropathies (sacroiliac joint X-ray, HLA-typing), sarcoidosis (CXR, serum calcium, serum ACE), etc.

M: Topical steroids: dexamethasone, prednisolone (drops for daytime and ointment for night-time), systemic steroids and immunosuppressants reserved for severe resistant cases.
Mydriatics (antimuscarinics, e.g. cyclopentolate) paralyse the papillary sphincter and ciliary muscle, ↓ pain and prevent posterior synechiae formation and 'pupil block' glaucoma.
Monitor intraocular pressure.

C: Cataracts, glaucoma (trabecular meshwork blocked by inflammatory cells or damaged by chronic inflammation), band keratopathy (band of calcium deposited in the cornea), posterior synechiae, rubeosis iridis (new vessels grown on the iris), vitreous opacities, cystoid macular oedema.

P: Prognosis is improved by screening for and treating the uveitis in juvenile chronic arthritis to prevent permanent ocular damage.

Note: posterior uveitis is an inflammation of choroid caused by infections, e.g. CMV, toxoplasma, TB or systemic inflammatory conditions (e.g. sarcoid or vasculitides). Posterior uveitis may present with floaters (caused by debris/inflammatory cells in the vitreous) and decreased vision.

D: Primary infection is called Varicella (chickenpox). Reactivation of the dormant virus in the dorsal root ganglia, causes zoster (shingles). Confusingly also known as herpes zoster in some texts.

A: VZV is an α-herpes dsDNA virus. Highly contagious, transmission is by aerosol inhalation or direct contact with the vesicular secretions.

A/R: Contact with individuals with active viraemia, immunosuppression, age (see Epidemiology).

E: Chickenpox peak incidence occurs at 4–10 years. Shingles peak incidence occurs at >50 years. About 90 % of adults are VZV IgG positive (previously infected).

H: Incubation period 14–21 days.
Chickenpox: Prodromal malaise, mild pyrexia, sudden appearance of intensely itchy spreading rash affecting the face and trunk more than the extremities, the oropharynx, conjunctivae and genitourinary tract. As vesicles weep and crust over, new vesicles appear. Contagious from 48 h before the rash and until all the vesicles have crusted over (within 7–10 days).
Shingles: May occur after a period of stress. Tingling/hyperaesthesia in a dermatomal distribution, followed by painful skin lesions. Recovery in 10–14 days.

E: **Chickenpox:** Macular papular rash evolving into crops of vesicles with areas of weeping (exudate) and crusting (vesicles, macules, papules and crusts may all be present at one time), skin excoriation (from scratching), mild pyrexia.
Shingles: Vesicular macular papular rash, in a dermatomal distribution, skin excoriation.

P: **Pathomechanism:** Viral inhalation and infection of upper respiratory tract. Viral replication in regional lymph nodes, liver and spleen. By week 2–3 infection spreads to skin producing rash then leading to clinical resolution. Virus remains latent in dorsal root ganglia (lifelong). Reactivation causes virus to travel down sensory axon to produce dermatomal shingles rash.

I: Both chickenpox and shingles are usually clinical diagnoses.
Vesicle fluid: Electron microscopy, direct immunofluorescence, cell culture, PCR.
In pregnancy, consider VZV serology (latex agglutination) or PCR for VZV DNA (see Management).

M: According to Department of Health UK Guidelines 2001 (http://www.prodigy.nhs.uk/ClinicalGuidance/).
Chickenpox (primary infection):
Children: Treat symptoms (calamine lotion, analgesia, antihistamines).
Adults: Consider aciclovir, valaciclovir or famciclovir if within 24 h of rash onset especially if elderly, smoker, immunocompromised or pregnant (especially second or third trimester).
Shingles (reactivation): Aciclovir, valaciclovir or famciclovir if within 72 h of appearance of the rash if elderly, immunocompromised or ophthalmic involvement. Low-dose amitriptyline may benefit those with moderate/severe discomfort. Simple analgesia (paracetamol).

Prevention: VZIG may be indicated in the immunosuppressed and in pregnant women exposed to Varicella zoster. Chickenpox vaccine was recently licensed in UK, but no guidelines available for appropriate use.

C: **Chickenpox:** Secondary infection, scarring, pneumonia, encephalitis, congenital varicella syndrome.*

Shingles: Postherpetic neuralgia, zoster opthalmicus (rash involves opthalmic division of trigeminal nerve), Ramsay Hunt's syndrome,† sacral zoster may lead to urinary retention, motor zoster (muscle weakness of myotome at similar level as involved dermatome).

P: Depends on the complications. Worse in pregnancy, the elderly and immunocompromised.

*Congenital varicella syndrome is characterized by scarring, ophthalmic defects, limb dysplasia and CNS abnormalities. Occurs in 1–2 % of offspring of mothers who developed chickenpox $\leq$ 20 weeks' gestation.

†Ramsay Hunt's syndrome is the reactivation of virus in geniculate ganglion causing zoster of the ear and facial nerve palsy. Vesicles may be seen behind the pinna of the ear or in the ear canal.

D: Vasculitis is the inflammation and necrosis of blood vessels. Primary vasculitides* are classified according to the main vessel size affected.
Large: Giant cell arteritis (GCA), Takayasu's aortitis (TA).
Medium: Polyarteritis nodosa (PAN), Kawasaki's disease (KD).
Small: Churg–Strauss syndrome (CSS), microscopic polyangiitis (MP), Henoch–Schönlein purpura (HSP), Wegener's granulomatosis (WG), mixed essential cryoglobulinaemia (MEC), relapsing polychondritis (RP).
The large vessel vasculitides have classical clinical patterns resulting from the vessels affected. Medium and small vessel vasculitides are characterized by multiorgan involvement with less specific clinical features.

A: Unknown. Postulated to be of autoimmune origin.

A/R: PAN is associated with hepatitis B infection. MEC is associated with hepatitis C infection. MP is associated with presence of p-ANCA. WG is associated with presence of c-ANCA.

E: Annual incidence of small vessel vasculitis is ~1 in 10 000.
TA is more common in Japanese young females, PAN may affect any age (♂ : ♀ = 2:1).

H & E: **Possible features of all diseases:**
General: Fever, night sweats, malaise, weight loss.
Skin: Rash (vasculitic, purpuric, maculopapular, livedo reticularis).
Joint: Arthralgia or arthritis.
GI: Abdominal pain, haemorrhage from mucosal ulceration, diarrhoea.
Kidney: Glomerulonephritis, renal failure.
Lung: Dyspnoea, cough, chest pain, haemoptysis, lung haemorrhage.
CVS: Pericarditis, coronary arteritis, myocarditis, heart failure, arrhythmias.
CNS: Mononeuritis multiplex, infarctions, meningeal involvement.
Eyes: Retinal haemorrhage, cotton wool spots.
Features characteristic of specific subtypes:
GCA: (see Giant cell arteritis).
TA: Constitutional upset, head or neck pain, tenderness over affected arteries (aorta and the major branches), dizziness, fainting, ↓ peripheral pulses, hypertension.
PAN: Microaneurysms, thrombosis, infarctions (e.g. causing GI perforations), hypertension, testicular pain.
KD: Age <5 years, fever of >5 days, fissured lips, red swollen palms and soles followed by desquamation, skin rash, inflamed oral cavity, conjunctival congestion, lymphadenopathy, coronary artery aneurysm.
CSS: Asthma, eosinophilia.
HSP: Purpura (leg and buttocks), arthritis, gut symptoms, glomerulonephritis with IgA deposition.
MP: Non-specific with multiple organs affected. Glomerulonephritis with no glomerular Ig deposits.
WG: Granulomatous vasculitis of upper and lower repiratory tract, nasal discharge, ulceration and deformity, haemoptysis, sinusitis, corneal thinning, glomerulonephritis.
RP: Affecting cartilage (e.g. ear pinna, nose, larynx) causing swelling, hoarse voice, tenderness, cartilage destruction and deformity (e.g. saddle nose).

*Vasculitis may also occur secondary to infections, abscesses, malignancies and connective tissue diseases (e.g. rheumatoid arthritis, SLE).

MEC: Arthritis, splenomegaly, skin vasculitis, renal disease, cryoglobulins (IgG and IgM mix).

P: Immune complex deposition in vessel walls triggers classical complement activation and inflammation.
Micro: Acute and chronic inflammatory cells in vessel wall. Some subtypes (GCA, WG, CS and PAN) have evidence of granulomatous inflammation.

I: **Blood:** FBC (normocytic anaemia, ↑ platelets, ↑ neutrophils), ↑ ESR/CRP.
Autoantibodies:
c-ANCA: Anti-proteinase 3, associated with WG.
p-ANCA: Anti-myeloperoxidase seen in MP and CSS but also IBD, primary biliary cirrhosis and chronic active hepatitis.
ANA: e.g. anti-dsDNA may suggest SLE instead.
Rheumatoid factor: Positive in 50 %.
Cryoglobulins: For cryoglobulinaemic vasculitis.
Urine: Haematuria, proteinuria.
CXR: Diffuse, nodular or flitting shadows. Atelectasia.
Biopsy: Renal, lung (transbronchial), temporal artery (in GCA).
Angiography: To identify aneurysms (in PAN).

M: **Medical:** Steroids (e.g. prednisolone, hydrocortisone) and immunosuppressants (e.g. cyclophosphamide, azathioprine). In fulminating vasculitis, plasma exchange and intravenous immunoglobulins may be warranted. In KD, aspirin is used in addition to the above therapies.

C: (see History and Examination).

P: Most remit on treatment or spontaneously (e.g. HSP), but up to 50 % of small vessel vasculitides may relapse.

Von Willebrand's disease

D: A common bleeding disorder caused by abnormalities in expression or function of von Willebrand's factor (vWF).

A: vWF is a plasma glycoprotein involved in blood clotting, and abnormal expression or functioning of it causes von Willebrand's disease. There are three subtypes.
Type 1: (>70 %): ↓ Levels of vWF, mode of inheritance often autosomal dominant.
Type 2: Relative reduction in vWF multimers and ↓ platelet binding ability of vWF. Mode of inheritance either autosomal dominant or recessive.
Type 3: ↓↓ Levels of vWF. Mode of inheritance autosomal recessive.

A/R: None.

E: Most common hereditary coagulopathy. Prevalence worldwide is ~1 %. Can present at any age.

H: May be asymptomatic (one-third of Type 1).
Mucocutaneous bleeding (mouth, epistaxis, menorrhagia).
↑ Bleeding after minor trauma, easy bruising, muscle bleeding and haemarthroses (rare).

E: Signs of anaemia (e.g. pallor), bruises.

P: vWF is composed of subunits linked by disulphide bonds to form multimers of low, intermediate and high molecular weight. vWF plays three important roles in haemostasis:

1. Acting as an adhesive bridge between platelets and damaged subendothelium of vessels by binding to platelet receptors (GP-Ib) and subendothelium collagen IV.
2. Mediating platelet–platelet binding.
3. vWF binds to factor VIII and prevents its degradation.

VWF gene is on chromosome 12 and is synthesized within vascular endothelial cells and megakaryocytes.

I: **Blood:** Clotting (↑ bleeding time, slightly ↑ APTT, ↓ factor VIII, ↓ vWF levels).
Other: Ristocetin cofactor assay (↓ platelet aggregation by vWF in the presence of ristocetin).

M: **Advice:** Avoid NSAIDs.
Medical: Usually none necessary. DDAVP or tranexamic acid (fibrinolytic inhibitor) for mild bleeding and in minor surgery. Intermediate purity factor VIII concentrate (containing vWF and factor VIII) or specific vWF may be another option.
Carrier detection: Usually unnecessary as von Willebrand's disease is usually inherited in a dominant fashion. In the rare cases of type 3 (autosomal recessive cases), carrier detection and prenatal diagnosis can be made.

C: The rare von Willebrand's disease type 3 can manifest with bleeding symptoms similar to severe haemophilia (e.g. haemarthrosis, intramuscular bleeding).

P: Variable morbidity. Many children are asymptomatic.

Wilson's disease

D: An autosomal recessive disorder characterized by ↓ biliary excretion of copper and accumulation in the liver and brain, especially in the basal ganglia.

A: The gene responsible is on chromosome 13, and codes for a copper-transporting ATPase (*ATP7B*) in hepatocytes. Mutations interfere with transport of copper into the intracellular compartments for incorporation into caeruloplasmin (and secretion into plasma) or excretion in the bile. Excess copper damages hepatocyte mitochondria, causing cell death and release of free copper into plasma, which is subsequently deposited in other tissues.

A/R: Family history, consanguinity.

E: Prevalence ~1 in 30 000, carrier frequency ~1 in 100. Liver disease may present in children (>5 year). Neurological disease usually presents in young adults.

H: **Liver:** May present with hepatitis, liver failure or cirrhosis. Jaundice, easy bruising, variceal bleeding, encephalopathy.
Neurological: Dyskinesia, rigidity, tremor, dystonia, dysarthria, dysphagia, drooling, dementia, ataxia.
Psychiatric: Conduct disorder, personality change, psychosis.

E: **Liver:** Hepatosplenomegaly, jaundice, ascites/oedema, gynaecomastia.
Neurological: (as above).
Eyes: Green or brown Kayser–Fleischer ring at the corneal limbus, sunflower cataract (copper accumulation in the lens, seen with slit lamp).

P: **Micro:** Excess copper seen on liver biopsy staining with rhodanine dye, with fatty change, hepatitis or cirrhosis.

I: **Blood:** FBC, LFT (↑ AST, ALT and AlkPhos), serum caeruloplasmin and copper (low but may be normal in active hepatitis as caeruloplasmin is an acute phase protein).
24-h urinary copper levels: Increased.
Liver biopsy: ↑ Copper content.
Genetic analysis: Particularly of family members.

M: **Medical:** Best managed by a specialist unit. Treat with copper chelators (e.g. D-penicillamine or trientine). Oral zinc (induces intestinal cell metallothionein which binds copper). Monitor urinary copper. General care for liver and neurological disease. Screen first-degree relatives.
Surgery: Liver transplantation may be necessary.

C: Cirrhosis, permanent CNS damage, gallstones (caused by haemolysis), copper-induced renal tubular damage causing hypercalciuria, phosphaturia and osteomalacia, renal tubular acidosis.

P: Severe liver disease and neurological damage have poor outcome. Early detection and treatment improves prognosis.

Wolff–Parkinson–White syndrome

D: Characterized by the presence of one or more accessory pathways (e.g. bundle of Kent) between atrium and ventricle, resulting in premature activation of ventricles (pre-excitation).

A: Accessory pathways may be a consequence of anomalous embryonic development of the myocardium.

A/R: May be associated with Ebstein anomaly (congenitally malpositioned tricuspid valve).

E: ~0.2 % of population (few are symptomatic), more common in young men.

H: Most asymptomatic.
Palpitation (atrial fibrillation or re-entry tachycardia).
Chest discomfort during tachycardia followed by dizziness or syncope.
Polyuria (in sustained tachycardia).

E: No signs if in sinus rhythm.
In tachycardia: often >200 bpm, hypotension.
In atrial fibrillation: tachycardia, irregular pulse, hypotension (see Atrial fibrillation).

P: **Pathophysiology:** Impulses conducted via the accessory pathway cause early activation of part of one ventricle, the remaining ventricular muscle receiving its impulse normally. This results in short PR interval, slurred initiation of the QRS and widening of the QRS complex. Wolff–Parkinson–White syndrome may be complicated by two types of tachycardia.

Re-entry tachycardia: Impulses are conducted anterogradely through the AV node and retrogradely via the accessory pathway, resulting in a short circuit.

Atrial fibrillation: Impulses can bypass the gating effect of the AV node and be rapidly conducted via the accessory pathway with shorter refractory period, potentially resulting in ventricular fibrillation.

I: **ECG:** Short PR interval, wide QRS that begins with a slurred upstroke (δ wave). Narrow QRS complex tachycardia during episodes of arrhythmia (see Pathology). Paroxysmal SVT (40–80 %), atrial fibrillation (10–20 %), atrial flutter (5 %).

Electrophysiology: Assess site and electrical characteristics, e.g. refractory period of accessory pathway.

M: **Acute tachycardia:**

Re-entry tachycardia: Vagal manoeuvres, IV adenosine or verapamil. Cardioversion if unstable.

Atrial fibrillation: Avoid digoxin as it worsens accessory pathway conduction (see Atrial fibrillation).

Chronic (symptomatic patients): Radiofrequency catheter ablation (curative treatment).

Surgical division of the accessory bundle (after repeated failure of radiofrequency ablation).

C: Atrial fibrillation, sudden death.

P: Good prognosis if asymptomatic. Radiofrequency ablation is curative and has very low risk.

Zollinger–Ellison syndrome

D: Severe peptic ulceration caused by a gastrin-secreting pancreatic islet cell tumour (gastrinoma).

A: The gastrinoma secretes large amounts of gastrin, a hormone that stimulates excessive acid secretion by the parietal cells in the stomach and may cause severe ulceration of the gastric and duodenal mucosa.

A/R: Zollinger–Ellison syndrome may be associated with hyperparathyroidism. 30 % of cases occur as part of multiple endocrine neoplasia (MEN type 1).

E: Annual incidence is 2–3 per million. Approximately 1 in every 1000 patients with duodenal ulcer.

H: Symptoms of peptic ulcer:

- Epigastric pain resistant to antacid treatment and worse during or after meals.
- Chronic heartburn.
- Steatorrhoea (↓ intestinal pH from gastric acid secretion denatures pancreatic enzymes).
- Complications such as GI haemorrhage, perforation.

E: Epigastric tenderness, there may be signs of anaemia.

P: These pancreatic islet cell tumours arise from the G cells of the pancreatic islets of Langerhans. Occasionally, they are found in the duodenum or stomach. 60 % of the tumours are malignant and may metastasize (e.g. liver). Severe peptic ulceration may be seen in the stomach, duodenum (first and second part) and also oesophagus and jejunum. Stomach may show hyperplasia of parietal cells.

I: **Blood tests:** *FBC* (may be anaemic), *amylase* (to differentiate from pancreatitis), clotting screen and cross-match blood if bleeding ulcers. Diagnosis by measurement of *fasting serum gastrin*. Also measure PTH, phosphate, Ca^{2+} if MEN is suspected.

Secretin provocation test: Slow IV infusion of secretin (hormone) on fasting patient. In normal individuals, plasma gastric concentration decreases. In patients with Zollinger–Ellison syndrome there is an immediate increase (after 1–2 min) in plasma gastrin concentration.

Endoscopy: Upper GI endoscopy and biopsy (to exclude malignancy).

Localization of tumour: CT, isotope scan, selective arteriography and local venous sampling for gastrin.

M: **Medical:** High-dose proton pump inhibitor treatment to reduce acid secretion. Regular follow-up endoscopy and biopsy to monitor hyperplasia in the gastric mucosa. In metastatic disease, chemotherapy with cytostatic agents such as streptozocin with or without 5-fluorouracil.

Surgery: Surgical removal of the tumour if it has been located may be curative, intraoperative ultrasonography may be of assistance.

C: Complications of peptic ulcer: haemorrhage (presenting with haematemesis, malaena or iron-deficiency anaemia), perforation (acute severe epigastric pain, collapse and peritonitis).

P: 5-year survival rate with metastasis is approximately 20 %.